Facets of Public Health in Europe

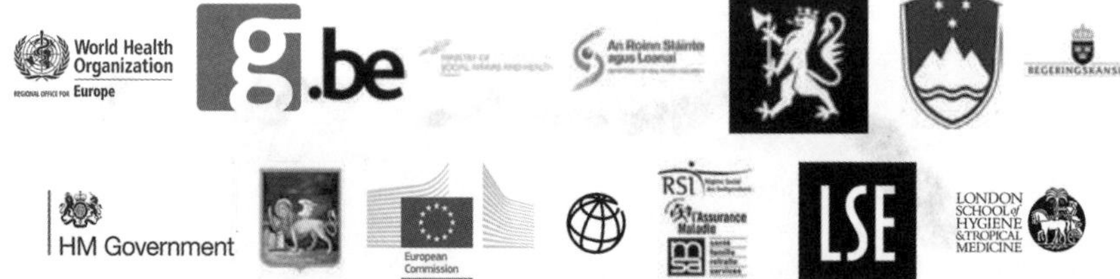

The European Observatory on Health Systems and Policies supports and promotes evidence-based health policy-making through comprehensive and rigorous analysis of health systems in Europe. It brings together a wide range of policy-makers, academics, and practitioners to analyse trends in health reform, drawing on experience from across Europe to illuminate policy issues.

The European Observatory on Health Systems and Policies is a partnership between the World Health Organization Regional Office for Europe, the Governments of Austria, Belgium, Finland, Ireland, Norway, Slovenia, Sweden, the United Kingdom, and the Veneto Region of Italy, the European Commission, the World Bank, UNCAM (French National Union of Health Insurance Funds), the London School of Economics and Political Science, and the London School of Hygiene & Tropical Medicine.

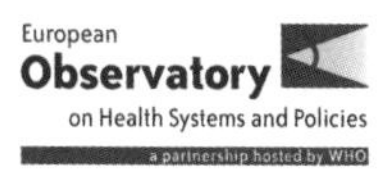

Facets of Public Health in Europe

Edited by

Bernd Rechel and Martin McKee

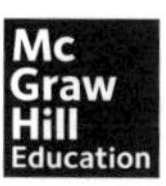

Open University Press

Open University Press
McGraw-Hill Education
McGraw-Hill House
Shoppenhangers Road
Maidenhead
Berkshire
England
SL6 2QL

email: enquiries@openup.co.uk
world wide web: www.openup.co.uk

and Two Penn Plaza, New York, NY 10121-2289, USA

First published 2014

A catalogue record of this book is available from the British Library

ISBN-13: 978-0-33-526420-9 (pb)
ISBN-10: 0-33-526420-4
eISBN: 978- 0-33-526421-6

Library of Congress Cataloging-in-Publication Data
CIP data applied for

Typesetting and e-book compilations by
RefineCatch Limited, Bungay, Suffolk

Printed by Bell & Bain Ltd, Glasgow

Fictitious names of companies, products, people, characters and/or data that may be used herein (in case studies or in examples) are not intended to represent any real individual, company, product or event.

European Observatory on Health Systems and Policies Series

The European Observatory on Health Systems and Policies is a unique project that builds on the commitment of all its partners to improving health systems:

- World Health Organization Regional Office for Europe
- Government of Austria
- Government of Belgium
- Government of Finland
- Government of Ireland
- Government of Norway
- Government of Slovenia
- Government of Sweden
- Government of the United Kingdom
- Veneto Region of Italy
- European Commission
- World Bank
- UNCAM
- London School of Economics and Political Science
- London School of Hygiene & Tropical Medicine

The series

The volumes in this series focus on key issues for health policy-making in Europe. Each study explores the conceptual background, outcomes, and lessons learned about the development of more equitable, more efficient, and more effective health systems in Europe. With this focus, the series seeks to contribute to the evolution of a more evidence-based approach to policy formulation in the health sector.

These studies will be important to all those involved in formulating or evaluating national health policies and, in particular, will be of use to health policy-makers and advisers, who are under increasing pressure to rationalize the structure and funding of their health system. Academics and students in the field of health policy will also find this series valuable in seeking to understand better the complex choices that confront the health systems of Europe.

The Observatory supports and promotes evidence-based health policy-making through comprehensive and rigorous analysis of the dynamics of healthcare systems in Europe.

Series Editors

Josep Figueras is the Director of the European Observatory on Health Systems and Policies, and Head of the European Centre for Health Policy, World Health Organization Regional Office for Europe.

Martin McKee is Director of Research Policy and Head of the London Hub of the European Observatory on Health Systems and Policies. He is Professor of European Public Health at the London School of Hygiene & Tropical Medicine as well as a co-director of the School's European Centre on Health of Societies in Transition.

Elias Mossialos is the Co-director of the European Observatory on Health Systems and Policies. He is Brian Abel-Smith Professor in Health Policy, Department of Social Policy, London School of Economics and Political Science and Director of LSE Health.

Richard B. Saltman is Associate Head of Research Policy and Head of the Atlanta Hub of the European Observatory on Health Systems and Policies. He is Professor of Health Policy and Management at the Rollins School of Public Health, Emory University in Atlanta, Georgia.

Reinhard Busse is Associate Head of Research Policy and Head of the Berlin Hub of the European Observatory on Health Systems and Policies. He is Professor of Health Care Management at the Berlin University of Technology.

European Observatory on Health Systems and Policies Series

Series Editors: Josep Figueras, Martin McKee, Elias Mossialos, Richard B. Saltman and Reinhard Busse

Published titles

Regulating entrepreneurial behaviour in European health care systems
Richard B. Saltman, Reinhard Busse and Elias Mossialos (eds)

Hospitals in a changing Europe
Martin McKee and Judith Healy (eds)

Health care in central Asia
Martin McKee, Judith Healy and Jane Falkingham (eds)

Funding health care: options for Europe
Elias Mossialos, Anna Dixon, Josep Figueras and Joe Kutzin (eds)

Health policy and European Union enlargement
Martin McKee, Laura MacLehose and Ellen Nolte (eds)

Regulating pharmaceuticals in Europe: striving for efficiency, equity and quality
Elias Mossialos, Monique Mrazek and Tom Walley (eds)

Social health insurance systems in western Europe
Richard B. Saltman, Reinhard Busse and Josep Figueras (eds)

Purchasing to improve health systems performance
Josep Figueras, Ray Robinson and Elke Jakubowski (eds)

Human resources for health in Europe
Carl-Ardy Dubois, Martin McKee and Ellen Nolte (eds)

Primary care in the driver's seat
Richard B. Saltman, Ana Rico and Wienke Boerma (eds)

Mental health policy and practice across Europe: the future direction of mental health care
Martin Knapp, David McDaid, Elias Mossialos and Graham Thornicroft (eds)

Decentralization in health care
Richard B. Saltman, Vaida Bankauskaite and Karsten Vrangbæk (eds)

Health systems and the challenge of communicable diseases: experiences from Europe and Latin America
Richard Coker, Rifat Atun and Martin McKee (eds)

Caring for people with chronic conditions: a health system perspective
Ellen Nolte and Martin McKee (eds)

Nordic health care systems: recent reforms and current policy challenges
Jon Magnussen, Karsten Vrangbæk and Richard B. Saltman (eds)

Diagnosis-related groups in Europe: moving towards transparency, efficiency and quality in hospitals
Reinhard Busse, Alexander Geissler, Wilm Quentin and Miriam Wiley (eds)

Migration and health in the European Union
Bernd Rechel, Philipa Mladovsky, Walter Devillé, Barbara Rijks, Roumyana Petrova-Benedict and Martin McKee (eds)

Health systems, health, wealth and societal well-being: assessing the case for investing in health systems
Josep Figueras and Martin McKee (eds)

Success and failures of health policy in Europe: four decades of divergent trends and converging challenges
Johan P. Mackenbach and Martin McKee (eds)

Health system performance comparison: an agenda for policy, information and research
Irene Papanicolas and Peter C. Smith (eds)

European child health services and systems: lessons without borders
Ingrid Wolfe and Martin McKee (eds)

Contents

List of contributors

Peter Achterberg is Senior Advisor at the Department for Public Health Forecasting, National Institute for Public Health and the Environment (RIVM), Bilthvoven, the Netherlands

Christoph Aluttis is researcher at Maastricht University, Faculty of Health, Medicine and Life Sciences, School for Public Health and Primary Care, Department of International Health, Maastricht, the Netherlands

Stefania Boccia is Associate Professor of Hygiene and Preventive Medicine and Deputy Director of the Section of Hygiene of the Institute of Public Health, Faculty of Medicine, Università Cattolica del Sacro Cuore (UCSC), Rome, Italy

Helmut Brand is Jean Monnet Chair in European Public Health and Head of the Department of International Health, Research School CAPHRI, Faculty of Health, Medicine and Life Science, Maastricht University, Maastricht, the Netherlands

João Breda is Programme Manager for Nutrition, Physical Activity and Obesity at the Division of Noncommunicable Diseases and Life-course, WHO Regional Office for Europe, Copenhagen, Denmark

Reinhard Busse is Associate Head of Research Policy and Head of the Berlin Hub of the European Observatory on Health Systems and Policies and Professor of Health Care Management at the Berlin University of Technology, Berlin, Germany

Cristina Catallo is Associate Professor at the Daphne Cockwell School of Nursing, Faculty of Community Services, Ryerson University Toronto, Toronto, Canada

Massimo Ciotti is Head of the Country Preparedness Support Section and Deputy Head of the Public Health Capacity and Communication Unit at the European Centre for Disease Prevention and Control (ECDC), Stockholm, Sweden

Katarzyna Czabanowska is Assistant Professor at the Department of International Health, Faculty of Health, Medicine and Life Sciences, Maastricht University, the Netherlands

Nichola Davies is Cardiac Community Manager at the Heart Foundation New Zealand, and was a Senior Policy Researcher at the United Kingdom Health Forum at the time of writing

Liam Donaldson is Professor of Health Policy at Imperial College, London, United Kingdom

EuroHealthNet is the European Partnership for improving health and equity, based in Brussels, Belgium

Dennis Faix is Medical Officer, Alert and Response Operations, Division of Communicable Diseases, Health Security & Environment, WHO Regional Office for Europe, Copenhagen, Denmark

Mojca Gabrijelčič is Senior Advisor at the Centre for Health Promotion and Disease Prevention at the National Institute of Public Health and Lecturer at the Medical Faculty, University of Ljubljana, Ljubljana, Slovenia

Paolo Guglielmetti is Administrator in the Health Threats Unit of the Health and Consumer (SANCO) Directorate General of the European Commission

Wiking Husberg is Ministerial Adviser at the Department of Occupational Safety and Health, Ministry of Social Affairs and Health, Helsinki, Finland

Elke Jakubowski is Acting Programme Manager for public health services at the WHO Regional Office for Europe, Copenhagen, Denmark, Research Associate at the European Observatory on Health Systems and Policies, and Lecturer on Comparative Public Health and Health Systems at the Hannover Medical School, Hannover, Germany

Josep Jansa is Head of the Section on Epidemic Intelligence and Response at ECDC, Stockholm, Sweden

Ilmo Keskimäki is Research Professor at the National Institute for Health and Welfare (THL), Division of Health and Social Services, Helsinki, Finland,

and Professor of Health and Social Policy at the School of Health Sciences, University of Tampere, Tampere, Finland

Rokho Kim is Specialist in Environmental and Occupational Health at the WHO Western Pacific Regional Office and former Scientist in Occupational Health at the WHO Regional Office for Europe

Hans Kluge is Director of the Division of Health Systems and Public Health, WHO Regional Office for Europe, Copenhagen, Denmark, and Special Representative of the WHO Regional Director to prevent and combat M/XDR-TB in the WHO European Region

Pieter Kramers is a freelance senior consultant on public health monitoring and reporting, and was formerly affiliated at the Institute for Public Health and the Environment (RIVM), the Netherlands

John Lavis is Director of the McMaster Health Forum, Associate Director of the Centre for Health Economics and Policy Analysis, Professor in the Department of Clinical Epidemiology and Biostatistics, and Associate Member of the Department of Political Science, McMaster University, Hamilton, Ontario, Canada. He is also Adjunct Professor of Global Health, Department of Global Health and Population, Harvard School of Public Health, Cambridge, MA, United States of America

Suvi Lehtinen is Chief of International Affairs at the Finnish Institute of Occupational Health, Helsinki, Finland

Giovanni Leonardi is Head of the Epidemiology Department, Public Health England, Centre for Radiation, Chemical, and Environmental Hazards, and Honorary Senior Lecturer, London School of Hygiene and Tropical Medicine, London, United Kingdom

Paul Lincoln is Chief Executive of the United Kingdom Health Forum

Martin McKee is Professor of European Public Health at the London School of Hygiene & Tropical Medicine, and Research Director at the European Observatory on Health Systems and Policies, London, United Kingdom

Claudia Bettina Maier is Programme Analyst at UNAIDS, Geneva, Switzerland and was Technical Officer at the European Observatory on Health Systems and Policies at the time of writing

Jose M. Martin-Moreno is Professor of Preventive Medicine and Public Health at the University of Valencia, Valencia, Spain, and the coordinator of the Quality Unit at the University Clinical Hospital, as well as Adviser to the WHO Regional Office for Europe

Jukka Pukkila is Programme Manager, Alert and Response Operations, Division of Communicable Diseases, Health Security & Environment, WHO Regional Office for Europe, Copenhagen, Denmark

Jorma Rantanen is Chairman of the Board, University of Jyväskylä, Jyväskylä, Finland, Director General and Professor Emeritus of the Finnish Institute of Occupational Health, and Past President of the International Commission on Occupational Health

Bernd Rechel is Researcher at the European Observatory on Health Systems and Policies and Honorary Senior Lecturer at the London School of Hygiene & Tropical Medicine, London, United Kingdom

Walter Ricciardi is Director of the Department of Public Health, Catholic University of the Sacred Heart, Rome, Italy

Guénaël R. Rodier is Director of the Division of Communicable Diseases, Health Security & Environment, WHO Regional Office for Europe, Copenhagen, Denmark

Cristiana Salvi is Communications Officer, Communicable Diseases, Health Security and Environment, WHO Regional Office for Europe, Copenhagen, Denmark

Francisco Santos-O'Connor is Specialist in Occupational Health and Safety, Labour Administration, Labour Inspection and Occupational Safety and Health Branch, International Labour Organization, Geneva, Switzerland, and at the time of writing was Expert in Public Health Preparedness, Public Health Capacity and Communication Unit, ECDC, Stockholm, Sweden

Louise Sigfrid is Honorary Research Fellow at the Department of Health Services Research and Policy, London School of Hygiene & Tropical Medicine, London, United Kingdom

Theodore Herzl Tulchinsky is Emeritus Associate Professor, Braun School of Public Health, Hebrew University-Hadassah, Ein Karem, Jerusalem, Israel and Deputy Editor of Public Health Reviews, Paris-Rennes, France

Stephan Van den Brouke is Professor of Health Psychology and Prevention, Université Catholique de Louvain, Louvain, Belgium

Thomas Van Cangh is Expert in Preparedness at the Public Health Capacity and Communication Unit at ECDC, Stockholm, Sweden

Hans van Oers is Chief Science Officer for Health System Assessment and Policy Support, National Institute for Public Health and the Environment (RIVM), Bilthvoven, the Netherlands and Professor in Public Health, Tranzo

Scientific Center for Care and Welfare, Tilburg University, Tilburg, the Netherlands

Carmen Varela Santos is Senior Expert and Group Leader of Training Network Strengthening in the Public Health Training Section at ECDC, Stockholm, Sweden

Marieke Verschuuren is Researcher at the National Institute for Public Health and the Environment (RIVM), Bilthoven, the Netherlands

Trudy Wijnhoven is Technical Officer for Nutrition Surveillance, at the Division of Noncommunicable Diseases and Life-course, WHO Regional Office for Europe, Copenhagen, Denmark

Matthias Wismar is Senior Health Policy Analyst at the European Observatory on Health Systems and Policies, Belgium

Phillip Zucs is Senior Expert in Communicable Disease Surveillance at the Surveillance and Response Support Unit at ECDC, Stockholm, Sweden

List of tables, figures, and boxes

Tables

Figures

Boxes

Foreword I

Governments across Europe are increasingly recognizing the need to strengthen essential public health functions so as to maximize their contribution to health, wealth, and societal well-being. This book brings together the most up-to-date evidence on public health practice in Europe, identifies areas where improvements are most urgently needed, and shows how these can be achieved. Leading experts throughout Europe address a broad range of topics, including health monitoring, health protection, healthcare, public health leadership and public health research. The chapters provide valuable insight for researchers and policy-makers seeking to understand the current situation and to identify future directions for public health.

A number of cross-cutting themes emerge from this volume. One is the importance of intersectoral working. The health sector can only address some of the determinants of health, and action by all sectors is required to improve the health of populations. As the contributions to this volume highlight, there are a number of strategies that can be used to achieve this aim, such as coalition-building across sectors, identifying shared objectives, and creating intersectoral governance structures.

Another key finding permeating this volume is the existence of wide inequalities between and within countries in Europe. Tackling these inequalities is of paramount importance for public health.

While this book makes an important contribution to our understanding of the state of public health in Europe, it also highlights an emerging research agenda. We still know too little about what public health policies and interventions are being implemented where and even less about which are most effective. Filling these knowledge gaps will be important for stepping up efforts to improve public health. This volume provides a fascinating account of how far we have come and provides some essential signposts of where we might go next.

Olivia Wigzell
Ministry of Health and Social Affairs, Sweden

Foreword II

Ever since the birth of public health in the seventeenth century, its success has depended on close interaction with society. Today we live in a globalized world undergoing changes more rapidly than ever before and this places increasing demands on the public health community. The scope of action goes far beyond health and medical care. Public health professionals must acquire skills to reach out to the whole of society where the significant determinants of health are located, including working conditions, education, and the environment, and offer practices and opportunities to establish new structures, partnerships and networks. Regulation and legislation are also necessary to limit the health-damaging impacts from certain environments, products and procedures.

This book aims to help establish a contemporary and forward-looking connection between health and society in the WHO European Region with its 53 member states. The main political tool for this is Health 2020, the new European policy framework and strategy for better and fairer population health in the region. This initiative was unanimously adopted by the 53 member states of the WHO European Region in 2012. Recognizing that Health 2020 is an umbrella policy and strategy that provides a common vision and includes key strategic directions, including for strengthening public health capacities, it acknowledges that every member state has to define its own starting point.

Health is also more and more frequently the subject of international law. Globally there are new and diverse political, technical and financial frameworks which are shaping how public health is understood, delivered and evaluated in our societies. This new governance architecture for public health has increased the number and diversity of stakeholders who are involved in shaping decisions that can have a direct or indirect impact on the health of the population. It is fair to say that in the twenty-first century there are few areas of public health for which an internationally adopted strategy with clear goals, and often an action plan, does not exist.

The major shortcoming is about implementation. Evidence-based strategies and interventions, like "best practices" or "good practices", have been high on the public health agenda since the turn of the last century. This book aims to help get closer to finding and implementing solutions. Over the past 15 years, the European Commission has played a significant role in developing best practices. These achievements could be of benefit for many countries, if adapted to their national contexts and circumstances. Yet, the WHO European Region is a divided region and the gradients from west to east and north to south are large. Another fact that cannot be hidden is that data and accessible scientific publications are biased towards the west and the north.

In many cases we need to strengthen the capacities of national public health systems. Significant investments in knowledge, human resources and structures may be required to enable public health systems across Europe to successfully fulfil their mission. But do we know where exactly to invest? What are the main challenges and how to prioritize? What are the structures, the methods of governance, funding and human resource development that provide the best results? Who are the providers, the key stakeholders and the allies of public health, and what are the relationships between them? What is the best way to get them on board for common action? What are the existing models, tools, measures and approaches and in which direction are they developing? How could research results and evidence be better used to support decision-making in public health? Some countries respond better than others, but what are the reasons behind this?

This new publication by the European Observatory on Health Systems and Policies attempts to answer these questions. The authors deserve recognition for their courage and perseverance as they break new ground in the field, which has so far only rarely been the subject of thorough analysis and where the publication bias in favour of the western and northern part of the WHO European Region is a considerable barrier to give justice to the eastern and southern parts. The book provides explanations on how we got to where we are and provides a critical view of where it would be most prudent to invest in the future so that public health could better tackle the constantly changing circumstances that determine the health of the population and have a significant impact on the development of society. At times provocative and challenging, we believe this book is going to be a welcome companion to many of us in public health.

Bosse Pettersson and Vesna-Kerstin Petrič

Bosse Petterson is Independent Public Health Consultant and former Deputy Dircector General of the Swedish National Institute of Public Health.

Vesna-Kerstin Petrič is Head of the Division for Health Promotion and Prevention of Noncommunicable Diseases at the Ministry of Health of Slovenia.

Acknowledgements

We are especially grateful to the authors of this book for their valuable contributions and their patience with developing various iterations of their chapters. First drafts were presented at an author workshop in Copenhagen in June 2011, which was kindly hosted by the World Health Organization Regional Office for Europe. We are grateful to those who participated there. In addition to the authors, they included Tit Albreht, Josep Figueras, Gauden Galea, Hans Kluge, Bosse Pettersson, Vesna Kerstin-Petrič, and Agis Tsouros.

We are very grateful for constructive comments on individual draft chapters by Tit Albreht, Claudia Bettina Maier, Ilmo Keskimäki, Richard Alderslade, Stefania Boccia, Christoph Aluttis, Helmut Brand, Stephan Van den Broucke, Ted Tulchinsky, Nichola Davies, Matthias Wismar, Cristina Catallo, Enrique Loyola, Claudia Stein, Ivo Rakovac, and Natela Nadareishvili, and to Bosse Petterson, Vesna Kerstin-Petrič, Elke Jakubowski and Hans Kluge for reviewing the whole volume.

Publication was managed by Jonathan North, assisted by Caroline White and with copy editing by Dave Cummings.

List of abbreviations

AIDS	acquired immunodeficiency syndrome
APHEA	Agency for Accreditation of Public Health Education in Europe
ASPHER	Association of Schools of Public Health in the European Region
BSE	bovine spongiform encephalopathy
CAP	Common Agricultural Policy
CDTR	Communicable Diseases Threat Report
CIHR	Canadian Institutes of Health Research
CIS	Commonwealth of Independent States
CISID	Centralized Information System for Infectious Diseases
COSI	WHO European Childhood Obesity Surveillance Initiative
CVS	chronic villous sampling
DALY	disability-adjusted life year
DHS	Demographic and Health Surveys
DMDB	European Detailed Mortality Database
DYNAMO-HIA	Dynamic Modelling for Health Impact Assessment Project
EAHC	European Agency for Health and Consumers
ECDC	European Centre for Disease Prevention and Control
ECHI	European Core Health Indicators
EEA	European Economic Area
EFTA	European Free Trade Association
EHEN	Environmental Health Economics Network
EHIS	European Health Interview Survey

EHMA	European Health Management Association
EIA	environmental impact assessment
ENHIS	Environment and Health Information System database
ENWHP	European Network for Workplace Health Promotion
EPAAC	European Partnership for Action Against Cancer
EPHA	European Public Health Alliance
EPHO	essential public health operation
EPIET	European Programme for Intervention Epidemiology Training
EPIS	Epidemic Intelligence Information System
ERA	European Research Area
ERC	European Research Council
EU	European Union
EUPHA	European Public Health Association
EUPHEM	European Programme for Public Health Microbiology Training
EuroFlu	European Influenza Network
Eva PHR	Evaluation of Public Health Reports Project
EWRS	Early Warning and Response System
FAO	Food and Agriculture Organization of the United Nations
GHO	Global Health Observatory
GISAH	Global Information System on Alcohol and Health
GLEWS	Global Early Warning System for Major Animal Diseases including Zoonoses
GOARN	Global Outbreak Alert and Response Network
HEIDI	Health in Europe: Information and Data Interface
HEN	Health Evidence Network
HIA	health impact assessment
HiAP	Health in All Policies
HiT	Health Systems in Transition
HIV	human immunodeficiency syndrome
HMDB	European Hospital Mortality Database
HSC	Health Security Committee
HTA	health technology assessment
IAEA	International Atomic Energy Authority
ICT4PHEM	Information and Communication Technologies for Public Health Emergency Management
IHR	International Health Regulations (2005)
IIA	integrated impact assessment
ILO	International Labour Organization
IMO	International Maritime Organization
INFOSAN	International Food Safety Authorities Network
IQWiG	Institute for Equality and Efficiency (Germany)
MDR-TB	multidrug-resistant tuberculosis
MediSys	Medical Information System
MERS-CoV	Middle East respiratory syndrome coronavirus
MICS	Multiple Indicator Cluster Survey

MMR	measles, mumps, and rubella
NCD	non-communicable disease
NFP	National IHR Focal Point
NGO	non-governmental organization
NHS	National Health Service (UK)
NICE	National Institute for Health and Care Excellence (UK)
NOPA	European Nutrition, Obesity and Physical Activity database
OECD	Organisation for Economic Co-operation and Development
PCBs	polychlorinated biphenyls
PCT	primary care trust
PHEIC	public health emergency of international concern
PIA PHR	Policy Impact Assessment of Public Health Reporting Project
PPP	private–public partnership
PROM	patient-reported outcome measure
PSA	prostate-specific antigen
PSSRU	Personal Social Services Research Unit (UK)
QALY	quality-adjusted life year
REACT	Response to Emergency infectious disease: Assessment and development of Core capacities and Tools Project
REMPAN	Radiation Emergency Medical Preparedness and Assistance Network
SA	sustainability assessment
SANEPID	Sanitary Epidemiological Service
SARS	severe acute respiratory syndrome
SCALE	Science, Children, Awareness, Legal Instrument, Evaluation initiative
SEA	strategic environmental assessment
SMEs	small and medium-sized enterprises
TB	tuberculosis
TEKES	Funding Agency for Technology and Innovation (Finland)
TESSy	The European Surveillance System
THE PEP	Transport, Health and Environment Pan-European Programme
UNAIDS	Joint United Nations Programme on HIV/AIDS
UNDP	United Nations Development Programme
UNEP	United Nations Environment Programme
UNICEF	United Nations Children's Fund
WHA	World Health Assembly
WHO	World Health Organization
WIND	Work Improvement in Neighbourhood Development programme
WTO	World Trade Organization

chapter one

Facets of public health in Europe: an introduction

Bernd Rechel, Martin McKee

Introduction

Over the past two centuries, public health has achieved tremendous successes, illustrated most strikingly by the remarkable reductions in deaths and disability from many infectious diseases. However, there is still much to be done, especially with regard to what has become the major component of the disease burden in the WHO European Region, non-communicable diseases (NCDs), many of which are due to lifestyle factors and amenable to public health action. The 2010 Global Burden of Disease Study reported that ischaemic heart disease was the leading cause of death in all parts of Europe in 2010 (Lozano, Naghavi et al. 2012) and the leading cause of disability-adjusted life years in central Europe, eastern Europe and central Asia, coming second in western Europe to lower back pain (Murray, Vos et al. 2012). Public health measures, such as tobacco control, salt reduction, improved diets and physical activity, and reduction in hazardous alcohol intake, are among the key actions that could help to accelerate progress in the struggle to reduce NCDs, both in Europe and beyond (Beaglehole, Bonita et al. 2011). There is a growing body of evidence to suggest that many of these interventions are cost-effective and of major long-term benefit to societies (McDaid and Suhrcke 2012).

The need for a sustained public health response to these epidemiological patterns has been recognized by a growing number of national and international organizations. The UN High-Level Meeting on Non-Communicable Diseases, in September 2011, has called attention to the urgent need for the prevention and control of non-communicable diseases worldwide. The new European health policy framework, Health 2020, adopted by the member states of the WHO European Region in September 2012 in Malta, has also emphasized the need for public health action, including through intersectoral policies (WHO 2012b). One of its main pillars is the European Action Plan for Strengthening Public Health Capacities and Services (WHO 2012a), also adopted in Malta, which in turn builds on the 2008 Tallinn Charter (WHO 2008).

Objectives of this book

This book seeks to underpin these efforts. It has two broad objectives: (1) to provide a description and analysis of existing public health structures, capacities, and services in Europe, and (2) to set out, as far as possible, which structures, capacities, and services would be needed to strengthen public health action.

While many public health textbooks have been published in recent decades, no book seems to have been devoted to a comprehensive description of public health practice in Europe. This book starts to fill this gap. It draws on published and grey literature, as well as several ongoing or recent European research projects. Key sources of information included European Union (EU) funded studies of public health capacity (Aluttis, Baer et al. 2013) and knowledge translation of public health information (Lavis and Catallo 2012), a study by the European Observatory on Health Systems and Policies on intersectoral governance (McQueen, Lin et al. 2012), and self-assessments of public health capacities and services, undertaken by several European countries with the support of the WHO Regional Office for Europe (Koppel, Leventhal et al. 2009; WHO 2009b; Ministry of Health of the Republic of Uzbekistan 2011). Finally, the Health Systems in Transition (HiT) country profiles of the European Observatory on Health Systems and Policies provided information on public health structures, capacities and services. Yet, as the contributions to this volume highlight, major gaps remain.

The second objective of this book is to set out which structures, capacities, and services countries in Europe should have to ensure the effective delivery of public health functions. In some cases, such as for dealing with public health emergencies, ensuring occupational health and safety, and other areas of health protection, these are set out in international agreements, conventions or, in the case of EU member states and those in the process of accession, by European directives. In other cases, such as for financing public health or ensuring the existence of a sufficiently large and well-trained public health workforce, European countries have made political commitments to improve the delivery of public health functions, in documents such as the 2012 European Action Plan for Strengthening Public Health Capacities and Services, which has been approved by all 53 member states of the WHO European Region.

The geographical scope of the book is, where relevant and possible, the entire WHO European Region, and it aims to reflect the very different situations in different parts of the region. Furthermore, the contributions to this volume strived to achieve an appropriate balance when discussing the work of various international organizations (EU, WHO and others), national governments, and sub-national and civil society actors.

The prospective audience for this book includes all those with an interest in understanding and improving public health practice in Europe. This includes researchers, professionals, managers, government advisers, policy-makers, and the general public. Naturally, the description and analysis of public health structures, capacities, and services might be of most interest to researchers, professionals, and recipients of services, while the description of what these structures, capacities, and services should look like, and what the policy options are, might be of most interest to those developing policies in the health and other sectors. We hope that the book will serve as a useful guide to both constituencies.

Conceptual framework

What is public health? Although the term is widely used, its meaning is not always clear. Crucially, understandings of public health vary among different countries in Europe and the term is difficult to translate into some other European languages (Kaiser and Mackenbach 2008; Tragakes, Brigis et al. 2008). Although there is no generally accepted definition, a concept paper of the WHO European Region concluded in 2011 that the definition of public health put forward in 1988 by Sir Donald Acheson, and based on an earlier definition by Winslow (1920), serves as a useful point of departure (Marks, Hunter et al. 2011). Acheson (1988) defined public health as "the science and art of preventing disease, prolonging life and promoting health through the organized efforts of society".

The next question, then, is what kinds of actions are needed to achieve these goals. What are the most important public health services and activities? A number of "essential public health functions" have been suggested in different parts of the world (WHO 2009a), including in the United States (US Department of Health and Human Services 1995) and the United Kingdom (Faculty of Public Health Medicine 2001). An international Delphi study conducted in 1997 produced another set of essential public health functions (Bettcher, Sapirie et al. 1998), which were subsequently modified by the Pan American Health Organization and the WHO Regional Office for the Western Pacific (WHO 2002, 2003).

An adaptation of these "essential public health functions" has been developed by the WHO Regional Office for Europe in the form of 10 essential public health operations (EPHOs). In line with the two objectives of this book, EPHOs can guide assessments of public health capacities and services, as well as the actions required to strengthen them (WHO 2012a). They also have the benefit of identifying horizontal activities across the whole political and administrative spectrum of policy-making, rather than focusing on the activities of specific institutions (Koppel, Leventhal et al. 2009).

The latest iteration of EPHOs was adopted by WHO in 2012 as an Annex to the European Action Plan for Strengthening Public Health Capacities and Services (WHO 2012a):

1. Surveillance of population health and well-being
2. Monitoring and response to health hazards and emergencies
3. Health protection, including environmental, occupational, food safety, and others
4. Health promotion, including action to address social determinants and health inequity
5. Disease prevention, including early detection of illness
6. Ensuring governance for health and well-being
7. Ensuring a sufficient and competent public health workforce

8. Ensuring sustainable organizational structures and financing
9. Advocacy, communication and social mobilization for health
10. Advancing public health research to inform policy and practice

EPHOs can be divided into core and enabling operations (WHO 2003). EPHOs 1–5 can be thought of as core public health operations, while EPHOs 6–10 are overarching operations that enable the delivery of public health activities (Figure 1.1). In practice, however, no public health system is organized according to these functions, elements of which can be found within many different activities and structures. Consequently, while the future accumulation of evidence may make it possible to structure a book according to these functions, this is not yet feasible, although some of the functions do map on to the ones examined in this book.

Structure of the book

This book is divided into four parts. Part 1 (Chapters 1 and 2) clarifies concepts and definitions, Part 2 (Chapters 3–13) explores how key public health functions are being delivered across Europe, Part 3 (Chapters 14–18) analyses the resources needed to deliver them, and Part 4 (Chapter 19) brings together key conclusions on the actions required for strengthening public health in Europe.

Following this introduction, Chapter 2 explores the changing context of public health in Europe. It reviews changing patterns of disease, the opportunities brought about by advances in information technologies, professional skills and qualifications, the increasing recognition of the social determinants of health, and the changing role of the state.

Chapter 3, which describes the monitoring of population health in Europe, is the first of the chapters exploring key public health functions. It argues that understanding population health is a crucial precondition for formulating

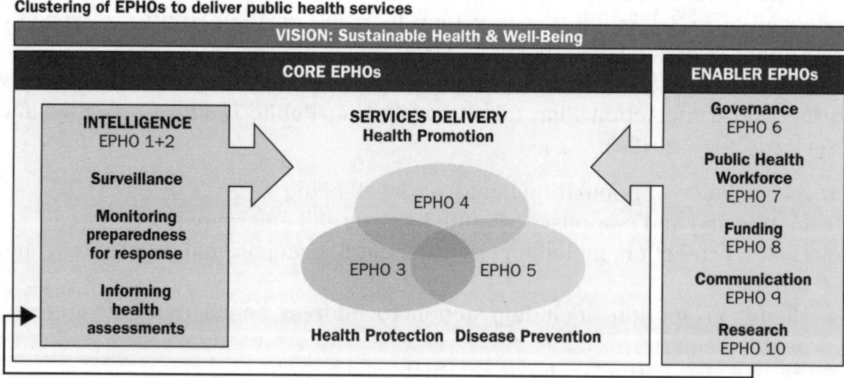

Figure 1.1   Ten essential public health operations

Source: WHO (2012a)

effective public health policy and action. The chapter reviews the very diverse health information systems in place in Europe for population-wide monitoring and surveillance. It describes available information sources on health and healthcare utilization and explores where and why routine data are not available or reliable. The chapter concludes by making the case for increased international cooperation and European harmonization of data collection systems.

Chapter 4 discusses the role of the WHO and the EU in responding to public health emergencies, including infectious disease outbreaks. Based on the conceptual framework of an event management cycle, the chapter reviews the origin and function of the 2005 International Health Regulations, and examines which core capacities for surveillance and response are required at the national level. The chapter then describes how the WHO and EU support each step of national event management and how they strengthen national capacity to deal with public health emergencies.

Chapters 5–7 are concerned with key aspects of health protection. Chapter 5 explores current programmes and structures for occupational health and safety in Europe. It starts by clarifying the sometimes confusing terminology of occupational health and safety and then discusses the major international instruments in place for advancing occupational health and safety in Europe. The chapter then assesses the diverging situation in different parts of the WHO European Region, the main challenges countries are facing in improving occupational health and safety systems, and which strategic directions they could follow. The chapter argues that modern public health services should include a strong programme for health and safety at work, strive for universal coverage and integration into primary health care, and in particular target vulnerable workers and high-risk sectors.

Chapter 6 begins by giving a brief overview of major environmental health hazards and the burden of disease that can be attributed to them. It then describes the main elements of environmental health services and the disciplines involved in this area. Actors and disciplines involved in delivering environmental health services in Europe vary widely, as does the training of professionals working in environmental health. The chapter identifies actions at the international, national, and local level to strengthen environmental health in Europe.

Chapter 7 addresses food and nutrition. Much of the disease burden in Europe is related to unhealthy nutrition, such as a high intake of foods rich in salt, added sugars, and saturated and trans-fatty acids, and an obesity epidemic is unfolding in most European countries. This chapter describes relevant international initiatives on food and nutrition, national policy actions, and efforts to improve surveillance, monitoring, and evaluation. It argues that primary health care should play a part in addressing obesity and malnutrition.

Chapter 8 assesses how health care can be informed by public health. Ideally, health systems should be geared towards the ultimate objective of improving population health. To achieve this goal, it is necessary to assess healthcare needs, effective and cost-effective interventions, and equitable allocation of resources. The chapter also considers how health services can become settings for health promotion activities.

Chapter 9 provides a review of cancer screening programmes in Europe. It begins by discussing criteria for implementing screening programmes. The chapter then explores the evidence for screening for cancer of the cervix, breast, and colon, including some of the current controversies. This is followed by a review of cancer screening practices across Europe. The chapter concludes that there were major improvements, but also much scope for further progress. It argues in favour of systematic, population-based screening activities, but also recognizes that financial and professional capacity differ widely across the WHO European Region.

Chapter 10 provides an overview of the organizational structures in place in Europe for health promotion activities, the integration of health promotion in health service provision, and the training of health promotion professionals. The chapter shows that countries in Europe differ widely in how far they promote the health of their populations. The scope for improvement seems to be largest in many of the countries of central and eastern Europe and the former Soviet Union, but there is also much room for improvements in western Europe.

Chapter 11 explores some of the ways to tackle the social determinants of health. There is overwhelming evidence on the impact of social, environmental, and economic factors on mortality, morbidity, and health inequalities in Europe. Yet, action is far from straightforward and often requires complex, multisectoral policies and programmes. This chapter sets out how the necessary practical steps are nevertheless achievable, giving examples from the local, national, and international level. It argues that actions to reduce inequities in health should be universal, but still target the most vulnerable groups of the population in particular. Examples include the enforcement of seatbelt legislation or traffic calming measures in densely populated neighbourhoods, which offer benefits for the majority, while tackling inequities especially.

Chapter 12 discusses intersectoral working for public health. It reviews experience of adopting intersectoral policies at the national and supranational level in Europe and explores structures for intersectoral governance, including ministerial linkages, cabinet sub-committees, public health ministers, parliamentary and intersectoral committees, joint budgets, and delegated finance. The chapter then sets out ways of putting intersectoral structures and strategies into action. It argues that there is substantial scope for "lesson-learning" across Europe.

Chapter 13 addresses the use of health impact assessments in Europe. It explains the purpose of these assessments, their key stages and the different forms they can take, including the trend towards integrated impact assessments and the use of rapid, community-led, and equity-focused health impact assessments. The chapter then discusses whether impact assessments should be mandated or voluntary. It concludes by arguing for the importance of embedding health in the decision-making processes of organizations and building relationships across sectors.

Chapters 14–18 discuss some of the key resources needed for public health. Chapter 14 explores the great diversity that exists in the organization and financing of public health in Europe. In terms of organization, countries differ in the balance between centralized and decentralized public health operations, and how they address the vertical and horizontal integration of public health activities across different programmes, sectors, and levels of care. In terms of financing, the share of total health expenditure devoted to public health and the mechanisms in place for raising revenues for public health activities differ widely. However, there tends to be a mix of sources of finance, with growing interest by health ministries, although not finance ministries, in taxes earmarked for public health purposes. The chapter concludes that it will be essential to maintain existing structures and levels of funding in the current economic climate.

Chapter 15 addresses the public health workforce. The delivery of public health services requires a well-trained and qualified health workforce, including both public health specialists and other health professionals. However, attempts to quantify the public health workforce have remained elusive. This chapter reviews the current structures in place in Europe for the education of public health workers. It starts by exploring existing definitions and common characteristics of the public health workforce in Europe, and then describes the current status of this workforce. The chapter concludes by outlining existing systems of education and professional development for public health in Europe and the measures needed for their further development.

Chapter 16 discusses public health leadership. Previously associated with a single person, position or institution, leadership in public health is now dispersed among local governments and communities, as well as other stakeholders. This chapter discusses what public health leadership is, what its functions are, and the forms it can take. It then reviews public health leadership in Europe at the national and international level and explores how it can be strengthened and developed. The chapter argues that public health leadership will increasingly have to reach out out to others, influence those that work beyond its control, and build coalitions and alliances.

Chapter 17 addresses public health research in Europe. It reviews existing EU-level structures to support public health research and then discusses recent EU-funded research projects that aimed to map public health research in the EU. The chapter then turns to a discussion of national structures to support public health research in Europe, with case studies of Italy, Finland, Poland, and Estonia. It argues that there is a need for national strategies for public health research, improved coordination between ministries of science, health, and finance, improved coordination across different research and innovation programmes within the EU, and better engagement with public health researchers, users, and partners, including civil society organizations.

Chapter 18 explores knowledge translation as it relates to public health information. It aims to encourage a discussion of the ways in which health information (including on health systems) is packaged for and interactively shared among public health policy-makers and stakeholders in Europe. The chapter draws on findings of a recent EU-funded research project that assessed contemporary efforts to broker information for public health policy and to bridge the gap between information and action in European public health. It argues that knowledge brokering can help to address the gap between knowledge and practice through an emphasis on innovative information packaging and interactive knowledge-sharing mechanisms.

Chapter 19 brings together the main conclusions from the contributions to this book. It argues that there is substantial scope for strengthening public health functions and resources in many countries of the WHO European Region. More research is needed to accurately map public health structures and capacities in Europe, but this should not preclude action based on what we know so far.

References

Acheson, D. (1988). *Public Health in England*. Report of the Committee of Inquiry into the Future Development of the Public Health Function. London, HMSO.

Aluttis, C. A., C. Chiotan, M. Michelsen, C. Costongs and H. Brand, on behalf of the Public Health Capacity Consortium (2013). *Reviewing Public Health Capacity in the EU*. Maastricht, Maastricht University.

Beaglehole, R., R. Bonita, R. Horton, C. Adams, G. Alleyne, P. Asaria, V. Baugh, H. Bekedam, N. Billo, S. Casswell, M. Cecchini, R. Colagiuri, S. Colagiuri and T. Collins (2011). "Priority actions for the non-communicable disease crisis." *The Lancet* **377**(9775): 1438–1447.

Bettcher, D., S. Sapirie and E. Goon (1998). "Essential public health functions: results of the international Delphi study." *World Health Statistics Quarterly* **51**: 44–54.

Faculty of Public Health Medicine (2001). *Strengthening Public Health Function in the UAE and EMR of the WHO*. London, Royal Colleges of Physicians of the United Kingdom.

Kaiser, S. and J. Mackenbach (2008). "Public health in eight European countries: an international comparison of terminology." *Public Health* **122**(2): 211–216.

Koppel, A., A. Leventhal and M. Sedgley, Eds. (2009). *Public Health in Estonia 2008: An analysis of public health operations, services and activities*. Copenhagen, WHO Regional Office for Europe.

Lavis, J. and C. Catallo, Eds. (2012). *Bridging the Worlds of Research and Policy in European Health Systems*. Copenhagen, WHO, on behalf of the European Observatory on Health Systems and Policies.

Lozano, R., M. Naghavi, K. Foreman, S. Lim, K. Shibuya, V. Aboyans, J. Abraham, T. Adair, R. Aggarwal and S. Y. Ahn (2012). "Global and regional mortality from 235 causes of death for 20 age groups in 1990 and 2010: a systematic analysis for the Global Burden of Disease Study 2010." *The Lancet* **380**: 2095–2128.

Marks, L., D. J. Hunter and R. Alderslade (2011). *Strengthening Public Health Capacity and Services in Europe: A concept paper*. Copenhagen, WHO Regional Office for Europe.

McDaid, D. and M. Suhrcke (2012). The contribution of public health interventions: an economic perspective. In *Health Systems, Health, Wealth and Societal Well-Being*. J. Figueras and M. McKee, Eds. Maidenhead, Open University Press: 125–152.

McQueen, D., V. Lin, M. Wismar, C. Jones, L. St.-Pierre and M. Davies, Eds. (2012). *Intersectoral Governance for Health in All Policies*. Copenhagen, WHO Regional Office for Europe on behalf of the European Observatory for Health Systems and Policies.

Ministry of Health of the Republic of Uzbekistan (2011). *Self-Assessment of Public Health Services in the Republic of Uzbekistan*. Technical Report. Copenhagen, WHO Regional Office for Europe.

Murray, C. J. L., T. Vos, R. Lozano, M. Naghavi, A. D. Flaxman, C. Michaud, M. Ezzati, K. Shibuya, J. A. Salomon, S. Abdalla and V. Aboyans (2012). "Disability-adjusted life years (DALYs) for 291 diseases and injuries in 21 regions, 1990–2010: a systematic analysis for the Global Burden of Disease Study 2010." *The Lancet* **380**: 2197–2223.

Tragakes, E., G. Brigis, J. Karaskevica, A. Rurane, A. Stuburs, E. Zusmane, O. Avdeeva and M. Schäfer (2008). "Latvia: health system review." *Health Systems in Transition* **10**(2): 1–253.

US Department of Health and Human Services (1995). *For a Healthy Nation: Returns on investment in public health* [http://books.google.co.uk/books?id=g0zWZ817UD IC&pg=PP1&dq=For+a+Healthy+Nation:+Returns+on+Investment+in+Public+Hea lth&ei=WTcESv-DKKTGzQT4vNj2Aw, accessed 30 April 2008]. Washington, DC, US Department of Health and Human Services.

Winslow, C.-E. A. (1920). "The untilled fields of public health." *Science* **51**(1306): 23–33.

World Health Organization (WHO) (2002). *Essential Public Health Functions: The role of ministries of health*. Manila, WHO Regional Office for the Western Pacific.

World Health Organization (WHO) (2003). *Essential Public Health Functions: A three-country study in the Western Pacific Region*. Manila, WHO Regional Office for the Western Pacific.

World Health Organization (WHO) (2008). *The Tallinn Charter*. Tallinn, WHO.

World Health Organization (WHO) (2009a). *Evaluation of Public Health Services in Slovenia*. Copenhagen, WHO Regional Office for Europe.

World Health Organization (WHO) (2009b). *Evaluation of Public Health Services in South-eastern Europe*. Copenhagen, WHO Regional Office for Europe.

World Health Organization (WHO) (2012a). *European Action Plan for Strengthening Public Health Capacities and Services*. Copenhagen, WHO Regional Office for Europe.

World Health Organization (WHO) (2012b). Health 2020 Policy Framework and Strategy. Copenhagen, WHO Regional Office for Europe.

chapter two

The changing context of public health in Europe

Martin McKee, Bernd Rechel, Hans Kluge, Ted Tulchinsky

Introduction

Public health in Europe should be in a state of continuous flux, as both the threats and the potential responses to those threats are changing. Yet, too often, it remains stuck in the past, lagging behind the curve. This chapter explores the evolving challenges and opportunities that face the public health community in Europe today. It identifies trends in six broad domains:

- *Epidemiological*: changing patterns of disease, including the emergence of new diseases and the re-emergence of ones that had seemed to have been eradicated, as well as the global epidemic of non-communicable diseases.
- *Informational*: manifest in the vast increase in computing power and the ability to obtain and link data from a wealth of diverse sources, but also the diversification of sources of information, such as social media, that are increasingly being exploited in ways that threaten population health.
- *Professional*: the increasing acceptance of a multidisciplinary approach to public health in place of the traditional medically dominated model.
- *Conceptual*: the growing recognition of the importance of upstream determinants of health, the so-called "causes of the causes", and the role played by modern vectors of disease, such as the multinational corporations selling tobacco, alcohol, and the energy-dense foods that are driving the global epidemic in non-communicable diseases.
- *Political*: changing beliefs about the relationship between the individual and the state.
- *Distributional*: the widening of the health gap in Europe from the 1960s onwards, which is only now beginning to close, albeit slowly, as well as the increasing economic, cognitive, and political distance between small but powerful global elites (the "one percent", as referred to by the Occupy Movement) and the mass of the population.

The epidemiological transition

In 1971, Omran described the epidemiological transition, whereby success in combating the traditional high level of infectious diseases gives way to a growing burden of non-communicable disease. He divided the development of societies into three distinct phases: the Age of Pestilence and Famine, characterized by high mortality and low population growth, the Age of Receding Pandemics, during which there is a progressive decrease in mortality and an increase in life expectancy, and finally the Age of Degenerative and Man-Made Diseases, when mortality continues to decline and eventually stabilizes at a low level.

While victory in the fight against infectious disease seemed imminent in the early 1970s (Fauci 2001), four decades later it is apparent that reality is more complicated, with the emergence of new and the re-emergence of "old" infectious diseases. There have certainly been many successes against infectious diseases, including the eradication of smallpox and the near eradication of polio. However, humans continue to be engaged in an evolutionary struggle against microorganisms, with no obvious signs of victory. Microorganisms and their vectors adapt to new ecological niches, taking advantage, for example, of how the mass production of food encourages the emergence of antibiotic resistances (Davis, Price et al. 2011). Microorganisms have also been able to exploit the increased pace of global movement, including the influenza virus and HIV, albeit moving in different ways (Macpherson, Gushulak et al. 2007; Bajardi, Poletto et al. 2011). As can be seen in the re-emergence of tuberculosis in the countries of the former USSR (Coker, McKee et al. 2006; Rechel, Roberts et al. 2013) and of malaria in Greece following austerity-induced cuts of vector control in 2010 (Kentikelenis, Karanikolos et al. 2011), any weakening in public health capacity can lead to the spread of infectious disease. There have been many public health responses to prevent this. For example, new organizational structures have emerged, such as UNAIDS, the Global Fund against AIDS, TB and Malaria, and GAVI, all at the global level, and the European Centre for Disease Prevention and Control, at the European level. Better understanding of the new threats posed by infectious disease has also boosted intersectoral action, such as in response to the AIDS epidemic where the health sector, the police, and the justice system must work together (see Chapter 12 on "Intersectoral working"). Yet the struggle continues.

Omran (1971) was more accurate in his prediction of a growth in what he termed "degenerative and man-made diseases". Although there have been major successes in advanced industrialized countries against many non-communicable diseases, exemplified by the 50% reduction in deaths from ischaemic heart disease in countries of north-western Europe in the 1980s and 1990s (Kuulasmaa, Tunstall-Pedoe et al. 2000; Tunstall-Pedoe, Vanuzzo et al. 2000), there have also been many failures. These include the dramatic increase in the prevalence of obesity in many European countries (see Chapter 7, "Food security and healthier food choices"), driven primarily by the consumption of energy-dense food and resulting in an increase in the prevalence of diabetes and its complications (Basu, Stuckler et al. 2013). At the same time, there is growing recognition of the burden of mental illness, which now accounts for 40% of all years lived with disability in Europe (Petrea and McCulloch 2013).

These developments have called for a new approach by public health. Some of the greatest achievements of the past were brought about by large-scale programmes to improve the environment, such as the creation of safe water supplies and improved sanitation, or by mass immunization campaigns. These examples required the implementation and scaling up of relatively simple and straightforward measures. Contemporary threats to public health are much more complex to address. The history of the USSR exemplifies this well. The communist system was successful in scaling up basic interventions, such as against infectious diseases, but failed to tackle the growing challenge of non-communicable diseases (McKee 2007a), a legacy that is still felt in many former Soviet countries today (Rechel, Roberts et al. 2013).

Many of the new threats to population health have been termed "lifestyle diseases", suggesting that the victims acquire these diseases because of the choices they make. This simplistic view fails to account for the constraints imposed by the circumstances in which people make their choices and ignores the highly addictive nature of substances such as alcohol or tobacco. If it is to be effective, a public health response must take account of these factors (see Chapter 11, "Tackling the social determinants of health"). This means that it will almost inevitably be multifaceted. The challenges can be exemplified by the burden of alcohol-related mortality that is rising in some European countries. Traditional public health responses, such as educating the public about the harmful effects of alcohol, are largely ineffective. What is instead required is a coordinated response tackling price, availability, and marketing (Holder and Edwards 1995).

Advances in information technology

Public health can benefit from the vast increase in the availability of information about how individuals live their everyday lives. Yet, the same information can also be used to the detriment of population health. Advances in computing power have been exploited widely by commercial organizations to capture detailed profiles of our everyday lives and consumption patterns. Individuals willingly sign up to supermarket club cards, airline frequent flyer cards, and credit cards, while mobile phones allow tracking of our movements, and Internet search engines can monitor what we are reading. All of these sources of information are used to optimize marketing efforts, in some cases promoting products that can be life-enhancing but all too often promoting those that are damaging to health (Dorotic, Bijmolt et al. 2012).

In contrast, the public health community has only scratched the surface of this rich stream of data (Kuh 2012), in part because of a lack of resources, but also due to data protection regulations that, in many countries, place those seeking to promote better health at a significant disadvantage compared with those seeking to undermine it. For example, it is now possible to track individuals using the geographical positioning system software within mobile phones, thereby tracking their patterns of physical activity and their use of different modes of transport (Palmer, Espenshade et al. 2012). This can be linked to the rapidly increasing volume of geo-coded data, as well as information on the built environment available from digital maps and imagery, such as that provided by Google Streetview. This will, however, require that public health systems in some countries markedly increase their capacity to analyse such data, subject to appropriate safeguards that guarantee the integrity of individuals and ensure the legitimacy of the state in the eyes of its citizens, something that has become much more difficult following revelations of the extensive covert surveillance being conducted by intelligence agencies in some countries that has fundamentally undermined trust in data protection safeguards.

Advances in technology also offer new opportunities for individualized public health interventions designed to change behaviour, such as text messaging as an aid to smoking cessation (Free, Knight et al. 2011). However, those promoting products that undermine health can exploit the same advances. The alcohol industry in particular has invested heavily in social media such as Facebook and Twitter, targeting young people with a continuing stream of promotional messages and using them as participants in its marketing activities (Hastings and Sheron 2013). These methods circumvent traditional restrictions on advertising, but so far the public health community has failed to mount an appropriate response, although measures such as standardized packaging of cigarettes, by breaking the link between these new forms of marketing and the final product, offer considerable promise and, at the time of writing, both Ireland and Scotland have committed to pursuing this approach.

Enhancing professional skills and qualifications

Traditionally, public health was undertaken by doctors and nurses, often wearing white coats and uniforms, while standing in front of school classes offering information on the health consequences of different behaviours. This approach has never been particularly effective but, in some countries, it remains in widespread use (see Chapter 15, "Developing the public health workforce").

A modern approach to public health requires individuals with a much wider range of skills in many different disciplines, as well as the ability to work with others in multiprofessional teams (see Chapter 12 on "Intersectoral working"). Alcohol control policies, for example, require a wide range of skills, in addition to traditional public health skills such as epidemiology, statistics, and sociology. These include skills in economics, to be able to explain concepts such as price elasticity to politicians (Lhachimi, Cole et al. 2012); social geography, to understand the geographical determinants of consumption patterns (Bryden, Roberts et al. 2012); and psychology and information sciences, to understand the sophisticated methods used by marketing organizations (Nicholls 2012). Public health also plays an increasingly important role in guiding the actions of the healthcare sector, for example in ensuring that services are configured in ways that reflect health needs, that they deliver effective and appropriate care, and that they respond to the legitimate expectations of the population (see Chapter 8, "Healthcare public health").

Yet, even where the need for a broad range of skills is now recognized, individuals from other disciplinary backgrounds are often relegated to a subordinate position under medical leadership. The United Kingdom offers one of the few exceptions to this, embracing multidisciplinary public health whereby public health professionals, whatever their primary degree, undertake the same training programme and obtain the same qualifications (Griffiths, Crown et al. 2007).

While the poor performance of some countries may be attributable in part to weaknesses in public health infrastructure, it is important to recognize that a well-trained public health workforce is only one of the many prerequisites for the development and implementation of successful health policies. Some European countries with well-trained public health workforces, such as Denmark or Lithuania, compare poorly with their neighbours in terms of health policy performance, which in some cases results from a lack of political will and in others from an inability to implement policies (McKee and Mackenbach 2013).

Looking upstream to the causes of the causes

Public health has traditionally been concerned with the immediate causes of disease. In the nineteenth century, many of these causes were infectious, as became increasingly recognized following Pasteur's development of the germ theory. Subsequently, Robert Koch set out his postulates to determine whether an infectious agent was the cause of a disease or not (Porter 1997). This basic model of causation was not, however, adequate to ascertain the causes of the growth in non-communicable diseases in the twentieth century, leading Bradford Hill to set out his nine criteria of causality (Hill 1965). These criteria recognized that, in the absence of randomly allocating individuals to be exposed to a potential risk factor, it would be necessary to draw on different types of information to make a judgement about the causes of disease. Throughout the second half of the twentieth century, the Bradford Hill criteria were applied to a rapidly increasing volume of risk factor epidemiology, identifying the role played by factors such as dietary fat and sugar, tobacco, hazardous alcohol consumption, and a wide range of environmental exposures.

Yet, while this research could explain why a particular individual contracted a disease, it failed to explain why so many diseases were socially patterned. In other words, the probability of contracting a particular disease was much more common in one social class or ethnic group than in others. Research undertaken in the 1960s and 1970s, initially largely in the United Kingdom and the United States, challenged the then prevailing view that rising prosperity would eliminate social inequalities (Filakti and Fox 1995). Indeed, there was evidence that inequalities were widening (Black and Whitehead 1988).

This focused attention on what has become termed the "social determinants of health" (see Chapter 11, "Tackling the social determinants of health"). This approach aims to look beyond the immediate causes of ill-health, such as diet and smoking, to understand the causes of the causes. In some ways, it is a return to the roots of public health in the nineteenth century, when Virchow identified the power structures in society as being at the root of the typhus epidemic in Silesia (Rather 1990). A social determinants perspective advocates policies that look upstream, in order to tackle the fundamental drivers of disease in the population. These include the distribution of resources, such as the way in which the system of tax and benefits redistributes resources from rich to poor (or vice versa), but also a life-course approach (Marmot, Allen et al. 2012), recognizing that the roots of adult ill-health often go back to experiences in utero or early life (Kuh and Ben-Shlomo 1997).

A strand of public health has also recognized explicitly that there are powerful forces in society that undermine health (see Chapter 19, "Drawing the lessons"). The tobacco industry produces a product that will kill 50% of its users when used as intended. Yet, despite being associated with more deaths in the twentieth century than Hitler and Stalin combined, the tobacco industry is still viewed by some European politicians as a legitimate business, as was apparent in the intensive (and extremely well-resourced) lobbying leading up to the 2013 European Parliament vote on the Tobacco Products Directive, where many Members of the European Parliament sided with the tobacco industry against the recommendations of the European Commission and the Council of Ministers. On the other hand, increasing numbers of national governments are adhering to provisions in the WHO Framework on Convention on Tobacco Control, which sets out principles for engagement with this widely discredited industry.

While there is no need for anyone to smoke, everyone does need to eat and drink. Yet the global food system is increasingly in the hands of a small number of multinational corporations who have the power to determine what we consume (Lock, Stuckler et al. 2009). For example, the extensive use of high fructose corn syrup in fast food is the consequence of a system that is designed to advance the interests of the large American grain producers (Lustig, Schmidt et al. 2012). Increasingly, multinational corporations are seen as the vectors of the epidemic in non-communicable diseases, in the same way that mosquitoes act as vectors of malaria (Geneau, Stuckler et al. 2010). Unlike mosquitoes, however, they are able to change the environment to advance their own interests. They do so by lobbying, to ensure that the rules within which they operate are as favourable as possible to them (Mindell, Reynolds et al. 2012), and by advocating for trade liberalization, so that their products can penetrate the markets in developing countries (Stuckler, McKee et al. 2012).

This shift in public health attention from proximal risk factors to more distal ones is also needed when considering the contemporary financial and economic crisis (see Chapter 19, "Drawing the lessons"). The health consequences of the austerity measures implemented by governments in some of the European countries worst affected are becoming increasingly apparent, with a rise in suicides, outbreaks of infectious disease, and shortages of essential medications (Karanikolos, Mladovsky et al. 2013). While accepting the need for measures that address these issues directly, such as increased investment in suicide prevention or needle exchange programmes, public health advocates have called for action to tackle the underlying causes, such as Europe-wide banking regulation and policies that promote rather than inhibit economic growth (Stuckler, Basu et al. 2010). In this way, public health is returning to the example of Virchow in the nineteenth century.

The changing role of the state

The post-war European welfare state was based on the principle of solidarity, according to which those fortunate enough to have resources would support those who lacked them. This model has come under increasing attack since the early 1980s, when politicians in some western European countries started to pursue a neoliberal agenda that would reduce significantly the scope of the welfare state. However, given overwhelming support for societies based on the notion of solidarity, they made only limited progress and, in most countries, swings in the electoral cycle did not veer far from the centre ground. The global financial and economic crisis that began in 2007 has, however, given a renewed impetus to the neoliberal agenda. As predicted by the Canadian author Naomi Klein (Klein 2007), the crisis has been used by some to argue that, in the face of sustained recession, the European welfare state was unsustainable, an ideological position unsupported by the evidence.

At the same time, neo-fascist parties aim to exploit the economic hardship in some European countries, such as Greece and Hungary, by promoting racist ideologies, in some cases drawing on the imagery of the 1930s. Increasingly in these countries, violent extremists are posing a threat to migrants from outside Europe. However, there is a broader backlash against the rights of migrants in many European countries (Rechel, Mladovsky et al. 2013). In some countries, such as the United Kingdom, mainstream politicians try to distract attention from their economic policy failures by blaming migrants from other European Union member states, in particular Romania and Bulgaria, for taking advantage of health and welfare benefits, again contrary to the evidence.

These political developments pose a major threat to population health. They directly challenge the values that underpin public health, such as equity and inclusion. It is essential to remember that public health, with its belief in collective action by society, is fundamentally political. However, recalling events in the first half of the twentieth century, public health has not always been on the side of the vulnerable and marginalized. Indeed, in the 1930s, many schools of public health taught what was termed "racial hygiene". This distorted approach saw certain minorities as a threat to public health, rather than as groups requiring protection (McKee 2007b). It is essential that lessons be learned from history and the mistakes of the past not repeated.

Another change is the shift of many aspects of health policy to the supranational level. This is most obvious for EU member states, where many aspects of health protection have been harmonized, with common standards for air and water quality and product safety. However, less well recognized is the growing role of global trade treaties, where powerful actors seek to remove what they portray as non-tariff barriers to trade but others view as necessary protections for health and social cohesion. An example is the highly controversial EU–US trade deal, negotiated largely in secret, and, in particular, the growth of investor–state dispute resolution mechanisms that undermine the democratic process. On the other hand, there are some areas where international action may deliver mechanisms that can protect health, in areas such as climate change (although much more remains to be done). At the same time, there is increasing recognition of the role that local, sub-national actors can play in addressing local, national, and global health challenges (see Chapter 6, "Environmental health"; Chapter 11, "Tackling the social determinants of health"; Chapter 12, "Intersectoral working"; and Chapter 16, "Developing public health leadership").

The widening health gap

The variation in life expectancy among European countries is wider now than it was four decades ago. A recent analysis has demonstrated how this reflects, at least in part, substantial differences in the adoption of public health policies known to be effective (Mackenbach and McKee 2013). Using a set of 27 "process" and "outcome" indicators, as well as a summary score indicating a country's overall success in implementing effective health policies in 10 different areas of health policy (tobacco; alcohol; food and nutrition; fertility, pregnancy and childbirth; child health; infectious diseases; hypertension detection and treatment; cancer screening; road safety and air pollution), major differences across countries emerged (Figure 2.1). Within Europe, Sweden and Norway stand out as the leaders in almost all areas of healthy public policy while others, especially those that emerged from the former Soviet Union, lag far behind. In part, this reflects differences in the means to adopt healthy policies but it is primarily a consequence of differences in public and political will. The best performing countries are those scoring highest on measures of self-expression on the World Values Survey – in other words, those countries where people no longer worry about having the basics for survival but instead can look ahead to a brighter future. Given the increasing opportunities to promote health, as discussed above, the public health community still has much to do to ensure public and political buy-in, as otherwise their absorption into routine policy and practice will, as in the past, be unconscionably slow (Tulchinsky and Varavikova 2010).

Conclusion

Europe is changing and with it both the threats to population health and the opportunities to respond to them. Yet so far, it has made only limited progress in protecting the health of the population, and unevenly so. This chapter has suggested key trends to consider and some of the avenues for future action. What is already clear is that European public health must take a broad

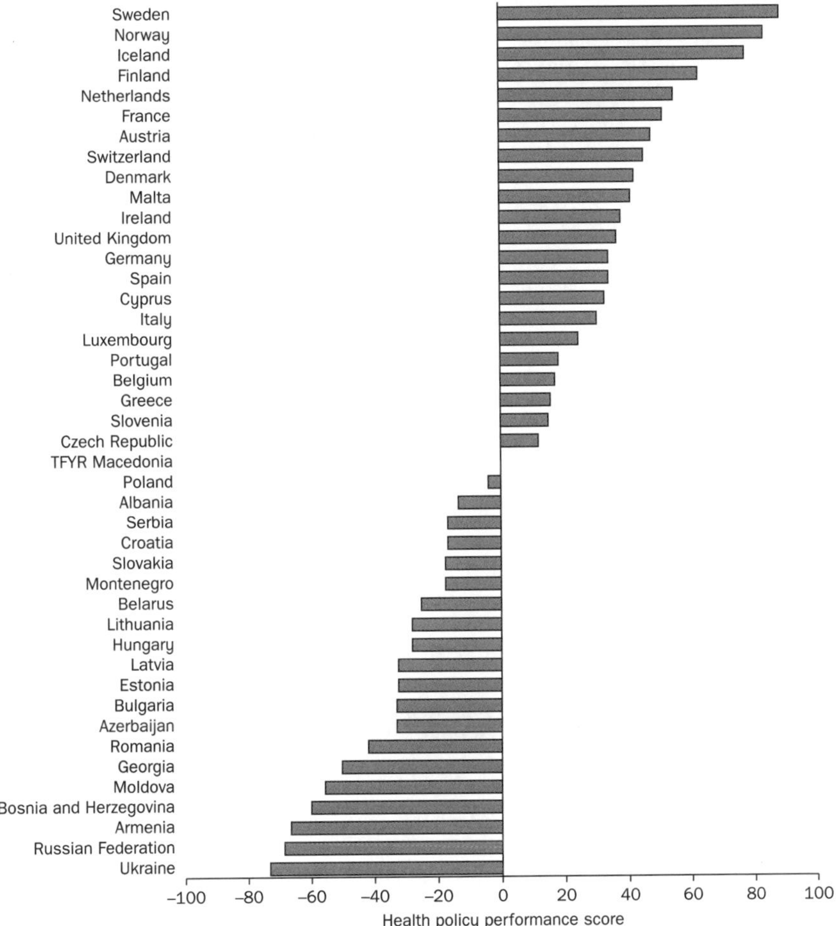

Figure 2.1 Performance on a composite measure of health policies in Europe

Source: Mackenbach and McKee (2013)

perspective, putting into practice its long-standing commitment to promote health in all policies.

References

Bajardi, P., C. Poletto, J. J. Ramasco, M. Tizzoni, V. Colizza and A. Vespignani (2011). "Human mobility networks, travel restrictions, and the global spread of 2009 H1N1 pandemic." *PLoS One* **6**(1): e16591.

Basu, S., D. Stuckler, M. McKee and G. Galea (2013). "Nutritional determinants of worldwide diabetes: an econometric study of food markets and diabetes prevalence in 173 countries." *Public Health Nutrition* **16**(1): 179–186.

Black, D. and M. Whitehead (1988). *Inequalities in Health: The Black Report and the health divide.* Harmandsworth, Penguin.

Bryden, A., B. Roberts, M. McKee and M. Petticrew (2012). "A systematic review of the influence on alcohol use of community level availability and marketing of alcohol." *Health and Place* **18**(2): 349–357.

Coker, R., M. McKee, R. Atun, B. Dimitrova, E. Dodonova, S. Kuznetsov and F. Drobniewski (2006). "Risk factors for pulmonary tuberculosis in Russia: case-control study." *British Medical Journal* **332**(7533): 85–87.

Davis, M. F., L. B. Price, C. M. Liu and E. K. Silbergeld (2011). "An ecological perspective on U.S. industrial poultry production: the role of anthropogenic ecosystems on the emergence of drug-resistant bacteria from agricultural environments." *Current Opinion in Microbiology* **14**(3): 244–250.

Dorotic, M., T. H. Bijmolt and P. C. Verhoef (2012). "Loyalty programmes: current knowledge and research directions." *International Journal of Management Reviews* **14**(3): 217–237.

Fauci, A. S. (2001). "Infectious diseases: considerations for the 21st century." *Clinical Infectious Diseases* **32**(5): 675–685.

Filakti, H. and J. Fox (1995). "Differences in mortality by housing tenure and by car access from the OPCS Longitudinal Study." *Population Trends* **81**: 27–30.

Free, C., R. Knight, S. Robertson, R. Whittaker, P. Edwards, W. Zhou, A. Rodgers, J. Cairns, M. G. Kenward and I. Roberts (2011). "Smoking cessation support delivered via mobile phone text messaging (txt2stop): a single-blind, randomised trial." *The Lancet* **378**(9785): 49–55.

Geneau, R., D. Stuckler, S. Stachenko, M. McKee, S. Ebrahim, S. Basu, A. Chockalingham, M. Mwatsama, R. Jamal, A. Alwan and R. Beaglehole (2010). "Raising the priority of preventing chronic diseases: a political process." *The Lancet* **376**(9753): 1689–1698.

Griffiths, S., J. Crown and J. McEwen (2007). "The role of the Faculty of Public Health (Medicine) in developing a multidisciplinary public health profession in the UK." *Public Health* **121**(6): 420–425.

Hastings, G. and N. Sheron (2013). "Alcohol marketing: grooming the next generation." *British Medical Journal* **346**: f1227.

Hill, A. B. (1965). "The environment and disease: association or causation?" *Proceedings of the Royal Society of Medicine* **58**(5): 295–300.

Holder, H. D. and G. Edwards (1995). *Alcohol and Public Policy: Evidence and issues.* Oxford, Oxford University Press.

Karanikolos, M., P. Mladovsky, J. Cylus, S. Thomson, S. Basu, D. Stuckler, J. P. Mackenbach and M. McKee (2013). "Financial crisis, austerity, and health in Europe." *The Lancet* **381**(9874): 1323–1331.

Kentikelenis, A., M. Karanikolos, I. Papanicolas, S. Basu, M. McKee and D. Stuckler (2011). "Health effects of financial crisis: omens of a Greek tragedy." *The Lancet* **378**(9801): 1457–1458.

Klein, N. (2007). *The Shock Doctrine: The rise of disaster capitalism.* London, Allen Lane.

Kuh, D. and Y. Ben-Shlomo (1997). *A Life Course Approach to Chronic Disease Epidemiology.* Oxford, Oxford University Press.

Kuh, K. F. (2012). "Personal environmental information: the promise and perils of the emerging capacity to identify individual environmental harms." *Vanderbilt Law Review* **65**: 1565–1629.

Kuulasmaa, K., H. Tunstall-Pedoe, A. Dobson, S. Fortmann, S. Sans, H. Tolonen, A. Evans, M. Ferrario and J. Tuomilehto (2000). "Estimation of contribution of changes in classic risk factors to trends in coronary-event rates across the WHO MONICA Project populations." *The Lancet* **355**(9205): 675–687.

Lhachimi, S. K., K. J. Cole, W. J. Nusselder, H. A. Smit, P. Baili, K. Bennett, J. Pomerleau, M. McKee, K. Charlesworth, M. C. Kulik, J. P. Mackenbach and H. Boshuizen (2012). "Health impacts of increasing alcohol prices in the European Union: a dynamic projection." *Preventive Medicine* **55**(3): 237–243.

Lock, K., D. Stuckler, K. Charlesworth and M. McKee (2009). "Potential causes and health effects of rising global food prices." *British Medical Journal* **339**: b2403.

Lustig, R. H., L. A. Schmidt and C. D. Brindis (2012). "The toxic truth about sugar." *Nature* **482**: 27–29.

Mackenbach, J. P. and M. McKee, Eds. (2013). *Successes and Failures of Health Policy in Europe: Four decades of diverging trends and converging challenges*. Maidenhead, Open University Press.

Macpherson, D. W., B. D. Gushulak and L. Macdonald (2007). "Health and foreign policy: influences of migration and population mobility." *Bulletin of the World Health Organization* **85**(3): 200–206.

Marmot, M., J. Allen, R. Bell, E. Bloomer, P. Goldblatt, on behalf of the Consortium for the European Review of Social Determinants of Health and the Health Divide (2012). "WHO European review of social determinants of health and the health divide." *The Lancet* **380**(9846): 1011–1029.

McKee, M. (2007a). "Cochrane on Communism: the influence of ideology on the search for evidence." *International Journal of Epidemiology* **36**(2): 269–273.

McKee, M. (2007b). "A crisis of governance?" *Journal of Public Health (Oxford)* **29**(1): 3–8.

McKee, M. and J. Mackenbach (2013). "Conditions for successful health policies." In *Successes and Failures of Health Policy in Europe: Four decades of divergent trends and converging challenges*. J. Mackenbach and M. McKee, Eds. Maidenhead, Open University Press: 331–355.

Mindell, J. S., L. Reynolds, D. L. Cohen and M. McKee (2012). "All in this together: the corporate capture of public health." *British Medical Journal* **345**: e8082.

Nicholls, J. (2012). "Everyday, everywhere: alcohol marketing and social media – current trends." *Alcohol and Alcoholism* **47**(4): 486–493.

Omran, A. R. (1971). "The epidemiologic transition: a theory of the epidemiology of population change." *Milbank Memorial Fund Quarterly* **49**(4): 509–538.

Palmer, J. R., T. J. Espenshade, F. Bartumeus, C. Y. Chung, N. E. Ozgencil and K. Li (2012). "New approaches to human mobility: using mobile phones for demographic research." *Demography* **50**: 1105–1128.

Petrea, I. and McCulloch, A. (2013). "Mental health." In *Successes and Failures of Health Policy in Europe: Four decades of divergent trends and converging challenges*. J. Mackenbach and M. McKee, Eds. Maidenhead, Open University Press: 193–213.

Porter, R. (1997). *The Greatest Benefit to Mankind: A medical history of humanity from antiquity to the present*. London, HarperCollins.

Rather, L. J. (1990). *A Commentary on the Medical Writings of Rudolf Virchow: Based on Schwalbe's Virchow-Bibliographie*. San Francisco, CA, Norman Publishing.

Rechel, B., P. Mladovsky, D. Ingleby, J. P. Mackenbach and M. McKee (2013). "Migration and health in an increasingly diverse Europe." *The Lancet* **381**(9873): 1235–1245.

Rechel, B., B. Roberts, E. Richardson, S. Shishkin, V. M. Shkolnikov, D. A. Leon, M. Bobak, M. Karanikolos and M. McKee (2013). "Health and health systems in the Commonwealth of Independent States." *The Lancet* **381**(9872): 1145–1155.

Stuckler, D., S. Basu, M. McKee and M. Suhrcke (2010). "Responding to the economic crisis: a primer for public health professionals." *Journal of Public Health (Oxford)* **32**(3): 298–306.

Stuckler, D., M. McKee, S. Ebrahim and S. Basu (2012). "Manufacturing epidemics: the role of global producers in increased consumption of unhealthy commodities including processed foods, alcohol, and tobacco." *PLoS Medicine* **9**(6): e1001235.

Tulchinsky, T. H. and E. A. Varavikova (2010). "What is the New Public Health?" *Public Health Reviews* **32**: 25–53.

Tunstall-Pedoe, H., D. Vanuzzo, M. Hobbs, M. Mahonen, Z. Cepaitis, K. Kuulasmaa and U. Keil (2000). "Estimation of contribution of changes in coronary care to improving survival, event rates, and coronary heart disease mortality across the WHO MONICA Project populations." *The Lancet* **355**(9205): 688–700.

Monitoring the health of the population

*Marieke Verschuuren, Peter W. Achterberg,
Pieter G. N. Kramers, Hans van Oers*

Introduction

Monitoring, evaluation, and analysis of health status are among the essential public health functions identified by Ramagen and Ruales (2008). Indeed, health monitoring is the first of the ten essential public health operations identified for the WHO European Region (see Chapter 1). Health monitoring is a prerequisite for good governance: effective provision of public health and health care requires information on the population's health and disease burden, as well as the underlying determinants. More specifically, monitoring population health provides insights into the magnitude and distribution of health inequalities and the magnitude, impact, and distribution of health determinants. In turn, these can be used to inform the planning of public health and healthcare services. Determinants of health include genetic, bio-physiological, behavioural, and environmental (social and physical) factors, in addition to prevention and health care.

As a concept, population health is always an aggregate of individual health data (Reidpath 2005). Thus, in practice, population health monitoring or public health monitoring is the regular collection and analysis of mostly individual data on relevant components of health and its determinants in the population or samples thereof. Reporting is an indispensable part of public health monitoring. If the outcomes of monitoring exercises are not reported, they will not reach policy-makers or other target audiences, and the policy cycle cannot be completed.

Population health monitoring can take a variety of approaches, which may differ widely in their scope and purpose. For instance, the scope can be either comprehensive or topical. A comprehensive approach aims to provide an overview of all components of health; a topical approach may, for example, focus on children's health, environmental health or diabetes. Population health monitoring can also take place at different geographical levels – international, national, regional or local. Sub-national or international comparisons can be valuable components of health reporting, introducing elements of benchmarking and identifying best practices. Finally, population health monitoring can be expanded to include integrative research such as modelling and forecasting, requiring the integration of a multitude of epidemiological, psychosocial, (bio) medical, and other research approaches.

A first step in developing public health monitoring is to identify the relevant components of health, health deficits, and health determinants – the factors that cause health to improve or deteriorate. This requires a conceptual approach, considering all elements consistently and with a view to possible actions and policy options that aim to improve population health. A well-defined and detailed conceptual model identifies general areas of interest (e.g. behavioural factors), specifies more detailed areas (e.g. smoking), and allows for precise definition of the data needed. The model needs to build on existing knowledge regarding associations and causal pathways linking health determinants and health outcomes and allow for further analyses, including mathematical modelling. Examples include the calculation of composite health measures, such as population-attributable risks, disability-adjusted life years (DALYs), estimates of avoidable mortality, and measures of health expectancy. Most conceptual approaches focus on negative aspects such as risk factors that lead to diseases, injuries or death. However, health-promoting determinants and positive notions of health can also be part of this approach. Generally, policies impact indirectly on population health, via one or more of the determinants of health (e.g. lifestyle, environment), and are moderated through health protection, prevention or care (see Chapter 11, "Tackling the social determinants of health" and Chapter 13, "Health impact assessment").

John Graunt's report, *Natural and Political Observations Made upon the Bills of Mortality* (1662), is an early example of a conceptual approach to public health monitoring. This report describes disease occurrence and death among the population of London, taking a broad perspective to examine poverty and environmental issues, with the aim of informing a policy-maker (adviser to the King of England). The Lalonde Report, *A New Perspective on the Health of Canadians* (1974), is a more recent example of a national health report employing a broad conceptual approach to population health. In fact, many public health monitoring models now being used at regional, national, and international level can be traced back to the Lalonde Report. One example is the model used in the Dutch public health status and forecast report (Figure 3.1).

Health system performance assessment is a concept that is closely related to, and partially overlaps, general public health monitoring (Derose and Petitti 2003; Arah, Westert et al. 2006; Westert, van den Berg et al. 2010). Here, the main question is how well health systems achieve their goals. These include health improvements concerning, for example, subjective health, disease burden, and accessibility of care. WHO's often-quoted *World Health Report 2000* set out three goals for health systems: (1) good health, (2) responsiveness to the expectations of the population, and (3) fair financial contribution. It also identified four key functions: (i) service provision, (ii) resource generation, (iii) financing, and (iv) stewardship (WHO 2000).

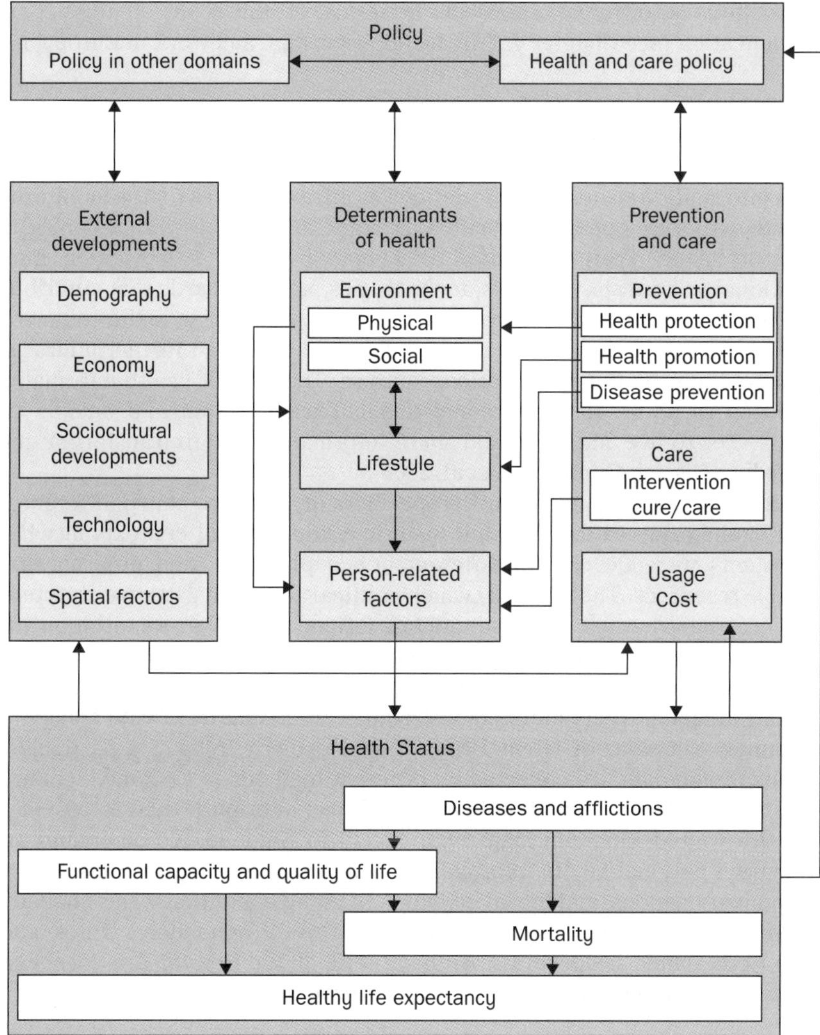

Figure 3.1 Conceptual model used for health monitoring in the Dutch public health status and forecast report

Source: Hollander, Hoeymans et al. (2007)

Infectious or communicable disease surveillance is another overlapping concept. This implies the continuous monitoring of the frequency and distribution of disease and death due to infections transmitted from humans, animals, food, water or the environment and related risk factors (Health Protection Agency 2011). Communicable disease surveillance differs from general public health monitoring because its aims are early detection and containment of outbreaks.

This requires a different approach in terms of timescale, analyses, and communication (see Chapter 4, "The health security framework in Europe").

Health information systems in Europe

Health information systems can be defined as infrastructures for the monitoring of health activities, population health outcomes, and policies with a significant impact on health. They encompass the people, institutions, legislation, inter-institutional relationships, values, technologies, and standards that contribute to the different stages of data processing. These stages include the collection, analysis, storage, transmission, display, dissemination, and further utilization of data and information from various sources. The goal of health information systems is to allow all professional and lay users within and outside the health sector to use, interpret, and share information and to transform it into knowledge (Gissler, Dumitrescu et al. 2006).

Health information systems in Europe show great intercountry differences. This is mainly due to the different historical and cultural contexts in which the systems were developed; different policy priorities; and differences in available resources. The extent to which political and administrative structures are decentralized can have a significant influence on the organization and functioning of health information systems. For example, Belgium is a federal state in which some data are collected at federal level, some at regional level. It is similar in Spain, where autonomous regions are in charge of data collection. The United Kingdom of Great Britain and Northern Ireland is particularly complex. Some data are collected by different methods in England, Scotland, Wales, and Northern Ireland and so, in practice, data purported to represent the entire United Kingdom may relate solely to England. A functioning and harmonized national health information system requires negotiations with all of a country's regions, and the involvement of many institutions. This challenge of scattered data ownership also applies to several non-federal states, such as the Netherlands (Kilpeläinen, Aromaa et al. 2008). Box 3.1 provides some examples of health information systems in Europe.

Box 3.1   Features of selected national health information systems in Europe

Azerbaijan: some key characteristics of the health information system

- No single health information system in place for the collection, reporting, and analysis of health data. Potentially useful information from different parts of the system is not shared.
- Significant amount of information is missing due to weak enforcement of reporting procedures for private healthcare providers outside the Ministry of Health remit.

- Financial disincentives discourage collection of data.
- Ministry of Health has developed a strategy for achieving an integrated health information system and envisages the introduction of new provider-payment mechanisms, providing incentives for data collection and reporting.

Belgium: main challenges of the health information system

- Poor international comparability (a lack of reporting data in line with international classifications and concepts).
- Lacking unique patient identification between available databases.
- Lacking data on several topics, including voluntary health insurance, extramural health care, and healthcare technologies.
- Data validity problems with diagnosis and treatment, particularly for co-morbidities and complications.

Czech Republic: example of a centralized system

- The Institute of Health Information and Statistics, the agency responsible for managing the national health information system, collects data for health policy and research.
- The system's functions include collection and processing of information on health status and health care; management of national health registries (15 in total, including the cancer registry and registry of hospitalized patients); and provision of information for the purpose of health research, while ensuring compliance with laws on data protection.
- All healthcare providers are required to send annual reports to the Institute of Health Information and Statistics.

Source: Ibrahimov, Ibrahimova et al. (2010), Gerkens and Merkur (2010), Bryndová, Pavloková et al. (2009)

Data

Routinely collected data are at the core of any health monitoring effort (Chan, Kazatchkine et al. 2010). For informing policy-making, data are usually summarized in the form of selected indicators (see sub-section below on "Indicators"). It is the effective presentation, analysis, and interpretation of data and indicators that results in health information (see next section on "Health reporting"). To obtain a comprehensive picture of population health, regular data from different types of sources are needed. The main types are vital statistics (births, deaths, causes of death), population surveys (using interviews or physical examinations), and registries. There are a wide variety of registries and the preferred sources may differ according to the health topic under consideration. For example, health interview surveys are the preferred source of information on lifestyle-related health determinants, such as smoking and alcohol use. Disease prevalence and incidence are assessed using information derived from healthcare utilization registries (e.g. hospital discharge registries, GP registries, insurance data) or specific disease registries (e.g. cancer registries), as these are based on confirmed diagnoses. Health examination surveys are preferable for estimating the occurrence of overweight and obesity, for example, as self-reported data tend to be underestimates. Sometimes, a topic requires parallel data collections using different sources – for example, to monitor trends in the self-reported and register-based occurrence of certain diseases, such as depression in the Netherlands (Schoemaker, Poos et al. 2013).

Although vital statistics (births, deaths, causes of death) are widely available in Europe, there is still considerable scope to improve coverage and comparability. For example, a 2005 study of causes of death found that 12 high-income countries in western Europe had data of only "intermediate quality" (Mathers, Fat et al. 2005). Differences between countries can arise due to a lack of systematic data quality assessments, different coding practices or health system-related factors, such as whether an autopsy is obligatory in cases of unexpected death.

Registry data for some health topics are available in Europe, mostly in EU member states, although again there is some concern about availability and comparability. Examples include cancer, diabetes, hospital discharges, and injuries. Data availability is very limited for other conditions and aspects of healthcare utilization, as only a few countries have dedicated registries. The Nordic countries (Denmark, Finland, Iceland, Norway, and Sweden) are an exception, with many population-based health registries established in the 1960s. These use unique personal identifiers that allow linkage between registries. In contrast, data protection regulations in many other European countries do not allow different sources to be linked, thus preventing full use of routinely collected health data. In the EU, the 1995 Data Protection Directive does not prohibit the processing (e.g. linkage) of personal health data for public health monitoring purposes. However, it does leave significant room for interpretation by individual member states and has resulted in large intercountry differences in data accessibility (Verschuuren, Badeyan et al. 2008). Some countries (e.g. Estonia) have adopted much more restrictive provisions (Rahu and McKee 2008) and improvement in this situation is a prerequisite for enhancing the availability of registry data at national and European level. A draft Data Protection Regulation that will supersede the Directive was published in January 2012, but it remains to be seen whether this will improve or worsen public health monitoring in the EU (Carinci, Di Iorio et al. 2011).

Regular, nationally representative health examination surveys are rare; Finland and the United Kingdom are exceptions (Kilpeläinen, Aromaa et al. 2008). In contrast, regular health interview surveys are undertaken in most EU member states, although intervals between survey rounds differ and are sometimes quite lengthy. Other surveys are conducted at regular intervals in many European countries outside the EU. These include USAID-funded Demographic and Health Surveys (DHS) and UNICEF's Multiple Indicator Cluster Survey (MICS) series.

The current development of a European health interview survey (EHIS) is an important step towards harmonizing public health monitoring in EU member states, based on earlier work by WHO and a group of national statistical offices (Bruin, Picavet et al. 1996). The European Commission plans to have completed a first full wave of the EHIS by 2014, based on the overarching Regulation on Community statistics on public health and health and safety at work (Regulation (EC) No. 1338/2008) and the specific Regulation relating to statistics based on the EHIS (Commission Regulation (EU) No. 141/2013). Efforts to implement an EU-wide health examination survey are also ongoing (European Commission 2013a), but full implementation will be a challenge in view of the high costs associated with such surveys.

Indicators

To support policy-making, health data and health information can be summarized in the form of indicators. An indicator can be defined as a concise definition of a concept meant to provide maximal information about an area of interest. This implies that an indicator should (Kramers 2005):

- tell us something about an area of interest for (policy) action, sometimes defined as a concrete policy target (e.g. reduce the percentage of smokers to less than 20%);
- do this in the most efficient way, i.e. provide the simplest possible numerical presentation, calculated from basic data, to give a robust view of the situation (e.g. life expectancy as a measure for overall age-specific mortality).

At the core of each health information system, there should thus be a set of carefully selected, policy-relevant and valid indicators. It is important to emphasize that the selection of indicators should be driven by needs rather than data. In practice, there will be limitations related to the availability of data and resources for improving data collection, but long-term management of health information systems requires recognition of the discrepancies between what we would like to know and what the available information can tell us. Meta-information on the indicators used in health information systems (e.g. selection rationale, precise definitions, problems with data quality) and keeping this meta-information up to date is of utmost importance for improving the effectiveness of health information systems.

The European Core Health Indicators (ECHI) (formerly: European Community Health Indicators) shortlist is an example of a set of indicators developed for general public health monitoring at international level. This was developed by collaboration of the European Commission, Eurostat, EU member states, the WHO Regional Office for Europe, the Organisation for Economic Co-operation and Development (OECD) and other international agencies. Based on explicit criteria (see Box 3.2), the selection process resulted in a comprehensive shortlist of 88 core indicators. Most EU member states are now working to integrate this shortlist into national health information systems.

Box 3.2   Criteria for selection of indicators for the ECHI shortlist

- List should cover the entire public health field, following the structure of the Lalonde model and including health status, determinants of health, health interventions and health services, and socioeconomic and demographic factors.
- Indicators should serve user needs and so should be linked to major public health policy issues, at both EU and member state level.
- Existing indicator systems (e.g. those of the OECD and WHO Regional Office for Europe) should be used as much as possible, but there should also be room for innovation.
- List should adopt viewpoint of the general public health official as its frame of reference.
- List should focus on significant public health problems, including health inequalities.
- List should focus on the greatest potential for effective policy action.

Source: Verschuuren, Kramers et al. (2010)

One of the first examples using ECHI indicators as an evidence base for national health policy is the Dutch report *Dare to Compare!*, in which the health of the population was benchmarked using the ECHI shortlist (Harbers, Van der Wilk et al. 2008). However, it should be noted that the ECHI indicators were primarily selected for international comparisons and therefore are not necessarily the most appropriate indicators for the purpose of national or subnational policy-making.

Health reporting

Health reporting is the art of presenting the results of health monitoring to a target audience. As with monitoring, the scope of reporting can be comprehensive or topical; target audiences range from policy-makers to the broader interested public. Reports can range from the simple listing of numbers to integrated analyses, making extensive use of research results. Examples of topical and general public health reports from the 1990s and 2000s have been brought together by the EU-funded Evaluation of Public Health Reports (Eva PHR) and the follow-up Policy Impact Assessment of Public Health Reporting (PIA PHR) Project (PIA PHR 2013).

Different types of reporting can be understood to relate to different levels of an information pyramid (Figure 3.2). The first level of the pyramid comprises data, the basis for all reporting efforts. However, such data are meaningless unless accompanied by contextual information (e.g. underlying definitions and calculations) and explanatory notes on data validity. The second (information) level requires the effective presentation, analysis, and interpretation of data. Comprehensive reporting efforts are needed to reach the third (knowledge)

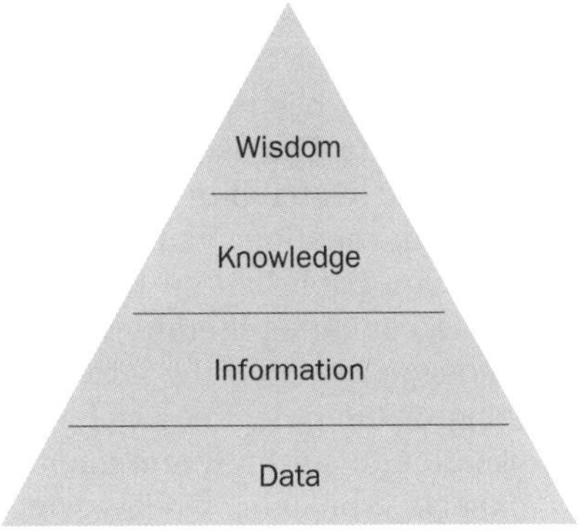

Figure 3.2 Information pyramid

level, placing the data into a broader policy-relevant perspective, including time-trends and societal context. Links between different parts of the conceptual public health model (see Figure 3.1) can be made by combining information from different areas (e.g. public health, health services research, clinical medicine, sociology). The fourth and highest (wisdom) level of the pyramid is the ability to make well-informed policy decisions.

Comprehensiveness, policy orientation, and an integrative approach are thus important elements in determining the effectiveness of health reporting. This was also a conclusion of the Eva PHR Project, which developed a set of quality criteria for health reports, based on a literature review and expert opinion. Other important criteria for effective health reports included a conceptual approach, a prospective approach, and high-quality data. The project also mapped the expectations of users of health reports and identified models of best practice for effective health reporting. It was found that health reporting is characterized by great heterogeneity, with most health reports applying a very broad scope and presenting all available data and indicators. In contrast, policy-makers required analysed information about health status and determinants, linked to the provision of health care and finances and to future health trends and evaluation of activities implemented (lögd 2003).

A Dutch study drew up quality criteria for regional public health reporting. This not only included the criteria emerging from the Eva PHR Project but also additional criteria related to the "position in the policy cycle" (Bon-Martens, Achterberg et al. 2012). This underlines the importance of considering timescales for policy-making when reporting health information (see Chapter 18, "Knowledge brokering in public health").

Health monitoring and reporting in Europe are increasingly taking place at the regional and local levels. For example, a growing number of Dutch regional health services are developing and maintaining comprehensive health reporting systems. These are based on the approach used by the national public health status and forecast report (Hollander, Hoeymans et al. 2007) – identified by the Eva PHR Project as one of the best practice models. Another example of advanced health reporting at regional level is the public health observatories in the United Kingdom. These provide indicator-based, comprehensive, and interactive health information (Public Health England 2013).

Health reports have traditionally been produced in printed forms such as reports, brochures, and policy briefs. The rise of the Internet has resulted in two main developments: (1) increased availability and accessibility of information, and (2) the possibility to make information available in dynamic and interactive ways. Hence, health information published on the Internet can now be used by almost everybody who is computer literate, has access to the Internet, and a command of the language in which the information is published. This has led to a vast broadening of the potential reach of health reports, and of efforts to adjust the information to suit different audiences (including policy-makers, public health experts, students, media, wider public). Increasing opportunities to receive feedback from a large pool of users can be helpful in keeping information complete and up-to-date (e.g. through discussion forums or wiki-like approaches). The Internet is full of inspiring examples of dynamic and interactive tools – well-known software packages for health information include InstantAtlas™ (Geowise 2013), Tableau© (Tableau 2013), and Gapminder (Gapminder 2013). Modern technologies also offer the possibility to set up links to information elsewhere on the Internet and to include analytical elements in data presentation tools to enable users to perform statistical analyses online. For example, the WHO Regional Office for Europe and the European Commission have developed interactive atlases to monitor and assess the association of health with different social determinants in 280 regions of the EU and neighbouring countries (WHO Regional Office for Europe 2013a). Figure 3.3 is an illustrative screenshot of data given in one of these atlases.

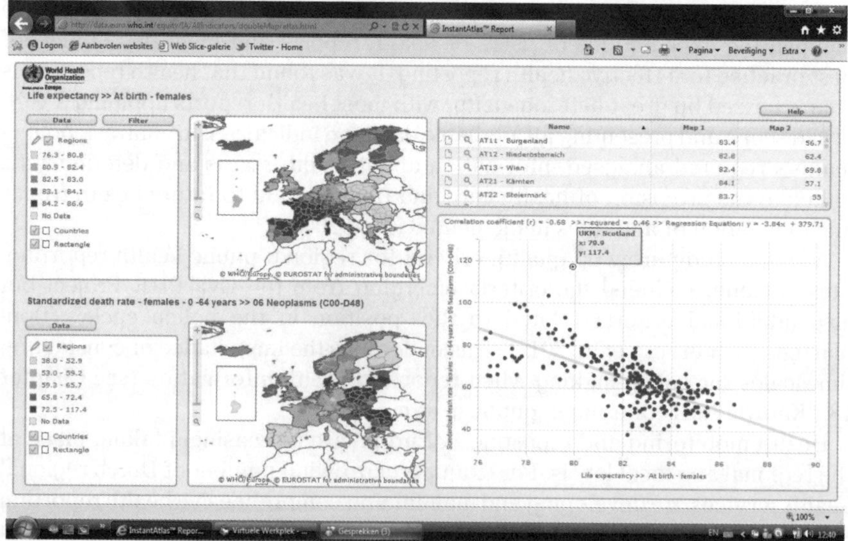

Figure 3.3   Screenshot of WHO correlation map atlas

Source: WHO Regional Office for Europe (2013a)

Forecasting

Historical time trends are a standard component of most health reporting but policy-makers often require projections of what could happen and forecasting is now a specialized branch of data analysis and reporting. Forecasting exercises are included in several health reports, most commonly projection of future population numbers. These demographic projections can be used as the basis for estimates of future incidence and prevalence rates of diseases, demand for health services, or overall health expenditure. Technically, forecasts range from simple extrapolation of trends (possibly age-adjusted) to complicated mathematical modelling. An example of the latter is the projection of cases of heart disease or cancer, and the resulting mortality, taking account of developments in smoking and alcohol consumption, which, in turn, are influenced by policy measures. Such models require many input variables, including (age-specific) relative risks and estimates of future health behaviours. Some of these variables can be based on sound epidemiological research, whereas others require assumptions or educated guesses. Forecasts often accommodate these uncertainties by varying the values of key parameters, resulting in different scenarios. Qualitative information may also be used in the development of these scenarios.

Scenarios can be very helpful in developing visions of the direction and magnitude of future changes, and provide insight into policy options. A 2010 study assessed whether existing models can be used as a standard tool for the quantification of health impact assessments of new policies. One of the assessment criteria was the ability to perform dynamic projections. The study found that none of the six generic models investigated fulfilled all the proposed criteria – they were either technically advanced with no or limited accessibility, or accessible but oversimplified (Lhachimi, Nusselder et al. 2010). To overcome these problems, a new model was developed within the EU-funded project Dynamic Modelling for Health Impact Assessment (DYNAMO-HIA 2013).

International actors in public health monitoring

One of WHO's core functions is shaping the research agenda and stimulating the generation, translation, and dissemination of valuable knowledge, including evidence on health trends and determinants (WHO 2006, 2011). Historically, WHO has been the leading international agency in the area of health data harmonization, collection, and dissemination. It has also supported countries in developing and upgrading their health monitoring systems. In the 1980s, the WHO Regional Office for Europe established the European Health for All database to support the monitoring of health trends, in line with WHO's Health for All strategy. Freely available online, and covering a broad range of topics, the database contains indicators on: demographic and socioeconomic statistics; mortality, morbidity, and disability; lifestyles; environment; healthcare utilization, resources and expenditure; and maternal and child health.

The WHO Regional Office for Europe maintains several other public health databases, such as the Environment and Health Information System (ENHIS) database, European Detailed Mortality Database (DMDB), European Hospital Morbidity Database (HMDB), European Nutrition, Obesity, and Physical Activity (NOPA) database, and the Centralized Information System for Infectious Diseases (CISID) (WHO Regional Office for Europe 2013b). At the global level, WHO maintains several health databases and information systems, most notably the Global Information System on Alcohol and Health (GISAH), the Global InfoBase – a data warehouse that collects, stores, and displays information on chronic diseases and their risk factors – and the Global Health Observatory (GHO) (WHO 2013).

Under Article 168 of the 2007 Lisbon Treaty on the Functioning of the European Union, the EU is bound to help attain a high level of health protection, improve public health, prevent disease, and obviate sources of danger to health (European Union 2007). The EU's actions for protecting and improving human health mainly take the form of European Commission health programmes. The Directorate General for Health and Consumers (DG SANCO) launched the first of these in the 1990s, one of which was the Health Monitoring Programme. This and two subsequent health programmes funded many projects dealing with various aspects of public health monitoring, including data collection and the development of indicators and guidelines (European Commission 2013b).

Other European Commission directorates are also involved in activities related to public health monitoring. The Directorate General for Research and Innovation has funded numerous relevant projects (European Commission 2013c); the Directorate General for Employment, Social Affairs, and Inclusion has funded work on indicators for social inclusion and protection, developed together with EU member states under the open method of coordination (European Commission 2013d). Overall, the European Commission has funded a range of short-term activities but has failed to create the mechanisms necessary for project results to be adopted into practice. This has caused problems for the sustainability of the health monitoring work initiated by the various projects.

For a long time, the legal basis for the European Commission's collection of health data was very narrow and data collection in the field of public health was mainly based on informal agreements. This changed following adoption of the 2008 *Regulation on Community statistics on public health and health and safety at work* (Regulation (EC) No. 1338/2008). The first implementing regulations on statistics on causes of death (Commission Regulation (EU) No. 328/2011) and accidents at work (Commission Regulation (EU) No. 349/2011) were adopted within this framework regulation in 2011. The implementing regulation on the EHIS followed in 2013 (Commission Regulation (EU) No. 141/2013). Thus, the collection of health data in the EU is becoming more and more obligatory. In addition to Eurostat, several other European agencies play a role in the collection of health information. These include the European Monitoring Centre for Drugs and Drug Addiction, the European Environment Agency, and the European Foundation for the Improvement of Living and Working Conditions.

With regard to health reporting, the European Commission funded a project for the development of a web-based pilot system for EU-wide flexible health reporting and monitoring – EUPHIX (Achterberg, Kramers et al. 2008). However, for technical and resource-related reasons, the pilot system was not followed up as intended. In 2011, the European Commission launched HEIDI (Health in Europe: Information and Data Interface), based on a wiki-like approach, with selected public health experts acting as authors (European Commission 2012). However, the HEIDI web site was closed in 2013, following a DG SANCO decision to reorganize all its public health-related websites.

The mission of the OECD is to promote policies that will improve the economic and social well-being of people around the world; collection and analysis of data is at the heart of this work. The OECD Health Data have been developed with the aim of comparing health systems across the 34 OECD countries and are used to generate regular *Health at a Glance* reports. The indicators mainly focus on healthcare activities and health expenditure – providing key indicators on health status, determinants of health, healthcare activities and health expenditure, and examining health system elements such as access to, and quality of, care (OECD 2011a).

Data harmonization between the major international actors involved in health monitoring has progressed through strategic collaboration between the European Commission, WHO, and OECD. This includes statistics on health expenditure, building especially on earlier OECD work and now laid down in a common System of Health Accounts (OECD 2011b). Within the broader WHO European Region there is now joint collection of other data on health systems, such as those on health workers and medical technologies. In September 2010, the European Commission and the WHO Regional Office for Europe signed a joint declaration which identifies several areas for closer collaboration, among them a single European health information system (Box 3.3).

Box 3.3 European Commission and WHO Regional Office for Europe: Joint Declaration

Modernizing and integrating the public health information system

Information and evidence for health policy- and decision-making in Europe is vital. Intercountry comparisons add a unique dimension to a country's own efforts and have been very effective in pinpointing areas for public health action, at both European and country level. This requires joint work to provide a common basis of information and evidence to ensure both the efficiency of our work and also its effectiveness.

Users of health information expect answers to questions about health at European level to be consistent, regardless of the source. Different answers to the same question undermine the credibility of both the Commission and the WHO. Working in partnership on the common collection and provision of information also reduces the burden on countries and makes

> best use of limited resources. We will therefore strengthen our cooperation in order to work towards a single integrated information system for health in Europe. This can build on existing cooperation, including expanding the use of shared data collection, collaborative analysis of health issues, and generation and dissemination of knowledge in support of health policy.
>
> *Source*: WHO Regional Office for Europe (2010)

Conclusions and policy recommendations

Many European countries have (sometimes long-lasting) experiences of setting up, reforming, and maintaining health monitoring systems. Instead of reinventing the wheel, it is better to share experiences and work together on new developments. Indeed, a recent article on the WHO perspective stated that:

> Countries would benefit most from [. . .] collaborative efforts that include support for data collections, sharing of data, development of scientific methods of estimation, publication of estimates, development of estimation tools and country capacity strengthening. (Boerma, Mathers et al. 2010)

Further alignment of the many systems of data collection that currently exist in Europe at regional, national, and international level would improve efficiency and data quality. A more coherent and collaborative European health information system would also help to overcome current variations in the availability of health data in Europe, where poorer countries often have poorer health information systems.

As already noted, some progress has been made. For example, the OECD, European Commission, and WHO Regional Office for Europe joint data collection on health expenditure according to the System of Health Accounts has relieved countries of the need to send similar data to three different data collectors. Furthermore, this will not only help to prevent different numbers appearing in different international databases on the same topic, but also enhance data quality and comparability through the use of common definitions and collection methods.

Notwithstanding these positive steps towards data harmonization, there is still a lot of work to be done. A central problem is the absence of a sufficiently detailed common European strategy and vision on health information and sustainable data collection. This challenge may be addressed to some extent by the recent agreement between the European Commission and the WHO Regional Office for Europe concerning closer collaboration on health information. In particular, WHO could play a more strategic role by helping to improve the sustainability of EU-initiated work in this area and by coordinating the expansion of initiatives to the rest of Europe.

Coordination of health reporting at international level can also be improved. A number of comprehensive European health monitoring reports have been produced in quick succession over the past few years; these were published, inter alia, by different Directorates General of the European Commission (e.g. 2009 Report on *The State of Health in the European Union*; 2010 *Health Trends in the EU*), WHO Regional Office for Europe (*European Health Report 2009*), and the OECD (*Health at a Glance: Europe 2010*). Many other, more topical, European health reports were published, often on very similar or even identical topics (e.g. chronic diseases; ageing and health). Most of these reports are based on the same set of data sources (for an overview, see ScotPHO 2013) and it is clear that closer collaboration between international organizations would yield much more efficient use of resources for health reporting. Establishment of an agreed core set of indicators for public health monitoring at European level would help to achieve minimum standards for public health reporting and reduce the costs of gathering data and information. It seems most logical to build on the ECHI work if we are to achieve this goal.

All of the aforementioned European health reports are informative in one way or another but they have had limited success in influencing European health policies, (re)setting the public health agenda, or changing research priorities. Policy practice always comprises a mixture of scientific evidence and more "irrational" elements of decision-making (see Chapter 18, "Knowledge brokering in public health"). Often, this makes it difficult to demonstrate the association between a health monitoring report and its policy impact, even when this impact seems clear to those involved. One example of a health report with direct policy implications was an international study on perinatal health that showed unexpected high perinatal mortality in the Netherlands. The findings not only influenced public and scientific opinions in the Netherlands (Sheldon 2008) but also led to a change in health policy (Merkus 2008), including the introduction of a national system of perinatal audit. More work is needed on the utilization of research to identify some of the barriers remaining between research, health reporting, and policy development (Goede, Putters et al. 2010).

Policy-makers face numerous challenges when setting up and maintaining health information systems. Technical and content-related issues are described in this chapter but politics and finances also matter. While the fluctuating political climate can undermine the sustainability of health information systems, resources may be too limited to ensure the continuity and comprehensiveness of the system. This holds especially true in the current economic crisis. Disease-specific registries (e.g. for diabetes or cardiovascular disease) are particularly expensive to maintain and this is the main reason why, with the exception of cancer registries, there are so few in European countries.

Another challenge is finding the right balance between rigidity (needed to produce solid time trends) and flexibility (needed to accommodate new public health problems and emerging policy needs). Furthermore, it can be difficult to meet the different and sometimes conflicting interests of different users of health information (e.g. advocacy groups, international donors, researchers, journalists). Finally, it is difficult to ensure that relevant and timely public health data find their way to the right target audiences, particularly in the light of specific rules and regulations governing data processors (Gissler, Dumitrescu et al. 2006).

Health monitoring is a prerequisite for evidence-informed policy-making and good governance. Despite all the difficulties involved, countries need to recognize the importance of the regular collection of health data and find sustainable ways to set up high-quality health information systems.

References

Achterberg, P. W., P. G. Kramers and J. A. M. van Oers (2008). "European community health monitoring: the EUPHIX model." *Scandinavian Journal of Public Health* **36**(7): 676–684.

Arah, O. A., G. P. Westert, J. Hurst and N. S. Klazinga (2006). "A conceptual framework for the OECD Health Care Quality Indicators Project." *International Journal for Quality in Health Care* **18**(Suppl. 1): 5–13.

Boerma, J. T., C. Mathers and C. Abou-Zahr (2010). "WHO and global health monitoring: the way forward." *PloS Medicine* **7**(11): e1000373.

Bon-Martens, M. J. H. van, P. W. Achterberg, L. A. M. van de Goor and J. A. M. van Oers (2012). "Towards quality criteria for regional public health reporting: concept mapping with Dutch experts." *European Journal of Public Health* **22**(3): 337–342.

Bruin, A. de, H. S. Picavet and A. Nossikov (1996). "Health interview surveys: towards international harmonization of methods and instruments." *WHO Regional Publications, European Series*, **58**(i–xiii): 1–161.

Bryndová, L., K. Pavloková, T. Roubal, M. Rokosová and M. Gaskins (2009). "Czech Republic: health system review." *Health Systems in Transition*, **11**(1): 1–122.

Carinci, F., C.T. Di Iorio, W. Ricciardi, N. Klazinga and M. Verschuuren (2011). "Revision of the European Data Protection Directive: opportunity or threat for public health monitoring?" *European Journal of Public Health* **21**(6): 684–685.

Chan, M., M. Kazatchkine, J. Lob-Levyt, T. Obaid, M. Sidibe, A. Veneman and T. Yamada (2010). "Meeting the demand for results and accountability: a call for action on health data from eight global health agencies." *PLoS Medicine* **7**(1): e1000223.

Commission Regulation (EU) No. 328/2011 of 5 April 2011 implementing Regulation (EC) No. 1338/2008 of the European Parliament and of the Council on Community statistics on public health and health and safety at work, as regards statistics on causes of death. *Official Journal of the European Union* L 90/22.

Commission Regulation (EU) No. 349/2011 of 11 April 2011 implementing Regulation (EC) No. 1338/2008 of the European Parliament and of the Council on Community statistics on public health and health and safety at work, as regards statistics on accidents at work. *Official Journal of the European Union* L 97/3.

Commission Regulation (EU) No. 141/2013 of 19 February 2013 implementing Regulation (EC) No. 1338/2008 of the European Parliament and of the Council on Community statistics on public health and health and safety at work, as regards statistics based on the European Health Interview Survey (EHIS). *Official Journal of the European Union* L 47/20.

Derose, S. F. and D. B. Petitti (2003). "Measuring quality of care and performance from a population health care perspective." *Annual Review of Public Health* **24**: 363–384.

DYNAMO-HIA (2013). Rotterdam, DYNAMO-HIA [http://www.dynamo-hia.eu/root/o14.html, accessed 29 August 2013].

European Commission (2009). *The State of Health in the European Union: Towards a healthier Europe.* EUGLOREH, EU Public Health Programme Project, Global Report on the Health Status in the European Union [http://www.eugloreh.it/ActionPagina_993.do].

European Commission (2010). *Health Trends in the EU.* Luxembourg, Directorate-General of Employment, Social Affairs and Equal Opportunities.

European Commission (2012). *Public Health: Highlights 2012.* Brussels, Directorate General for Health and Consumers [http://ec.europa.eu/health/highlights/2012/news_20120504_heidi_wiki_en.htm, accessed 2 September 2013].

European Commission (2013a). *The European Health Examination Survey.* Brussels, Directorate General for Health and Consumers [http://ec.europa.eu/health/

data_collection/tools/mechanisms/index_en.htm#fragment1, accessed 29 August 2013].

European Commission (2013b). *Health Programme: Policy.* Brussels, Directorate General for Health and Consumers [http://ec.europa.eu/health/programme/policy/index_en.htm, accessed 29 August 2013].

European Commission (2013c). *Health: Public health.* Brussels, Directorate General for Research and Innovation [http://ec.europa.eu/research/health/public-health/index_en.html, accessed 2 September 2013].

European Commission (2013d). *Social Protection and Social Inclusion.* Brussels, Directorate General for Health and Consumers [http://ec.europa.eu/social/main.jsp?langId=en&catId=750, accessed 2 September 2013].

European Union (2007). Treaty of Lisbon amending the Treaty on European Union and the Treaty establishing the European Community, signed at Lisbon, 13 December 2007. *Official Journal of the European Union* C 306/1.

Gapminder (2013). Stockholm, Gapminder [http://www.gapminder.org/, accessed 2 September 2013].

Geowise (2013). *InstantAtlas™.* Edinburgh, Geowise Ltd. [http://www.instantatlas.com/public-health_background.xhtml, accessed 2 September 2013].

Gerkens, S. and S. Merkur (2010). "Belgium: health system review." *Health Systems in Transition* **12**(5): 1–266.

Gissler, M., A. Dumitrescu and V. Addor (2006). *Improving the Performance of National Health Information Systems: The 2002–2003 reform in Finland from an international perspective.* Copenhagen, WHO Regional Office for Europe.

Goede, J. de, K. Putters, T. van der Grinten and Hans A. M. van Oers (2010). "Knowledge in process? Exploring barriers between epidemiological research and local health policy development." *Health Research Policy and Systems* **8**: 26.

Graunt, J. (1662). *Natural and Political Observations Made upon the Bills of Mortality.* E. Stephan [http://www.edstephan.org/Graunt/bills.html, accessed 2 September 2013].

Harbers, M. M., E. A. Van der Wilk, P. G. N. Kramers, M. M. A. P. Kuunders, M. Verschuuren, H. Eliyahu and P. W. Achterberg (2008). *Dare to Compare! Benchmarking Dutch health with the European Community Health Indicators (ECHI).* Bilthoven, National Institute for Public Health and the Environment (RIVM Report No. 270051011).

Health Protection Agency (2011). [http://www.hpa.org.uk/Topics/InfectiousDiseases/InfectionsAZ/Surveillance, accessed 12 August 2011].

Hollander, A. E. M. de, N. Hoeymans, J. M. Melse, J. A. M. van Oers and J. J. Polder, Eds. (2007). *Care for Health: The 2006 Dutch public health status and forecasts report.* Bilthoven, National Institute for Public Health and the Environment [http://www.rivm.nl/bibliotheek/rapporten/270061004.pdf, accessed 2 September 2013].

Ibrahimov, F., A. Ibrahimova, J. Kehler and E. Richardson (2010). "Azerbaijan: health system review." *Health Systems in Transition,* **12**(3): 1–117.

Kilpeläinen, K., A. Aromaa and the ECHIM Core Group, Eds. (2008). *European Health Indicators: Development and initial implementation. Final report of the ECHIM Project.* Helsinki, National Public Health Institute [http://www.echim.org/docs/ECHIM_final_report.pdf, accessed 2 September 2013].

Kramers, P. G. N. (2005). *Public Health Indicators for Europe: Context, selection, definition.* Bilthoven, National Institute for Public Health and the Environment (RIVM Report No. 271558006).

Lalonde, M. (1974). *A New Perspective on the Health of Canadians: A working document.* Ottawa, Government of Canada [http://www.phac-aspc.gc.ca/ph-sp/pdf/perspect-eng. pdf, accessed 2 September 2013].

Landesinstitut für den Öffentlichen Gesundheitsdienst NRW (lögd) (2003). *Evaluation of National and Regional Public Health Reports (Eva PHR). Final report to the European Commission.* Bielefeld, Institute of Public Health North Rhine Westphalia [http://www.pia-phr.nrw.de/Eva_Final_Report.pdf, accessed 2 September 2013].

Lhachimi, S. K., W. J. Nusselder, H. C. Boshuizen and J. P. Mackenbach (2010). "Standard tool for quantification in health impact assessment: a review." *American Journal of Preventive Medicine* **38**(1): 78–84.

Mathers, C. D., D. M. Fat, M. Inoue, C. Rao and A. D. Lopez (2005). "Counting the dead and what they died from: an assessment of the global status of cause of death data." *Bulletin of the World Health Organization* **83**(3): 171–177.

Merkus, J. M. (2008). "De verloskundige zorg in Nederland opnieuw de maat genomen" ["Obstetric care in the Netherlands under assessment again"]. *Nederlands Tijdschrift voor Geneeskunde [Dutch Journal of Medicine]* **152**(50): 2707–2708.

OECD (2010). *Health at a Glance 2010: Europe.* Paris, OECD Publishing [http://ec.europa.eu/health/reports/docs/health_glance_en.pdf].

OECD (2011a). *Health at a Glance 2011: OECD indicators.* Paris, OECD Publishing [http://www.oecd.org/health/health-systems/49105858.pdf, accessed 2 September 2013].

OECD (2011b). *Health Policies and Data: A system of health accounts.* Paris, OECD Publishing [http://www.oecd.org/els/health-systems/asystemofhealthaccounts.htm, accessed 2 September 2013].

PIA PHR (2013) Düsseldorf, Policy Impact Assessment of Public Health Reporting [http://www.pia-phr.nrw.de/index.html, accessed 2 September 2013].

Public Health England (2013). *Network of Public Health Observatories.* London, Public Health England (http://www.apho.org.uk/, accessed 2 September 2013).

Rahu, M. and M. McKee (2008). "Epidemiological research labelled as a violation of privacy: the case of Estonia." *International Journal of Epidemiology* **37**(3): 678–682.

Ramagen C, Ruales J (2008). The essential public health functions as a strategy for improving overall health systems performance: trends and challenges since the public health in the Americas initiative, 2000–2007. Washington DC, Pan American Health Organization (http://www1.paho.org/english/DPM/SHD/HR/EPHF_2000-2007.pdf, accessed 2 September 2013).

Regulation (EC) No. 1338/2008 of the European Parliament and of the Council of 16 December 2008 on Community statistics on public health and health and safety at work. *Official Journal of the European Union* L 354/70.

Reidpath, D. D. (2005). "Population health: more than the sum of the parts?" *Journal of Epidemiology and Community Health* **59**(10): 877–880.

Schoemaker, C., M. J. J. C. Poos, J. Spijker, C. H. van Gool and B. W. Penninx (2013). *Neemt het aantal mensen met depressie toe of af? [Is the Number of People with Depression Increasing or Decreasing?].* Bilthoven, National Institute for Public Health and the Environment [http://www.nationaalkompas.nl/gezondheid-en-ziekte/ziekten-en-aandoeningen/psychische-stoornissen/depressie/trend/, accessed 2 September 2013].

ScotPHO (2013). *Overview of Key Data Sources.* Edinburgh, Scottish Public Health Observatory [http://www.scotpho.org.uk/publications/overview-of-key-data-sources/introduction, accessed 2 September 2013].

Sheldon, T. (2008). "Perinatal mortality in Netherlands third worst in Europe." *British Medical Journal* 337: a3118.

Tableau© (2013). *Visual Gallery.* Seattle, Tableau Software [http://www.tableausoftware.com/learn/gallery, accessed 2 September 2013].

Verschuuren, M., G. Badeyan, J. Carnicero, M. Gissler, R. P. Asciak, L. Sakkeus, M. Stenbeck and W. Devillé (2008). "The European data protection legislation and its consequences for public health monitoring: a plea for action." *European Journal of Public Health* **18**(6): 550–551.

Verschuuren, M., P. Kramers, G. Gudfinnsdóttir and A. Aromaa (2010). "Providing a solid evidence base for policy makers: ECHI initiative." *EuroHealth* **16**(3): 4–7.

Westert, G. P., M. J. van den Berg, S. L. N. Zwakhals, J. D. de Jong and H. Verkleij (2010). *Dutch Health Care Performance Report 2010*. Bilthoven, National Institute for Public Health and the Environment (RIVM Report No. 260602006 [http://www.gezondheidszorgbalans.nl/object_binary/o10298_dhCPR2010.pdf, accessed 2 September 2013].

World Health Organization (WHO) (2000). *The World Health Report 2000 – Health systems: Improving performance*. Geneva, WHO [http://www.who.int/whr/2000/en/index.html, accessed 2 September 2013].

World Health Organization (WHO) (2006). *Engaging for Health: Eleventh general programme of work 2006–2015*. Geneva, WHO [http://whqlibdoc.who.int/publications/2006/GPW_eng.pdf, accessed 2 September 2013].

World Health Organization (WHO) (2011). *WHO Reforms for a Healthy Future. Report by the Director-General*. Geneva, WHO [http://apps.who.int/gb/ebwha/pdf_files/EBSS/EBSS2_2-en.pdf, accessed 2 September 2013].

World Health Organization (WHO) (2013) *Global Health Observatory*. Geneva, WHO [http://www.who.int/gho/en/, accessed 2 September 2013].

World Health Organization (WHO) Regional Office for Europe (2009). The European Health Report 2009. Geneva, WHO [http://www.euro.who.int/__data/assets/pdf_file/0009/82386/E93103.pdf].

World Health Organization (WHO) Regional Office for Europe (2010). *Annex 2: European Commission and WHO Regional Office for Europe: Joint declaration*. Copenhagen, WHO [http://www.euro.who.int/__data/assets/pdf_file/0011/121601/RC60_edoc12add1.pdf, accessed 2 September 2013]: 3.

World Health Organization (WHO) Regional Office for Europe (2013a). *What We Do: Equity in health. Interactive atlases*. Copenhagen, WHO [http://www.euro.who.int/en/what-we-do/data-and-evidence/equity-in-health/interactive-atlases, accessed 2 September 2013].

World Health Organization (WHO) Regional Office for Europe (2013b). *What We Do: Data and evidence*. Copenhagen, WHO [http://www.euro.who.int/en/what-we-do/data-and-evidence, accessed 2 September 2013].

chapter four

The health security framework in Europe

*Francisco Santos-O'Connor,
Jukka Pukkila, Carmen Varela Santos,
Cristiana Salvi, Dennis Faix,
Thomas Van Cangh, Josep Jansa,
Phillip Zucs, Paolo Guglielmetti,
Massimo Ciotti, Guénaël Rodier*

Introduction

The monitoring of and response to health hazards and emergencies is one of the essential operations of public health (see Chapter 1, "Facets of public health in Europe: an introduction"). In our present world, shaped by global travel and trade, pathogens can spread more rapidly than ever, increasing the likelihood that infectious disease outbreaks will involve more than one country. The preparation for, investigation of, and response to such outbreaks and other public health emergencies requires the coordination of national and international organizations (MacLehose, Brand et al. 2001).

This local, national, and international response can be conceptualized as an event management cycle (Figure 4.1). Event management is an iterative process that begins with the detection of events, followed by successive rounds of risk assessment, the implementation of control measures, and evaluation, supported by underlying preparedness efforts to strengthen the ability to perform all of these activities. Event management may take place at the local, national, regional, or global level. Regardless of the level at which an event is managed, communication – both internal and external – is a key component. When an event is potentially of international public health concern, additional communication is mandated by the 2005 International Health Regulations and, inside the EU, by the Decision of the European Parliament and of the Council on serious cross-border threats to health.

Event detection usually takes place through surveillance or notification. The initial effort is to assess the risk to public health and to recommend control measures. After these are implemented, ongoing surveillance and evaluation

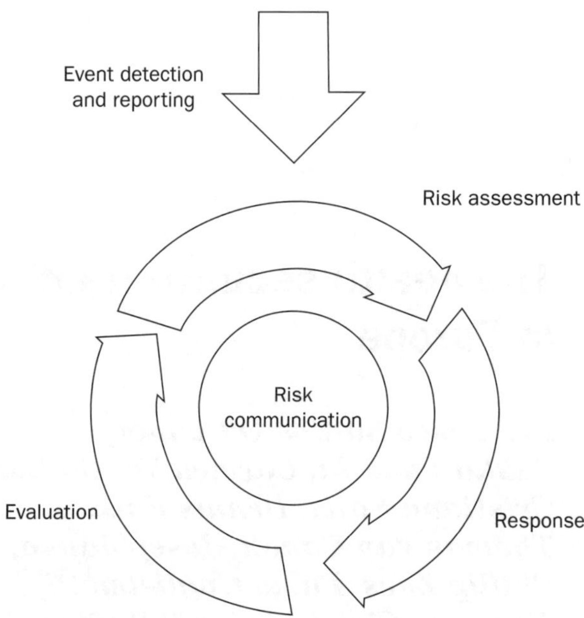

Figure 4.1 The event management cycle
Source: Author's compilation, based on WHO (2012b)

allow public health authorities to ascertain the effectiveness of control measures and establish that the outbreak has peaked and ended.

This chapter reviews the role of international organizations, in particular the World Health Organization (WHO) and the European Union (EU), in preparing for, detecting, and responding to events of public health importance. It starts by setting out the event management cycle, reviews the origin and function of the 2005 International Health Regulations, and explores which core capacities for surveillance and response are required at national level, and how WHO and EU support each of the steps of event management. Finally, the chapter discusses the involvement of WHO and EU in activities to strengthen national capacity to deal with public health threats and emergencies.

The International Health Regulations

The international response to public health events in the WHO European region may consist of voluntary requests for support from a country to a bilateral partner, regional surveillance networks, the European Centre for Disease Prevention and Control (ECDC) or WHO. Under the 2005 International Health Regulations (IHR), certain events of potential international public health concern are required to be reported to WHO. Similarly, if WHO is aware of a potential event, it may request verification from a country.

The IHR form the legal framework for collective responsibility for global health security and the international response to potential public health events of international concern (WHO 2005b). They originate in the International Sanitary Regulations, adopted in 1851. Following the 1969 revision of the IHR, the advent of emerging or re-emerging infectious diseases – such as plague in India in 1994 and Ebola in Zaire in 1995, along with non-infectious public health events, such as the nuclear disaster in Chernobyl in 1986 – led to a growing recognition that public health responses need to encompass all hazards rather than focus on a few specific diseases. The revised IHR were agreed upon at the World Health Assembly in 2005, after 10 years of development and following the 2003 outbreak of severe acute respiratory syndrome (SARS) and the pandemic threat caused by the avian influenza A(H5N1). The 2005 IHR entered into force on 15 June 2007 and (as of April 2012) legally bind all 193 WHO member states (Figure 4.2), plus the Holy See and the Principality of Liechtenstein.

The aim of the IHR is to prevent and respond to the international spread of disease, commensurate with public health risks, while avoiding unnecessary interference with international traffic and trade (WHO 2005b). Unlike the 1969

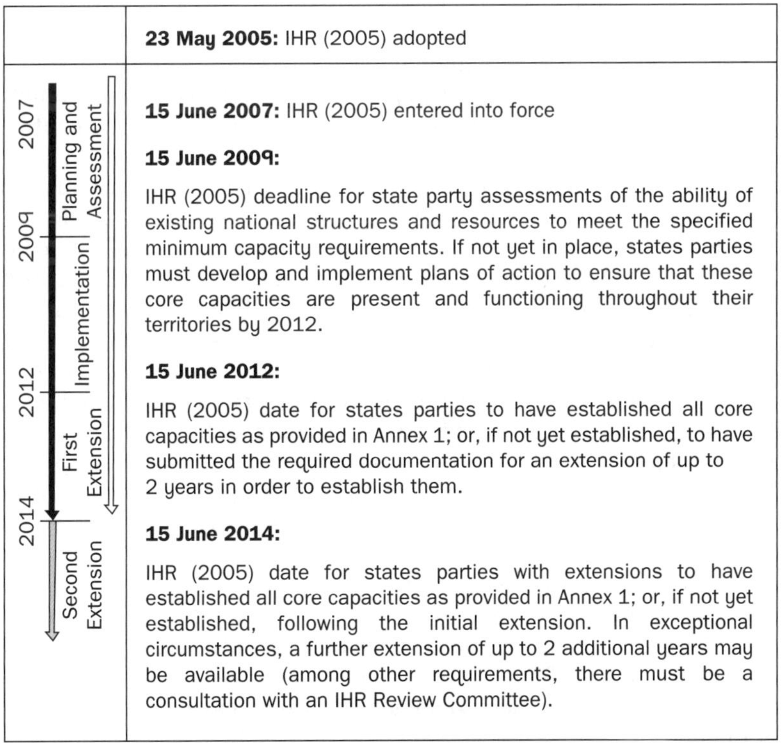

Figure 4.2 Timeline for implementation of the International Health Regulations (2005)

Source: Authors' compilation, adapted from WHO (2012a)

version of the IHR, the revised IHR include much more than a list of specific infectious diseases, and instead cover a wide range of public health risks of potential international concern. States parties to the IHR are now obliged to timely assess and notify WHO of any event of potential international public health concern, irrespective of its cause (whether chemical, biological or radio-nuclear) and origin (whether accidental or deliberate). This paradigm shift, from a list of diseases to an all-hazards approach, has been accompanied by two other paradigm shifts: moving from containment at borders to containment at source, and from pre-defined public health measures to responses adapted to the particular event.

The criteria for assessing the public health implications of any given event are outlined in the algorithm (decision instrument) presented in Annex 2 of the IHR. These include:

- health-related events that are unusual or unexpected,
- may have a significant impact on public health,
- may spread across borders,
- and may affect freedom of movement (of goods or people).

The decision instrument provides clear criteria for when an event may constitute a potential "public health emergency of international concern" (PHEIC), which the state party must assess within 24 hours and report to WHO within a further 24 hours. In addition to events fulfilling at least two of the four criteria given in Annex 2, all cases of the following four diseases must always be notified to WHO: smallpox, poliomyelitis due to wild-type poliovirus, human influenza caused by a new subtype, and SARS.

After an event is communicated to WHO, a joint risk assessment takes place to establish whether there is the need for response, assistance or information sharing. In extraordinary contexts involving major international public health concerns, the WHO Director General decides if the event formally constitutes a PHEIC. Between June 2007 (when the revised IHR entered into force) and March 2014, only one event was defined as a PHEIC – the influenza A(H1N1) pandemic, which was declared a PHEIC by the WHO Director General on 25 April 2009, after the first ever meeting of the IHR Emergency Committee.

When WHO receives an unofficial report of a public health event with potentially significant international implications, it is mandated to request verification of the event and its status from the respective country. WHO is further mandated to recommend and coordinate measures that will help prevent and respond to the international spread of disease, including public health actions at ports, airports, and land borders (so-called "points of entry"), and on means of transportation that involve international travel. When the WHO Director General has determined that the event constitutes a PHEIC, WHO will also issue "Temporary Recommendations" of appropriate health measures for states and others to implement, which have additional authority under the IHR.

The IHR (2005) oblige all state parties to designate "National IHR Focal Points" (NFPs), which have to be available at all times as the communication and information link for notification and other urgent IHR event-related communications with WHO. The NFPs also share information with other stakeholders and sectors in their country. The NFPs are often, but not always, the same as the designated Early Warning and Response System (EWRS) contact points in EU member states. The EWRS information technology platform provides an instrument for EWRS members to notify events to WHO, if the state party wishes to avoid double reporting.

The EU decision on serious cross-border threats to health

To better protect the population in the EU from a wide range of health threats, and provide for a fully coordinated response in the event of a crisis, Decision No. 1082/2013/EU of the European Parliament and the European Council of 22 October 2013 on serious cross-border threats to health, repealing Decision No. 2119/98/EC, has been adopted (European Union 2013). Building on lessons learned from past outbreaks and health crises, this new legal instrument aims to:

- extend the existing coordination mechanism for communicable diseases to cover serious cross-border threats to health caused by biological, chemical, and environmental events;
- strengthen preparedness and response planning for crises;
- enable a joint procurement procedure of medical countermeasures, including vaccines;
- enhance the current EWRS with new capabilities to communicate and exchange information on alerts from chemical, environmental, and unknown origin;
- recognize a situation of public health emergency for the purpose of making medicines available faster;
- formalize the mandate of the Health Security Committee (HSC), and thereby establish closer information exchange and coordination mechanisms between the EU and its member states.

This decision is a powerful instrument to respond in a coherent way to possible emergency situations in the EU that go beyond communicable disease outbreaks, and to align the EU legal framework on public health emergencies with the IHR. The decision adopts an all-hazards approach, expanding the existing instruments in the field of communicable diseases to cover other biological threats, as well as threats of chemical, environmental, and unknown origin. It repealed Decision No. 2119/98/EC on surveillance and control of communicable diseases.

Detection of public health events

To provide timely and validated intelligence on events of public health interest that may require an internationally coordinated response, countries and international organizations (including WHO and ECDC) have implemented

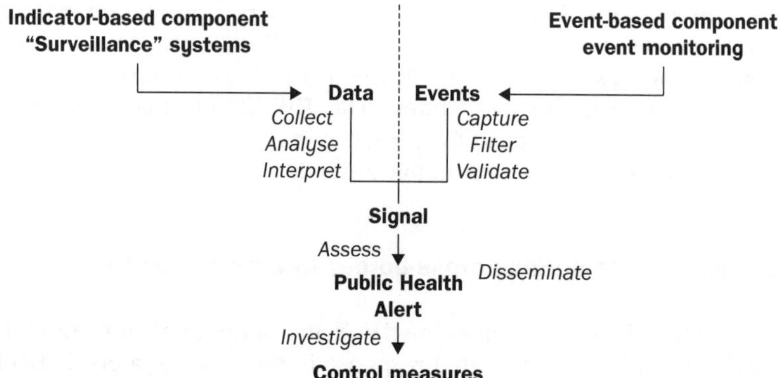

Figure 4.3 Epidemic intelligence framework

Source: Epidemic intelligence – a new framework for strengthening disease surveillance in Europe (Paquet, Coulombier et al. 2006)

epidemic intelligence activities. Paquet and colleagues define epidemic intelligence as the early identification, verification, assessment, and investigation of potential health hazards, in order to recommend public health control measures (Paquet, Coulombier et al. 2006).

The process starts with the identification of public health threats through an early warning system with two main sources of information: the "traditional" or indicator-based surveillance systems, collecting routine data about disease occurrence, and the event-based component, which involves the active review of unstructured information. While very different in nature, these two components follow similar processes: data collection vs. capture of events, data analysis vs. filtering of events, and interpretation of indicators vs. validation of events. Both components of epidemic intelligence are depicted in Figure 4.3.

Indicator-based surveillance

Indicator-based surveillance consists of the collection of structured data through routine operations, with specific data streams for particular diseases or syndromes. Indicator-based surveillance is the traditional surveillance tool of public health, designed to track trends in diseases or conditions over time and establish baseline rates of disease, burden of disease, morbidity, and mortality (see Chapter 3, "Monitoring the health of the population"). Indicators for surveillance may be based on clinical diagnoses, laboratory confirmation or other data, including information on, for example, school absenteeism, ambulance calls or sales of pharmaceuticals. Each disease or syndrome may have one or more indicators of varying sensitivity and specificity. For instance, multiple indicators have been used to track local and national trends in influenza, including the percentage of outpatient visits with influenza-like illness, the rate of laboratory-confirmed influenza cases, sales of over-the-counter medicines for colds, prescriptions for antiviral drugs, school absenteeism, and the use of certain search terms on the Internet. As some of these indicators are more specific and others more sensitive, a combination of indicators provides a more accurate overall picture.

Each country needs to establish a list of national priority diseases with the highest public health significance. The priority list has to include the key diseases listed in the IHR (smallpox, poliomyelitis due to wild-type poliovirus, novel influenza, and SARS). EU member states and other countries of the European Economic Area (EEA) also have to report to ECDC any diseases from the EU list of diseases. Each disease or condition requires a case definition on which to base surveillance efforts. The indicators for public health surveillance in a given country should be designed to give an overall picture of priority diseases, including baseline estimates, as well as trends and thresholds for alert and action.

Indicator-based surveillance also needs to include an early warning function for the early detection of public health events, such as an outbreak of a priority disease. A designated group or office at the national level needs to be responsible for the regular (at least weekly) review of surveillance data. The timeliness of various data streams may vary, but reporting units or systems have to report on time to facilitate the early warning function. Furthermore, when deviations or values above certain thresholds are detected, appropriate action, such as an outbreak investigation, needs to be taken by the public health system at the community level.

In addition to early warning alerts, indicator-based surveillance should also produce regular feedback to all levels and relevant stakeholders. Such feedback is generally in the form of epidemiological briefs or bulletins, electronic summaries or surveillance reports. It is also necessary to evaluate the surveillance systems for each disease or condition regularly and also if data streams or processes change.

In the WHO European region, there are many examples of indicator-based surveillance. During each influenza season, the WHO European Influenza Network (EuroFlu) collects weekly data from national sentinel surveillance networks of primary care practitioners to monitor outpatient visits with influenza-like illness or acute respiratory infection, virus type and subtype distribution, antiviral susceptibility, and vaccine match of circulating viruses. In addition, EuroFlu data inform WHO's annual selection of strains for the seasonal influenza vaccine. Indicators for many other communicable and vaccine-preventable diseases from all member states of the WHO European region are collected, analysed, and presented in the Centralized Information System for Infectious Diseases (CISID), accessible on the website of the WHO Regional Office for Europe (http://data.euro.who.int/cisid/).

For EU/EEA countries, The European Surveillance System (TESSy) provides a one-stop-shop for case-based reporting for the routine surveillance of 49 communicable diseases, including the 46 diseases listed in EU Decisions No. 2002/253/EC and No. 2003/534/EC, plus SARS, West Nile fever, and avian influenza (European Commission 2002, 2003; Ammon and Faensen 2009).

ECDC also collects case-based data on healthcare-associated infections, antimicrobial resistance, and antimicrobial consumption. The basis for EU-wide surveillance was Decision No. 2119/98/EC of the European Parliament and the Council of the EU in 1998 (European Union 1998), repealed in 2013 by the EU Decision on serious cross-border threats to health. According to its founding regulation (European Union 2004), from May 2005, the ECDC took on the task to standardize European surveillance by coordinating and further developing the pre-existing European surveillance networks that had developed separately. To harmonize procedures, EU case definitions were agreed jointly by member states and the European Commission (European Commission 2002, 2008a) and their use, where applicable, is mandatory for reporting to ECDC under the Decision on serious cross-border threats to health.

Event-based surveillance

Event-based surveillance is the organized and rapid capture of information about events that are a potential risk to public health (Bohigas, Santos-O'Connor et al. 2009). This information includes rumours and other ad hoc reports transmitted through formal (i.e. established routine reporting systems) and informal channels (i.e. the media, health workers, and reports from non-governmental organizations). This approach for detecting outbreaks and other relevant public health events allows the timely detection of health threats, which is not always achieved by traditional surveillance systems.

Event-based surveillance by WHO

Official information on public health events can reach WHO in different ways at all three levels of the organization (country offices, regional offices, and headquarters). The National IHR Focal Point (NFP) is the principal channel of official information to WHO on public health emergencies of potential international concern. As described above, each IHR state party has one NFP, which is an institution with an identified responsible person. In WHO, each regional office has established an IHR contact point for communications with NFPs.

WHO also receives official or unconfirmed information on public health events through its country offices (including the 29 WHO country offices in the WHO European region), technical programmes, various networks (such as EpiSouth, EpiNorth, and the European Network for Diagnostics of "Imported" Viral Diseases), health professionals, web sites of ministries, national, and sub-national institutions, and the media.

A large number of unofficial sources of information are continuously monitored by WHO. This monitoring is done at the global level by WHO headquarters, by the regional IHR contact points, and by WHO staff from various technical programmes. Many WHO country offices monitor the local media more or less systematically. In accordance with internal procedures of the WHO Regional Office for Europe, all WHO staff are obliged to bring information that signals a potential public health emergency to the attention of the IHR contact point as soon as possible.

The events that are officially reported to WHO, or when the information comes from official governmental sources (e.g. official web sites), are considered verified. When WHO becomes aware of a possible public health emergency of potential international concern through media monitoring, any other informal source or reports from another state party, the WHO IHR contact point makes a formal verification request to the respective state party where the event is allegedly occurring. The IHR require an acknowledgement or initial response to the verification request within 24 hours. Therefore, countries need to maintain the ability to respond rapidly to verification requests, collect relevant public health information, conduct a risk assessment, and communicate all of this to WHO within 24 hours. At the same time, WHO is obliged to offer collaboration and assistance.

Event-based surveillance by ECDC

ECDC also routinely searches information from event-based surveillance and filters it for potential public health events of European concern (i.e. affecting more than one EU member state), having the potential to do so, or requiring a coordinated response (Bohigas, Santos-O'Connor et al. 2009). So-called formal or official sources, such as the EU EWRS (see below), WHO through the IHR, and institutional web sites, always report validated events. Moreover, EU member states communicate validated events that could affect other countries through the EWRS, based on an assessment by public health authorities using established notification criteria (European Commission 2000, 2008b). However, unofficial sources (such as media reports) require validation (i.e. confirmation of authenticity) through cross-checking against independent sources of information or the active search for additional information.

The systematic screening of different sources of information includes preparing a document to be discussed at the daily round table organized every morning in ECDC with experts from different diseases and core functions. After that daily session, a new document is produced including the main aspects and actions to take for the selected threats. This daily round table report is shared with the Commission, some member states, other partners such as US CDC, and will shortly be shared with all member states. In the same sense, a weekly Communicable Diseases Threat Report (CDTR) is prepared and distributed, in order to summarize the most relevant topics discussed and threats systematically reviewed during the week.

Event-based surveillance by other institutions

Globally, there are a number of institutions constantly screening an exhaustive number of media sources for signals of potential public health emergencies or disasters. Some of these processes are fully automated (Brownstein and Freifeld 2007; Collier, Doan et al. 2008; Linge, Steinberger et al. 2009), while others include various levels of moderation by experts (Madoff 2004; Mykhalovskiy and Weir 2006; Wilson 2007). In addition to screening, automated systems conduct different levels of analysis and differ in the number of sources, languages covered, and frequency of scanning. Key words are used to recognize terms for names of diseases, symptoms, countries, and agencies. Editors in moderated systems may consider signals from individual web sites and automatic systems, as well as other formal and informal sources.

WHO and ECDC cooperate with many of these institutions and networks, including through the Information and Communication Technologies for Public Health Emergency Management (ICT4PHEM) initiative. In Europe, relevant institutions and networks include:

- the Europe Media Monitor (http://emm.newsbrief.eu/overview.html) of the European Commission Joint Research Centre;
- the Global Disaster Alert and Coordination System (http://www.gdacs.org/) of the European Commission Joint Research Centre;
- the Medical Information System (MediSys) (http://medusa.jrc.it/);
- the Pattern-based Understanding and Learning System (http://puls. cs.helsinki.fi/medical/);
- BioCaster Global Health Monitor (http://biocaster.nii.ac.jp/);
- the Global Public Health Intelligence Network (http://www.phac-aspc.gc.ca/ gphin/);
- HealthMap (http://www.healthmap.org/);
- the Hungarian National Association of Radio Distress-Signalling and Infocommunications (http://hisz.rsoe.hu/alertmap/);
- the Program for Monitoring Emerging Diseases (ProMED-mail; http://www. promedmail.org/), including editions in English and Russian.

Triage and recording of signals on public health events

Not all reports and alerts ("signals") generated through indicator- and event-based surveillance systems describe real events, and not all real events are of public health importance. The number of "false positives" (i.e. reported events that cannot be confirmed as real or when alert thresholds of indicator-based surveillance systems are exceeded but an outbreak is not confirmed) depends on the objectives and the design of surveillance systems, and the organizational level at which the event is assessed (WHO 2012b).

After detecting and validating public health events of potential European concern, further information from available sources is used to characterize the reported outbreaks by time, place, and persons affected and to analyse the risk for public health. Daily meetings take place in ECDC and WHO to review and preliminarily assess monitored events and threats. Member state authorities and experts can take part in this process. Signals considered relevant generate public health alerts that are then investigated, controlled, and communicated.

Event triage uses the same principles for assessing the risk an event may pose to public health as the more formal risk assessment described below. The WHO IHR Contact Point for Europe often uses the IHR Annex 2 decision instrument in the triage of signals on public health events. Actions from the IHR Contact Point for Europe include forwarding information to technical programmes, WHO country offices or headquarters, follow-up of an evolving event, and initiation

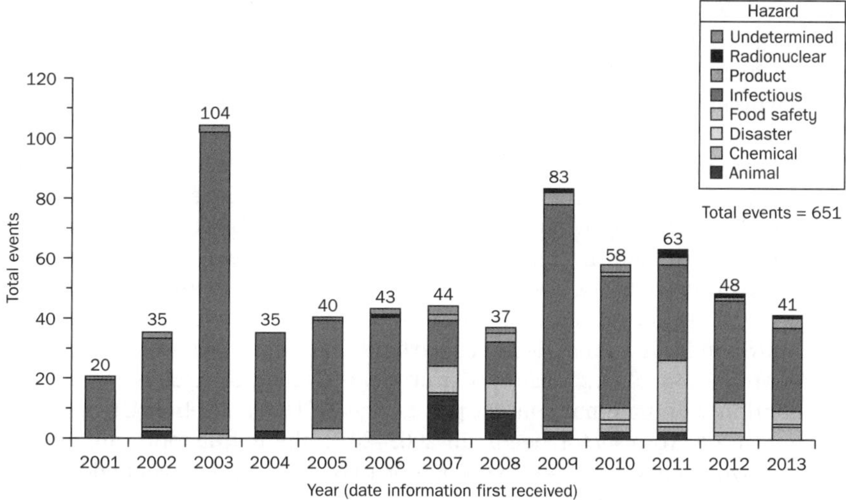

Figure 4.4 Public health events in the WHO European Region by hazard in 2001–2013 (as recorded in the WHO Event Management System)

of a communication with the affected state party. Public health events that require more actions from WHO than simply sharing information with others are recorded in the internal global WHO Event Management System, where all relevant information is collected and kept up-to-date. During the period 2001–2013, about 651 events with potential public health significance were recorded and followed up by the Alert and Response Operations in the WHO Regional Office for Europe (Figure 4.4). Of these events, 92 were significant enough to be recorded in the internal, global WHO Event Management System (EMS) and triggered IHR communications between WHO (IHR Contact Point for the European Region) and the National IHR Focal Point in the affected IHR States Parties.

ECDC also has a recording system for public health threats and related activities that are documented in the Threat Tracking Tool database, an IT platform specifically designed to keep track of verified events with a known or possible impact on public health. This facilitates information-sharing internally, as well as with the member states, the European Commission and other partners, and allows for auditing and evaluation of activities. Validated threats are actively followed up and all related relevant information documented until the threat has subsided or all appropriate measures have been implemented.

The Early Warning and Response System

The Early Warning and Response System (EWRS), operational since 1998, based on Decision No. 2119/98/EC of the European Parliament and the Council of the EU (European Union 1998), is a dedicated network for information exchange between public health authorities in EU member states, countries of the European Free Trade Association (EFTA) and the EEA, and the European Commission. WHO has also been part of the network since adoption of the IHR in 2005. The EWRS aims to support the planning and implementation of measures to respond to health threats due to communicable diseases of relevance to more than one member state.

Legal provisions set out the criteria for notifying outbreaks and acute events with potential impact on the EU, including agreed procedures for consultation and coordination. Following notification through the EWRS of an outbreak or an event matching the reporting criteria, the European Commission asks the ECDC to prepare an assessment of the situation, including the potential impact of the event on the EU. This risk assessment is then shared through the EWRS, and if the event deserves particular attention in terms of follow-up and coordination of response, the European Commission calls for ad hoc consultation with national contact points, the ECDC, and other EU agencies in the case of cross-sector needs. In 2002–2012, the notification rate was on average two events per week, with one or two of every ten events deserving special consultation for coordination purposes.

In case of need (e.g. in the response to the 2009 influenza A(H1N1) pandemic), the European Commission calls an EWRS teleconference to support the coordination of the risk management at EU level in close contact with ECDC, WHO, and other stakeholders. To ensure a coordinated approach, such consultations through teleconferences take place regularly to cover and update risk assessment, management, and communication issues.

The reports of the European Commission to the European Parliament and the European Council on the operation of the EWRS provide information on specific events of particular significance. In addition, specific post-event assessments and analyses have been carried out on the most recent outbreaks of *Escherichia coli* O104:H4, H1N1 pandemic influenza, MERS CoV, influenza H7N9, and polio. All these assessments are available on the Internet.

A number of elements have proved crucial for a robust coordination of the EU response to outbreaks. The existence of a formal network has been pivotal in bringing together appropriate actors. The rapid notification of events through the EWRS has allowed the ECDC to prepare rapid threat assessments, including the evaluation of potential risks for the EU. The EWRS application has worked well and could be adapted to different needs in diverse emergency situations. During recent years, the European Commission and the network have strengthened the coordination with other sectors (e.g. food, feed, and animal health sectors), developing procedures and links with other EU agencies and the European Commission. The entry into force of the new IHR in 2007, together with the influenza pandemic in 2009, have prompted a further upgrade of the EWRS informatics tool and of communication procedures.

The mechanism in place is adaptable so as to be able to respond to new legislation, as well as new technical developments in informatics technology. Article 168 of the Lisbon Treaty introduced new powers for the EU to combat serious cross-border health threats, in addition to communicable diseases and complementing national policies.

Between 1998 and December 2005, public health authorities notified 396 events and circulated 583 messages through a specifically developed web-based informatics tool. Since April 2005, the EWRS has been operated by the ECDC to assist members of the network in the area of risk assessment (Guglielmetti, Coulombier et al. 2006).

Cox and colleagues analysed the activity of the EWRS by incidence. Of a total of 917 "new events" (messages posted for all members by any member) aggregated on monthly intervals from May 2004 to September 2009, there was a seasonal pattern in the average number of new events, with more new events being posted between June and October (Cox, Guglielmetti et al. 2009). These authors also described a sharp increase in several months of 2009, corresponding to the start of the H1N1 influenza pandemic and a smaller increase during the first six months of 2006, corresponding to the detection of avian influenza A(H5N1) in Europe. This suggests that the notification process can indicate situations requiring the extensive mobilization of public health resources.

Decision No. 1082/2013/EU expands the scope of the EWRS beyond communicable diseases to cover all types of cross-border threats to health.

Reporting

Countries define their own reporting requirements for communicable diseases, including which diseases need to be reported, case definitions, if case-based or event-based reporting is required, and the frequency of reporting. As mentioned above, certain diseases need to be reported to WHO or ECDC. Countries report polio surveillance data to WHO on a weekly basis, and case-based data on measles and rubella on a monthly basis. The 16 member states of the WHO European region, in which diphtheria is endemic, report cases on a monthly basis. EU/EEA countries report cases of travel-associated Legionnaires' disease to ECDC daily, influenza data weekly, measles and rubella data monthly, food and waterborne disease surveillance data quarterly, and data for most other diseases annually. There is a growing number of examples of joint reporting to ECDC and the WHO Regional Office for Europe (influenza, tuberculosis, and HIV/AIDS) or data forwarding from the former to the latter (measles, rubella) to avoid duplication of work for the data providers. Annual data on all reportable communicable disease from WHO member states is collected using a UNICEF-WHO Joint Reporting Form. However, not only do the lists of reportable diseases vary between countries, but also their case definitions, and data collected through the Joint Reporting Form are often not comparable between countries.

As mentioned above, the IHR oblige states parties to notify WHO of all events that may constitute a public health emergency of international concern within 24 hours. Notification may be required for:

- events caused by biological agents (of infectious or non-infectious nature), chemical agents or radio-nuclear materials;
- events where the underlying agent, disease or mode of transmission is new, newly discovered or as yet unknown at the time of notification;

- events involving transmission or potential transmission through persons, vectors, cargo or goods (including food products) and environmental dispersion;
- events that have a potential future impact on public health and require immediate action;
- events arising outside of their known usual occurrence patterns.

Such potentially notifiable events extend beyond communicable diseases and include such issues as contaminated food or other products, including pharmaceuticals, and the environmental spread of toxic, infectious material or other contaminants. In addition to notifying WHO about events occurring within their own territories, IHR states parties are required to inform WHO about a public health risk identified outside their territory that may cause the international spread of disease.

Risk assessment

Risk assessment is a crucial step in managing public health events. The risk assessment of any event is demanding, especially in the early phases of the event when information is usually limited, incomplete or even controversial. In events where available information does not allow for proper assessment, the IHR provides an option for countries to keep WHO informed about the event in a confidential manner through "consultation", which can include discussion of appropriate follow-up and response measures to be taken, and offers an opportunity for a joint risk assessment.

Rapid risk assessment is a systematic process that facilitates risk management during an acute public health event, and allows defensible and evidence-based decision-making, improved operational and risk communication, and increased preparedness. To facilitate communication and understanding of rapid risk assessment results, it is important that these are performed systematically, with standard definitions of hazard severity and likelihood, as well as clear identification of assumptions and certainty of confidence in those assumptions. Ideally, it is conducted jointly between ECD and/or WHO and the affected member states. The rapid risk assessment documents what risks and control measures were assessed, the methods used for assessment, why they were considered important, and their relative priority. WHO and ECDC have both published guidance on rapid risk assessment for acute public health events.

According to the ECDC operational guidance on rapid risk assessment methodology, rapid risk assessment is a core part of the public health response and thus widely undertaken by public health professionals (ECDC 2011). Formal systems that are used to grade evidence and recommendations, such as the systematic methods used in evidence-based medicine, rely on published research evidence, and studies are graded according to design and susceptibility to bias. However, as time and evidence are limited, a rapid risk assessment may need to rely at least in part on specialist expert knowledge, and these formal systems are not directly applicable. However, the same principles of transparency, explicitness, and reproducibility also apply to a rapid risk assessment.

For the rapid risk assessment of most infectious disease threats, observational data are often the only available and obtainable source of information. Expert knowledge is also important if there is lack of time and evidence. In such cases, it is important to "unpack" and make explicit the expert knowledge and distinguish between knowledge based on good research, and experience and opinion-based knowledge. Serious attempts should be made to assess the quality of the evidence, based on the source, design, and quality of each study or piece of information. Uncertainties should be identified, clearly documented and communicated, and the assessment updated in light of new evidence over time. A rapid risk assessment includes the approach and tools required at each stage of the process: stage 0 is the preparation stage; stage 1 is the collection of event information; stage 2 is the literature search and systematic collection of information about the aetiological agent; stage 3 focuses on the extraction of evidence; stage 4 conducts an appraisal of the evidence; and stage 5 estimates the risk. Transparency and sharing of information is essential at every stage. This document incorporates a step-by-step guide through each stage with examples and checklists of the resources and evidence required. Advance preparation and planning saves time and is vital to ensure that potential threats are identified, assessed, and managed effectively. Ideally, the following should be in place: evidence-based protocols and guidance for responding to incidents, protocols for identifying sources of key information for rapid risk assessment, strategies for literature searches, and lists of relevant contacts including named experts.

Rapid risk assessments of potential communicable disease threats can be complex and challenging, as they must be produced within a short time when information is often limited and circumstances can evolve rapidly. The rapid risk assessment methodology described in this document enables the structured identification of key information using systematic appraisal of the best scientific evidence and/or specialist expert knowledge available at the time to provide a clear estimate of the scale of the health risk. This is important in not only communicating the potential magnitude of the risk in a systematic and transparent way, but allows documentation of evidence and gaps in knowledge at the time when the assessment is made.

Examples of infectious disease outbreaks affecting the WHO European region

Measles outbreaks

Since 2002, when the WHO Regional Office for Europe developed a strategic plan for the elimination of measles by 2010, progress has been made and vaccination coverage for measles, mumps, and rubella (MMR) has increased. Nevertheless, outbreaks are still being reported across Europe. An ECDC rapid risk assessment in March 2010 acknowledged the risk for a further spread of measles to susceptible individuals. Preliminary data as of February 2011 submitted to the Surveillance Community Network for vaccine-preventable infectious diseases (EUVAC.NET) indicated a total of 28,421 measles cases reported in EEA member states for 2010. Only eight EEA countries reported no cases at all for 2010 (EUVAC.NET 2010). This situation led the WHO Regional Office for Europe in September 2010 to set a new target date for eliminating measles and rubella in the European region by 2015 (WHO Regional Office for Europe 2010).

Pandemic influenza A(H1N1)

Upon the confirmation of swine influenza in two children in California (United States), coinciding with the recognition of increased influenza deaths in Mexico due to the same strain, WHO declared a public health event of international concern on 25 April 2009, which was later acknowledged as the beginning of the influenza A(H1N1) pandemic. ECDC published an initial rapid risk assessment on the situation on 23 April 2009 (ECDC 2009). Although the regular influenza season was considered to be over, a 99% increase in recorded cases of pandemic influenza A(H1N1) infections in the WHO European region was observed from calendar week 22 to week 23, bringing the total number of cases to 937 as of 4 June 2009. On 11 June 2009, the WHO headquarters in Geneva declared the epidemic "the first pandemic of the 21st century", based on its geographic distribution. Lessons learned from this event (http://www.ecdc.europa.eu/en/healthtopics/ pandemic_preparedness/pandemic_2009_evaluations/Pages/pandemic_2009_ evaluations.aspx; http://www.who.int/ihr/review_committee/en/) fed into the development of the EU decision on cross-border threats to health.

MERS CoV

In June 2012, a case of fatal respiratory disease in a previously healthy 60-year-old man was reported from Saudi Arabia. The cause was subsequently identified as a new coronavirus that has been named Middle East respiratory syndrome coronavirus (MERS-CoV). Retrospective investigations revealed that the first cases of the disease had occurred previously in a cluster of hospital-associated cases in Jordan in April 2012. By 9 January 2014, 178 laboratory-confirmed cases of MERS had been reported. All cases had either occurred in the Middle East or had direct links to a primary case infected in the Middle East.

Risk communication

Under the IHR, WHO member states have committed to develop and strengthen their capacity for risk communication. During an emergency, risk communication is a key public health tool to manage risks. Effective communication messages will increase the population's acceptance of the guidance given by health authorities, reduce behaviours that might lead to risk exposure, and improve surveillance (WHO 2005a, 2005c).

Developing a risk communication plan is the first step towards building the required capacity. While not all European countries have the resources to put in place an elaborate communication system, all have the capacity for basic planning. The following key capacities of a risk communication plan will need to be considered (elaborated from WHO 2008):

- **Assessment:** each country needs a "critical mass" of expert risk communicators. Countries should conduct an assessment of communication plans and capacity at different levels, train the required risk communication practitioners, and take advantage of the capacity of partner organizations. This would need to take into account peak times when surge capacity is needed.
- **Transparency:** regular and transparent communication with the public reduces anxiety and increases trust in state authorities. Countries should develop a system for the first announcement in the event of a verified or suspected risk and for the ongoing release of information as part of the risk communication plan, including proper tools and channels.
- **Coordination:** coordination is paramount during an emergency, both intersectorally and among different levels, and with international partners and other countries. Countries should identify coordination mechanisms, including those related to the release of information, message sharing, streamlined clearance procedures, and identification of spokespersons. National and international communication partners should be identified and a list developed and maintained.
- **Listening:** risk communication will not be effective without an understanding of the public's risk perception. Listening is a prerequisite for learning how people perceive and react to risks, how they trust the responders, and what beliefs and practices can prevent adoption of a protective behaviour. This will allow the formulation of effective messages. Countries should develop a system to assess existing community profiles (i.e. through public opinion surveys), gather information during an emergency (i.e. through community advisory panels, door-to-door visits, hotlines, media monitoring) and integrate findings into decision-making.
- **Information dissemination:** health crises are characterized by time pressure, high demand for information, and need of advice to minimize a public health threat; this makes the rapid and effective dissemination of information crucial. Mass media relations remain a pillar of efficient information dissemination. However, it is increasingly important to access other channels that the population uses and trusts, including social media, mobile phones, networks, and health workers.
- **Evaluation:** it is vital to understand the effectiveness of communication strategies in order to identify gaps and address them as appropriate. Countries need to put in place an evaluation mechanism during and after the emergency to assess the impact of communication interventions.

The risk communication plan should describe the functions and roles required to implement the above-listed components, as well as the needed activities and products. It should break down implementation into the following stages of an emergency: pre-event, initial phase of the emergency, peak of the emergency, and resolution. Finally, it needs uptake by the highest political levels of the country that would take decisions on communication during an emergency.

In the EU, public health authorities exchange information on potential threats, possible clusters, and uncommon events from communicable diseases through the Epidemic Intelligence Information System (EPIS), a real-time European web-based communication platform, which offers a valuable tool for experts from member states to exchange information on outbreak identification, validation, and assessment (Gossner 2013). Specific reporting and information on control measures is exchanged through the EWRS platform and public health authorities coordinate when, how, and by whom information about the event should be made public. Factors to consider include media or public opinion risks associated with the event and the development of appropriate media messages, in coordination with the affected member state and other stakeholders, to ensure consistency. An ad hoc communication team may be identified for this purpose. It regularly produces situation reports and updated rapid risk assessments that are shared through the EWRS and, if adequate, made public by different means, including press releases, TV/radio, and the Internet.

Response

The primary responsibility for investigating and responding to public health emergencies lies with the health authorities and professionals in the communities where the event occurs. However, the regional and national authorities need to be made aware as early as possible of any event that might go beyond previously affected areas and require the involvement of higher levels of administration. Functioning mechanisms for information sharing between different administrative levels and between sectors are needed in every country, as well as mechanisms for mobilizing an appropriate, sufficient, and timely response. As described above, under the IHR, the national authorities (especially the National IHR Focal Point institution) have the responsibility to inform the international community through WHO of all events that may constitute a public health emergency of international concern. These communications form the basis for requesting and offering international assistance for event investigation and response. Similar mechanisms apply between the EU and its member states under the Decision for serious cross-border threats to health.

In cases of infectious disease outbreaks, the following minimum steps are often undertaken concurrently (Gregg 2008; Heymann 2008):

- verifying that the threat exists and establishing a clear case definition;
- confirming the existence of an outbreak;
- establishing an outbreak control team that should meet regularly;
- identifying affected persons and their epidemiological characteristics;
- recording typical case histories;
- identifying additional cases;
- defining the population at risk;
- investigating the outbreak and formulating a hypothesis as to its source and spread;

- testing the hypothesis;
- determining control measures;
- containing or mitigating the outbreak;
- managing cases;
- implementing control measures;
- establishing regular communications, including with the affected population;
- conducting ongoing disease surveillance (also called active surveillance);
- preparing a report and auditing the response.

Many of these steps are also undertaken in the response to public health emergencies caused by non-infectious hazards. Furthermore, in the beginning of a public health event the causative hazard is often unknown.

Capacity-building

The WHO Regional Office for Europe developed a set of ten essential public health operations (EPHOs) to serve as a useful guide for strengthening public health services and capacity in the region (see Chapter 1, "Introduction"). EPHO 2, *Monitoring and response to health hazards and emergencies*, directly points towards the development of core capacities under the IHR.

The IHR define core public health capacity requirements for all states parties for disease surveillance, detection, assessment, and response at all levels, as well as for designated international points of entry. These requirements aim at ensuring that all states have the ability to meet their obligations under the IHR, so that events of public health importance can be prevented or controlled locally at source before spreading nationally or internationally.

At the community level, capacities to perform the following activities are required:

- detection of events involving disease or death above expected levels;
- immediate reporting of all essential information to the appropriate level of health care;
- immediate implementation of preliminary control measures.

The intermediate level is required to be able to:

- confirm the status of reported events and support or implement additional control measures;
- immediately assess reported events and, if found urgent, report all essential information to the national level.

At the national level, required core capacities include the capability to assess all reports of urgent events within 48 hours and to notify WHO immediately when the assessment indicates that the event is notifiable under IHR. The national level has to be able to rapidly determine the control measures required to prevent domestic and international spread, and to provide support through specialized staff, laboratory analysis of samples, logistical assistance, and on-site assistance to supplement local investigations. It also has to be capable of providing a direct operational link with senior health and other officials to rapidly approve and implement the required containment and control measures, and to provide direct liaison with other relevant government ministries. Furthermore, the national level is required to provide links with hospitals, clinics, airports, ports, ground crossings, laboratories, and other key operational areas for the dissemination of information and recommendations received from WHO.

Finally, states parties are obliged to ensure that their legislation supports the implementation of and compliance with the IHR by national public health authorities. They are also required to be able to establish, operate, and maintain a national public health emergency response plan, including the creation of multidisciplinary and multisectoral teams for response. Under the EU Decision on serious cross-border threats to health, additional information exchange requirements apply to EU member states to further coordinate their preparedness and response planning efforts. These aim to enhance the sharing of good practices, the homogenous implementation of core capacity requirements, and the interoperability of national preparedness planning.

The ECDC, the European Commission, EU and WHO member states, and WHO are involved in a great variety of activities to strengthen public health capacity across Europe to foster timely detection, effective and coordinated disease surveillance, adequate assessment, and an efficient response to expected and unexpected health threats through scientific studies and guidance, technical assistance, and training.

WHO has developed global and region-specific tools for the assessment, implementation, and monitoring of IHR core capacities. The IHR web site (http://www.who.int/ihr) provides access to both general publications and guidelines and specific assessment and monitoring tools. These include in-depth assessment protocols, specific assessment tools (e.g. for points of entry, laboratory capacities, risk communications, and legislation), monitoring checklists, states parties questionnaires, and other guidance.

During the biennium 2010–11, the WHO Regional Office for Europe mobilized field missions to nine public health events (six infectious disease events, two events of civil unrest leading to refugee influxes, and one chemical spill). During this period, the WHO Regional Office for Europe recorded and assessed 122 public health events that were considered to be of concern, while hundreds of events were screened, but did not lead to communications with the involved member states.

When mobilizing field missions, the newly adopted global WHO Emergency Response Framework sets internal performance standards for WHO. According to these standards, the timeline for establishing WHO presence on site, when WHO's assistance in public health emergencies is requested and required, is 24 hours in those countries where WHO is already present. The timeline for the arrival of an international response team is 72 hours.

Examples of capacity strengthening activities in the EU

Building and improving public health capacity is a key strategy to respond to public health emergencies. In the case of the 2009 influenza pandemic, for example, specific preparedness plans were put in place at national and EU level (Health Protection Agency 2010). On 28 November 2005, the European Commission adopted a generic preparedness plan to address threats and emergencies affecting or likely to affect public health in more than one EU country, providing a foundation on which national authorities could build their own generic or disease-specific plans (European Commission 2005).

Following its mandate (European Union 2004), ECDC organizes courses for senior public health professionals from EU member states, EEA and EFTA countries, and EU candidate and potential candidate countries. Most courses address technical aspects (including health threat detection, risk assessment, outbreak investigation, and risk communication). One of the courses focuses on the acquisition of managerial skills, targeting coordinators of outbreak investigation teams. The European Programme for Intervention Epidemiology Training (EPIET) and the European Programme for Public Health Microbiology Training (EUPHEM) are two-year "learning by doing" fellowships with an exchange component that contribute to capacity strengthening in Europe.

The European Commission, ECDC, and WHO also regularly organize simulation exercises to test EU and national preparedness plans and ensure their inter-operability, working together with national authorities, other institutions, and international organizations. Experience has shown the need for closer intersectoral collaboration and public health preparedness increasingly includes multidisciplinary teams and partnerships, not only through the above-mentioned disease-specific surveillance networks, but also through non-disease-specific public health networks [e.g. EUVAC.NET (Glismann, Ronne et al. 2001)] and non-public health networks [including virologists, such as ENIVD (Niedrig, Donoso-Mantke et al. 2007); entomologists, such as VBORNET (VBORNET 2009); and travel medicine physicians, such as EUROTRAVNET (Schlagenhauf, Santos-O'Connor et al. 2010)].

A good example of the added value of EU level preparedness activities is the public health response to outbreaks in mass gatherings, as was seen with the measles outbreak in Austria and Switzerland during the 2008 European Football Championship (Kreidl, Buxbaum et al. 2008). ECDC published a risk assessment before the championship, which concluded that ongoing measles outbreaks in both countries could have the potential for international spread, and so immunization was recommended for those planning to attend. During the event, epidemic intelligence and response activities were coordinated at European level. Low-level measles transmission occurred, but no cases associated with the event were reported.

International health assistance to outbreak response

Since its foundation in 1948, preventing the international spread of infectious disease has been one of WHO's core responsibilities, as set out in Article 21(a) of its constitution. WHO offers assistance to affected member states in the form of technical advice, supplies, and in a number of cases, by mounting coordinated international investigations or responses. The entry into force of the revised IHR on 15 June 2007 further expanded WHO's mandate in assisting its member states in their response. In its assistance, WHO draws on the resources from a large number of partner institutions and networks. So-called WHO Collaborating Centres have existed since 1948. As of 2012, they included more than 800 highly regarded academic and scientific institutions in over 80 countries, supporting WHO with time, expertise, and funding. Many of these institutions have resources that can be mobilized to support investigations of and response to all types of public health emergencies.

In April 2000, the Global Outbreak Alert and Response Network (GOARN) was established. GOARN is a technical collaboration of existing institutions and networks that pools human and technical resources for the rapid identification, confirmation, and response to outbreaks of international importance. Over time, GOARN has expanded to include over 300 partner institutions. An independent evaluation of GOARN analysed 75 documented field missions between June 2000 and March 2009. Altogether, 125 GOARN partners participated in these missions, including 48 institutions (38%) from the WHO European region. Of the 75 analysed field missions, 7 (9%) took place in the WHO European region, 5 of which were responses to avian influenza outbreaks in 2006. The 75 missions varied greatly in duration and number of staff involved (with between 2 and 114 staff deployed per mission).

In food-borne outbreaks, another valuable resource is the International Food Safety Authorities Network (INFOSAN). This is a joint initiative between WHO and the Food and Agriculture Organization of the United Nations (FAO). INFOSAN is a global network and currently includes 177 member states. Each has a designated INFOSAN emergency contact point for communication between national food safety authorities and the INFOSAN secretariat regarding urgent events. To help respond to country requests for assistance during food safety emergencies, INFOSAN partners with GOARN. It also works with the Global Early Warning System for Major Animal Diseases, including Zoonoses (GLEWS) to promote seamless action throughout the food-chain continuum.

Reports on communicable diseases – be they routine reporting or ad hoc reports on unusual events – originate mostly from front-line health workers. Ensuring complete and timely notifications therefore depends on reports of unusual events reaching national public health authorities. To assist national public health authorities in Europe to achieve this, a toolkit has been created by the European Commission-funded REACT (Response to Emerging infectious disease: Assessment and development of Core capacities and Tools) Project, based at the Norwegian Institute of Public Health. The toolkit offers suggestions on how to improve the reporting of public health events from clinicians and laboratory staff to the first level of public health authorities, and from there to the national public health authority (Norwegian Institute of Public Health 2011). At EU level, the ECDC may be requested by the European Commission, the member states, third countries, and international organizations to provide expert assistance or mobilize and coordinate teams to investigate communicable disease outbreaks (European Union 2004).

International health assistance in response to chemical releases

Chemical releases arising from technological incidents, natural disasters, conflicts, and terrorism are common. The International Federation of Red Cross and Red Crescent Societies has estimated that globally between 2000 and 2009, there were nearly 3200 technological disasters, with approximately 100,000 people killed, and more than 1.5 million people affected (International Federation of Red Cross and Red Crescent Societies 2010). Through the International Programme on Chemical Safety, WHO aims to create capacity to rapidly detect, assess, verify, alert, and respond to chemical events of international public health concern as part of the obligations under the IHR. WHO provides guidance for strengthening the role of public health in the prevention, preparedness, detection, alert, response, and recovery to chemical incidents and emergencies, particularly for developing countries and countries in transition.

International health assistance in response to radio-nuclear emergencies

The Radiation Emergency Medical Preparedness and Assistance Network (REMPAN) was established in 1987 in order to fulfil WHO's responsibility under the 1986 Convention on Assistance in Case of a Nuclear Accident or Radiological Emergency and the 1986 Convention on Early Notification of a Nuclear Accident. REMPAN currently includes 40 medical and research institutions specializing in diagnosis, monitoring, dosimetry (measurement of radiation doses), treatment, and long-term follow-up of radiation injuries, acute radiation syndrome, internal contamination, and other radio-pathology. The network is designated to provide emergency medical and public health assistance to people overexposed to radiation. It also facilitates long-term care and follow-up of victims of radiation accidents and conducts research in radiation emergency medicine, radiotherapeutics, bio-dosimetry, and radiation epidemiology. Assistance provided by REMPAN institutions in radiation emergencies may include:

- human resources and specialists: including specialists in radiation medicine, health physics, radiology, haematology, and other appropriate specialities (such as burn departments), as well as skilled nurses and technicians;
- equipment: most centres are well-equipped to provide special medical assistance to overexposed persons; they also have portable equipment for radiation monitoring;
- medical services: assistance is provided for the diagnosis, prognosis, medical treatment, and medical follow-up of persons affected by radiation;
- scientific services: expertise can be provided to assess radiation doses to exposed persons (most of the REMPAN institutions have bio-dosimetry laboratories);
- transportation: advice on the transportation of affected persons;
- specialized teams: WHO can organize multinational teams for providing medical assistance on site.

Under the Convention on Early Notification of a Nuclear Accident, the International Atomic Energy Agency (IAEA) is the designated international organization that has to be officially notified by the affected country and provided with relevant information. WHO, as well as other international organizations, are notified and provided with relevant information through the IAEA.

Conclusion

This chapter has reviewed the role of the WHO Regional Office for Europe and the European Union (European Commission and ECDC) in the management of events of public health importance in Europe. Although the primary responsibility for investigating and responding to public health emergencies lies with national health authorities, international organizations increasingly play a vital role in supporting national and sub-national actors. This relates particularly to information-sharing, cooperation, and technical assistance and supports all key steps of the event management cycle, including verification, reporting, risk assessment, and response. International legal instruments (in particular the IHR and the EU Decision on serious cross-border threats to health) prescribe core capacities at national level, including indicator- and event-based surveillance systems for the detection of public health events, as well as systems for assessment, risk communication, and response, and international agencies are involved in a variety of activities to strengthen capacity in European countries to respond to public health emergencies. Within the EU, the member states consult each other and coordinate their efforts to develop, strengthen, and maintain their capacities for the monitoring, early warning, and assessment of and response to serious cross-border threats to health. The consultation aims at sharing best practice and experience in preparedness and response planning. There is a clear trend in both WHO and the EU to go beyond the traditional focus on infectious diseases and instead cover a wide range of events of potential international concern. The IHR reinforced the coordination among states parties, including all EU member states, in the preparedness for and response to a public health emergency of international concern. EU legislation takes this development into account, including WHO's integrated all-hazards approach, covering all categories of threats independently of their origin.

Preparedness and response planning is an essential element allowing for the effective monitoring, early warning, and combating of serious cross-border threats to health. Such planning includes adequate preparedness of critical sectors of society, such as energy, transport, communications, and civil protection, which rely, in a crisis situation, on well-prepared public health systems. The latter in turn depend on the functioning of critical sectors and on the maintenance of essential services at an adequate level. Establishing the necessary structures and capacities at the intergovernmental, international, national, and sub-national level will be crucial for dealing successfully with future public health emergencies in Europe.

References

Ammon, A. and D. Faensen (2009). "[Surveillance of infectious diseases at the EU level]." *Bundesgesundheitsblatt Gesundheitsforschung Gesundheitsschutz* **52**(2): 176–182.

Bohigas, P., F. Santos-O'Connor and D. Coulombier (2009). "Epidemic intelligence and travel-related diseases: ECDC experience and further developments." *Clinical Microbiology and Infection* **15**(8): 734–739.

Brownstein, J. S. and C. C. Freifeld (2007). "HealthMap: the development of automated real-time internet surveillance for epidemic intelligence." *Eurosurveillance* **12**(48): art. 3322.

Collier, N., S. Doan, A. Kawazoe, R. M. Goodwin, M. Conway, Y. Tateno, Q. H. Ngo, D. Dien, A. Kawtrakul, K. Takeuchi, M. Shigematsu and K. Taniguchi (2008). "BioCaster: detecting public health rumors with a Web-based text mining system." *Bioinformatics* **24**(24): 2940–2941.

Cox, A., P. Guglielmetti and D. Coulombier (2009). "Assessing the impact of the 2009 H1N1 influenza pandemic on reporting of other threats through the Early Warning and Response System." *Eurosurveillance* **14**(45): art. 19397.

European Centre for Disease Prevention and Control (ECDC) (2009). *Human Cases of Swine Influenza without Apparent Exposure to Pigs, United States and Mexico.* Stockholm, ECDC [http://ecdc.europa.eu/en/healthtopics/Documents/090424_Influenza_AH1N1_TA_Swine_influenza_US-Mexico.pdf, accessed 15 March 2010].

European Centre for Disease Prevention and Control (ECDC) (2011). *Operational Guidance on Rapid Risk Assessment Methodology.* Stockholm, ECDC [http://ecdc.europa.eu/en/publications/Publications/1108_TED_Risk_Assessment_Methodology_Guidance.pdf].

European Commission (2000). Commission Decision of 22 December 1999 on the early warning and response system for the prevention and control of communicable diseases under Decision No. 2119/98/EC of the European Parliament and of the Council. *Official Journal of the European Communities* L 21/32–L 21/35.

European Commission (2002). 2002/253/EC: Commission Decision of 19 March 2002 laying down case definitions for reporting communicable diseases to the Community network under Decision No. 2119/98/EC of the European Parliament and of the Council. *Official Journal of the European Communities* L 86/44–L 86/62.

European Commission (2003). 2003/534/EC: Commission Decision of 17 July 2003 amending Decision No. 2119/98/EC of the European Parliament and of the Council and Decision 2000/96/EC as regards communicable diseases listed in those decisions and amending Decision 2002/253/EC as regards the case definitions for communicable diseases. *Official Journal of the European Union* L 184/135–L 184/139.

European Commission (2005). Communication from the Commission to the Council, the European Parliament, the European Economic and Social Committee and the Committee of the Regions on strengthening coordination on generic preparedness planning for public health emergencies at EU level. COM (2005) 605 final [http://eur-lex.europa.eu/LexUriServ/LexUriServ.do?uri=CELEX:52005DC0605:EN:NOT].

European Commission (2008a) Commission Decision (2008/426/EC) of 28 April 2008 amending Decision 2002/253/EC laying down case definitions for reporting communicable diseases to the Community network under Decision No. 2119/98/EC of the European Parliament and of the Council. *Official Journal of the European Union* L 159/46–L 159/90.

European Commission (2008b). Commission Decision of 28/IV/2008 amending Decision 2000/57/EC as regards events to be reported within the early warning and response system for the prevention and control of communicable diseases. C (2008) 1574 final [http://ec.europa.eu/health/ph_threats/com/docs/1574_2008_en.pdf].

European Union (1998). Decision No. 2119/98/EC of the European Parliament and of the Council of 24 September 1998 setting up a network for the epidemiological surveillance and control of communicable diseases in the Community. *Official Journal of the European Communities* L 268/201–L 268/207.

European Union (2004). Regulation (EC) No. 851/2004 of the European Parliament and of the Council of 21 April 2004 establishing a European Centre for Disease Prevention and Control. *Official Journal of the European Union* L 142/141–L 142/111.

European Union (2013). Decision No. 1082/2013/EU of the European Parliament and of the Council of 22 October on serious cross-border threats to health and repealing Decision No. 2119/98/EC. *Official Journal of the European Union* L 293/1–L 293/15.

EUVAC.NET (2010). *Status of Measles Surveillance Data 2010*. Copenhagen, Staten Serum Institute.

Glismann, S., T. Ronne and A. Tozzi (2001). "The EUVAC-NET project: creation and operation of a surveillance community network for vaccine preventable infectious diseases." *Eurosurveillance* **6**(6): 94–98.

Gossner, C. M. (2013). "ECDC launches the second version of the EPIS-FWD platform." *Eurosurveillance* **18**(27): art. 20517.

Gregg, M. B. (2008). *Field Epidemiology*. Oxford, Oxford University Press.

Guglielmetti, P., D. Coulombier, G. Thinus, F. Van Loock and S. Schreck (2006). "The early warning and response system for communicable diseases in the EU: an overview from 1999 to 2005." *Eurosurveillance* **11**(12): 215–220.

Health Protection Agency (HPA) (2010). *Assessment Report on the EU-Wide Response to Pandemic (H1N1) 2009*. London, HPA.

Heymann, D. L., Ed. (2008). *Control of Communicable Disease Manual*, 19th edition. Washington, D.C., American Public Health Association.

International Federation of Red Cross and Red Crescent Societies (2010). *World Disasters Report: Focus on urban risk*. Geneva, International Federation of Red Cross and Red Crescent Societies.

Kreidl, P., P. Buxbaum, F. Santos-O'Connor, L. Payne, R. Strauss, H. Hrabcik, H. C. Matter, A. Dreyfus and P. Arias (2008). "2008 European Football Championship – ECDC epidemic intelligence support." *Eurosurveillance* **13**(32): art. 18946.

Linge, J. P., R. Steinberger, T. P. Weber, R. Yangarber, E. van der Goot, D. H. Al Khudhairy and N. I. Stilianakis (2009). "Internet surveillance systems for early alerting of health threats." *Eurosurveillance* 14(13): art. 19162.

MacLehose, L., H. Brand, I. Camaroni, N. Fulop, O. N. Gill, R. Reintjes, O. Schaefer, M. McKee and J. Weinberg (2001). "Communicable disease outbreaks involving more than one country: systems approach to evaluating the response." *British Medical Journal* **323**(7317): 861–863.

Madoff, L. C. (2004). "ProMED-mail: an early warning system for emerging diseases." *Clinical Infectious Diseases* **39**(2): 227–232.

Mykhalovskiy, E. and L. Weir (2006). "The Global Public Health Intelligence Network and early warning outbreak detection: a Canadian contribution to global public health." *Canadian Journal of Public Health* **97**(1): 42–44.

Niedrig, M., O. Donoso-Mantke and R. Schadler (2007). "The European Network for Diagnostics of Imported Viral Diseases (ENIVD) – 12 years of strengthening the laboratory diagnostic capacity in Europe." *Eurosurveillance* **12**(4): art. 3180.

Norwegian Institute of Public Health (2011). *Toolkit for Local Implementation of the International Health Regulations (2005)*. Oslo, Norwegian Institute of Public Health.

Paquet, C., D. Coulombier, R. Kaiser and M. Ciotti (2006). "Epidemic intelligence: a new framework for strengthening disease surveillance in Europe." *Eurosurveillance* **11**(12): 212–214.

Schlagenhauf, P., F. Santos-O'Connor and P. Parola (2010). "The practice of travel medicine in Europe." *Clinical Microbiology and Infection* **16**(3): 203–208.

VBORNET (2009). *Network of Medical Entomologists and Public Health Experts (VBORNET)* [http://ecdc.europa.eu/en/activities/diseaseprogrammes/emerging_and_vector_borne_diseases/pages/vbornet.aspx, accessed 24 February 2013].

Wilson, J. (2007). "Argus: a global detection and tracking system for biological events." *Advances in Disease Surveillance* 4(21).

World Health Organization (WHO) (2005a). *Effective Media Communication during Public Health Emergencies: A WHO handbook*. Geneva, WHO.

World Health Organization (WHO) (2005b). *Revision of the International Health Regulations*. Geneva, WHO: 58.

World Health Organization (WHO) (2005c). *WHO Outbreak Communication Guidelines*. Geneva, WHO.

World Health Organization (WHO) (2008). *World Health Organization Outbreak Communication Planning Guide*. Geneva, WHO.

World Health Organization (WHO) (2012a). *Information to States Parties Regarding Determination of Fulfilment of IHR Core Capacity Requirements for 2012 and Potential Extensions*. Geneva, WHO.

World Health Organization (WHO) (2012b). *Rapid Risk Assessment of Acute Public Health Events*. Geneva, WHO.

World Health Organization (WHO) Regional Office for Europe (2010). *Resolution: Renewed commitment to elimination of measles and rubella and prevention of congenital rubella syndrome by 2015 and Sustained support for polio-free status in the WHO European Region*. Copenhagen, WHO Regional Office for Europe.

chapter five

Occupational health and safety

*Rokho Kim, Jorma Rantanen,
Suvi Lehtinen, Wiking Husberg*

Introduction

Employment and working conditions are major social determinants of health (CSDH 2008). While those in employment are often healthier than the unemployed, they risk being exposed to various health and safety hazards at work. The International Labour Organization (ILO) estimates that each year about 2.3 million men and women worldwide die from work-related accidents and diseases, with close to 360,000 fatal accidents and an estimated 1.95 million fatal work-related diseases (ILO 2009). The 880 million people in the WHO European Region include about 400 million workers. Occupational disease and injury ranks among the top ten risk factors responsible for the total disease burden in the WHO European Region (Concha-Barrientos, Imel Nelson et al. 2004). More than 300,000 lives are lost in Europe each year due to work-related diseases and accidents. Adverse health effects of poor working conditions are resulting in an economic cost of 4–5% of GDP (Takala, Hämäläinen et al. 2009). Persons with insecure jobs are at an increased risk of poor health (László, Pikhart et al. 2010). The protection of workers from sickness, disease, and injury is not only a fundamental human right, but also one of the main goals of the World Health Organization (WHO) and ILO, as set out in their constitutions.

Although there have been consistent improvements in health and safety at work in the WHO European Region, large disparities remain between and within countries with regard to the health status of workers, their exposure to occupational risks, and access to occupational health services. Workers in vulnerable or underserved groups (such as young or older people, pregnant women, people with disabilities, migrants) and those in high-risk sectors (such as mining, construction, health care, agriculture, small and medium-sized enterprises, informal employment, the self-employed) are more likely to suffer from occupational diseases and injuries (WHO 2007).

Following the example of Germany, where Bismarck introduced an industrial accident insurance system in 1884, most industrialized countries in Europe established occupational health services and workers' compensation systems. In parallel, industrial medicine emerged as a distinct medical specialty, incorporating preventive medicine and public health as well as clinical medicine. Industrial medicine then evolved into occupational medicine and, by the late twentieth century, occupational medicine and occupational hygiene became the two principal disciplines of modern occupational health. Occupational health and safety programmes have become an important part of modern public health services addressing the wider social and environmental determinants of health.

This chapter explores current challenges and opportunities for occupational health and safety in the WHO European Region. We first provide some terminological clarifications and then review the main international instruments for advancing occupational health and safety in Europe. This is followed by an overview of the situation in different parts of the region and an analysis of the main challenges today. The next section discusses strategic directions for the future. We conclude that modern public health services should include a substantive programme for health and safety at work, particularly targeting vulnerable workers and high-risk sectors.

Terminological clarifications

Occupational health

According to the twelfth session of the Joint ILO/WHO Committee on Occupational Health in 1995, "occupational health" concerns (Joint ILO/WHO Committee on Occupational Health 1995):

> the promotion and maintenance of the highest degree of physical, mental and social well-being of workers in all occupations; the prevention amongst workers of departures from health caused by their working conditions; the protection of workers in their employment from risk resulting from factors adverse to health; the placing and maintenance of workers in an environment adapted to their physiological and psychological capabilities; and, to summarize, the adaptation of work to workers and of each worker to his or her job.

The main foci of occupational health are maintaining and promoting workers' health and working ability, ensuring work and the working environment are conducive to safety and health, and developing work organizations and working cultures so that they support health and safety at work.

Occupational safety

Occupational safety focuses primarily on the prevention of occupational accidents and injuries in all types of industries and services. Recognizing that unsafe workplaces and work practices can also cause work-related diseases, the term "occupational safety" is often combined with the term "occupational health". In certain cases, a broader definition of occupational safety embraces the area of occupational health.

Occupational health and safety, and occupational safety and health

A healthy workplace should be a safe one, and a safe workplace should be a healthy one. Occupational health, occupational safety, occupational health and safety, and occupational safety and health are thus used interchangeably. Occupational health, as defined by WHO and ILO (see above), is often referred to as occupational health and safety in the health sector (e.g. by ministries of health, occupational health physicians and nurses, occupational hygienists), whereas it is often referred to as occupational safety and health in the labour sector (e.g. by ministries of labour, labour inspectors, safety engineers). The expression "occupational health and safety" is favoured by WHO, but "occupational safety and health" by ILO. Both are also referred to as "Health and Safety at Work" or "Safety and Health at Work" in EU legislation and policy documents (see below).

Occupational health services

The ILO has defined occupational health services as (ILO 1985):

> services entrusted with essentially preventive functions and responsible for advising the employer, the workers and their representatives in the undertaking, on the requirements for establishing and maintaining a safe and healthy working environment which will facilitate optimal physical and mental health in relation to work, and the adaptation of work to the capabilities of workers in the light of their state of physical and mental health.

Modern occupational health services include: improvement of work organization; workplace and health surveillance; risk assessment, management, and communication; first aid and accident management; and workplace health promotion.

Basic occupational health services

Universal coverage of all workers in all occupations with occupational health services has been recommended by WHO and ILO. However, workers in small and medium-sized enterprises and informal sectors often receive minimal occupational health services. To make the goal of "Occupational Health for All" more feasible, the concept of basic occupational health services emerged and was endorsed by the 13th ILO/WHO Joint Committee on Occupational Health in December 2003. Basic occupational health services are an application of the Alma Ata principles on primary health to occupational health. They can be defined as essential services for the protection of people's health at work, the promotion of health, well-being and work ability, and the prevention of ill-health and accidents, using scientifically sound and socially acceptable occupational health methods, through a primary healthcare approach (Rantanen 2005).

Workplace health promotion

Workplace health promotion has been defined as (ENWHP 2013):

> the combined efforts of employers, employees and society to improve the health and wellbeing of people at work. This can be achieved through a combination of: improving the work organization and working environment; promoting active participation; encouraging personal development.

The workplace is an excellent setting that can promote the physical, mental, economic, and social well-being of workers, and in turn enhance the health of their families, communities, and society at large.

International commitments and instruments

A number of international commitments and instruments have been adopted at the global and European level on health and safety at work.

Resolutions of the World Health Assembly

The World Health Assembly (WHA) is the decision-making body of WHO, and its resolutions constitute "soft law" in international relations (Fidler 2003). In 1996, it adopted Resolution WHA49.12, endorsing the Global Strategy on Occupational Health for All (WHO 1996). It urged member states to devise national programmes on occupational health for all, with special attention to the underserved working population, including migrant workers, workers in small industries and the informal sector, and other occupational groups at high risk or with special needs, including child workers. In a follow up, the 2007 World Health Assembly adopted Resolution WHA60.26, endorsing the Global Plan of Action on Workers' Health 2008–2017, with five objectives for actions (see Box 5.1).

Box 5.1   The five objectives of the 2007 WHO Global Plan of Action on Workers' Health

- to devise and implement policy instruments on workers' health;
- to protect and promote health at the workplace;
- to improve the performance of and access to occupational health services;
- to provide and communicate evidence for action and practice;
- to incorporate workers' health into other policies.

Source: WHO (2007)

ILO conventions

A key function of the ILO is to develop international standards on occupational safety and health. It has so far adopted approximately 70 conventions in this area. ILO conventions are legally binding international law for those countries that have signed and ratified them. The 1981 Occupational Safety and Health Convention (No. 155) and Recommendation No. 164 established the duty of employers to provide safe work conditions, the need for enterprise-based cooperation between workers and employers in occupational safety and health, and the right of workers to be informed about and decline dangerous work. The 1985 Occupational Health Services Convention (No. 161) and Recommendation No. 171 set out principles for the protection of workers against sickness, disease, and injury arising out of work and established the preventive function of occupational health services (Box 5.2). It further clarified that occupational health and safety policies should be adopted at the national level, based on tripartite collaboration between government, employers, and employees.

Box 5.2 Functions of occupational health services according to ILO Convention No. 161

- Identifying and assessing the risks related to health hazards in the workplace.
- Advising on planning and organization of work and working practices.
- Providing advice, information, training and education on occupational health, safety, and hygiene, and on ergonomics and protective equipment.
- Surveillance of workers' health in relation to work.
- Contributing to occupational rehabilitation and maintaining people of working age in employment, and assisting in the return to employment of those who are unemployed for reasons of ill health or disability.
- Organizing first aid and emergency treatment.

European Social Charter

The European Social Charter, adopted in 1961 by the Council of Europe and revised in 1996, guarantees social and economic human rights, and most of the 47 member states of the Council of Europe have agreed to be bound by it.

Article 2 on "the right to just conditions of work" mandates states parties to eliminate risks in inherently dangerous or unhealthy occupations.

Article 3 on "the right to safe and healthy working conditions" specifies the responsibilities of governments, including the progressive development of occupational health services for all workers with essentially preventive and advisory functions. The potential for recognized entities and non-governmental organizations (NGOs) to take legal action against non-compliant governments makes the European Social Charter a powerful instrument to promote occupational health and safety in Europe.

EU directives and strategies

EU directives on safety and health at work have their legal foundation in Article 153 of the Treaty on the Functioning of the European Union (Treaty of Rome; effective since 1958), which gives the EU the authority to adopt directives for improving safety and health at work. The EU Framework Directive on Safety and Health at Work (Directive 89/391/EEC) guarantees minimum safety and health requirements throughout the EU (Council of the European Communities 1989). The framework directive also established general principles, including risk assessment, avoidance, substitution, and prevention. It specifically prioritizes collective protective measures through the participation of health and safety representatives, and obliges employers to take appropriate preventive measures to make working safer and healthier.

The framework directive made widespread changes to occupational safety and health legislation in some EU member states. It also gave rise to "daughter directives", applying its general principles to specific areas and aspects of health and safety at work (European Agency for Safety and Health at Work 2013). These directives contributed to instilling a culture of prevention throughout the EU, as well as simplifying national legislative systems. However, various flaws were highlighted in the application of the legislation (European Commission 2004). One major challenge is poor compliance in small and medium-sized enterprises (SMEs), especially as regards risk assessment, workers' participation and training, and in the traditionally high-risk sectors of agriculture and construction. Following a first EU Strategy on Health and Safety at Work for 2002–2006, the EU adopted a second strategy for 2007–2012, which aimed to cut by a quarter work-related accidents (European Commission 2007). These strategies were an important policy signal and driver for national action on occupational safety and health and facilitated useful coordination with respect to public health initiatives. A new strategy was recommended for musculoskeletal disorders, stress, and occupational cancer deaths that ought to target in particular the challenges related to the implementation of the legal framework, with an explicit focus on SMEs and micro-enterprises (European Commission 2013).

Situation in the WHO European Region

Legislation on occupational health and safety differs greatly across the WHO European Region, ranging from legal requirements for every enterprise to provide occupational health services, through legal requirements only for large- and medium-sized enterprises, to no legal requirements at all. As a consequence, the coverage of occupational health services varies from less than 10% of the workforce in some countries to more than 90% in others.

Mortality related to work-related accidents is a good indicator of the effectiveness of occupational health and safety systems, because deaths are less likely to be under-reported than injuries and diseases. According to the

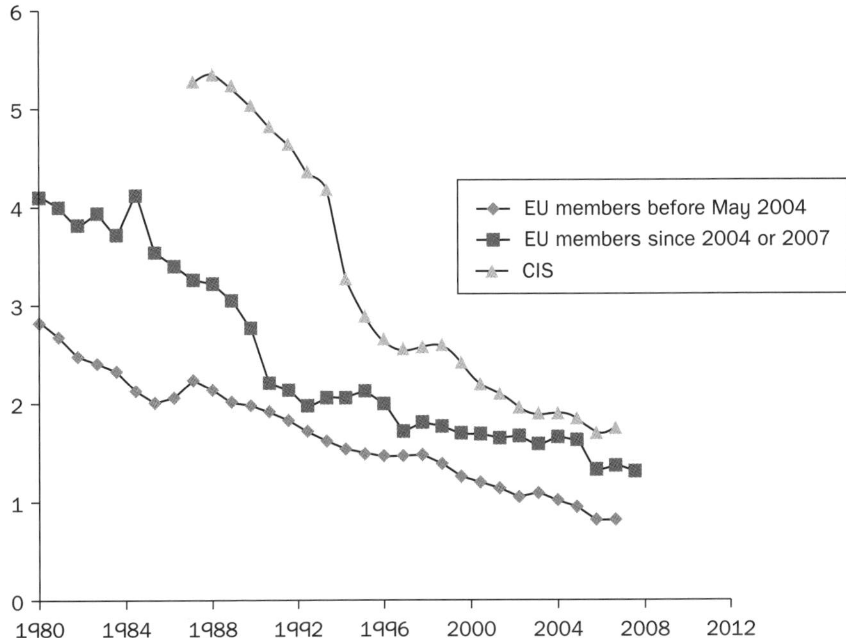

Figure 5.1   Deaths due to work-related accidents per 100,000 population (CIS: Commonwealth of Independent States)

Source: WHO (2013)

official data reported to WHO's European Health for All database, mortality rates from work-related accidents have decreased consistently since 1980 (Figure 5.1). However, there are persisting disparities between different parts of the region, with higher death rates in the countries of central and eastern Europe and the former Soviet countries.

Figure 5.2 shows trends in non-fatal injuries due to work-related accidents. In striking contrast to mortality rates, the countries of central and eastern Europe and the former Soviet Union report much lower rates of non-fatal work-related injuries than the EU member states before May 2004. This paradox is likely due to a severe under-detection and under-reporting of non-fatal work-related injuries in these countries.

EU member states

Figures 5.1 and 5.2 illustrate the gap that exists between different parts of Europe in terms of occupational health and safety. The progress in many "old" EU member states (as well as countries such as Norway or Switzerland) is largely due to continuous dialogue between the social partners, as well as the efforts of trade unions and providers of occupational health services. However, even in some of these countries, such as Greece, occupational health and safety

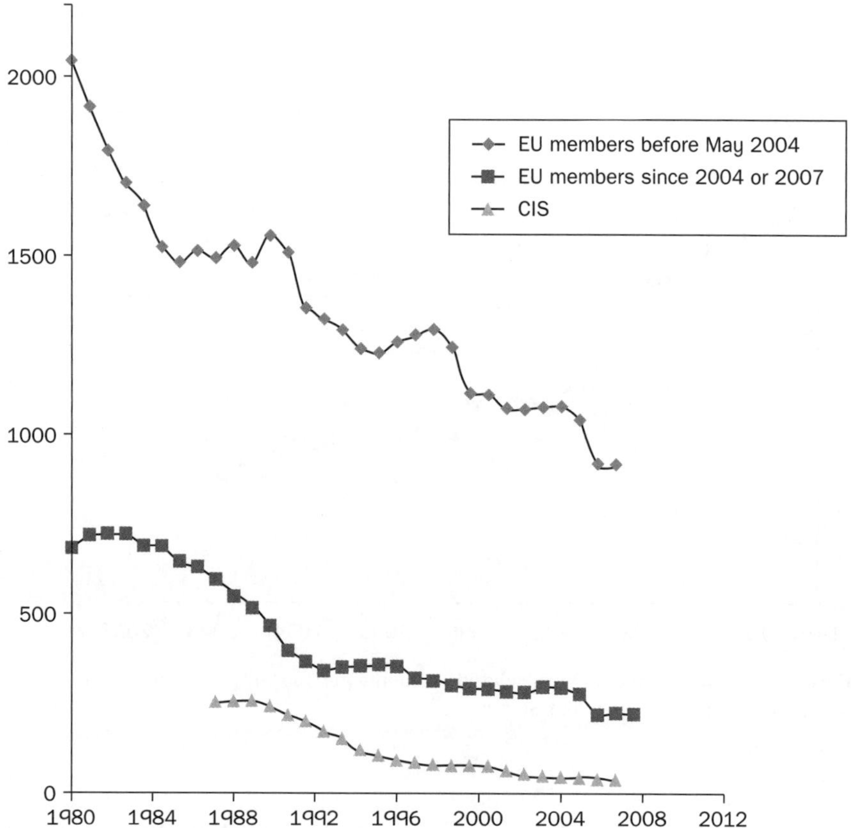

Figure 5.2   Persons injured due to work-related accidents per 100,000 population (CIS: Commonwealth of Independent States)

Source: WHO (2013)

is only accorded a low priority and under-reporting of occupational mortality and morbidity is considerable (Rachiotis, Alexopoulos et al. 2010).

The twelve "new" EU member states adopted EU directives on occupational safety and health during their accession period. However, they still lag behind their western neighbours in reducing work-related mortality. Reasons include weak enforcement, a lack of capacity, and insufficient involvement of social partners.

As of 2013, there was no specific EU directive on occupational health services, and quality and coverage differ greatly across and within EU member states. Except in those countries with a legislative requirement for universal or near-universal coverage (e.g. the Netherlands, Belgium, France, Finland, and Luxembourg), occupational health services coverage is well below 60% (WHO 2007). Furthermore, in most EU member states, workers in micro-enterprises and the informal sector often do not have access to occupational health services.

According to the Fifth European Survey of Working Conditions, covering 44,000 workers from 34 European countries in 2010, more than one in three manual workers and almost one in five non-manual workers thought that their health or safety was at risk because of their work, and that their work affects their health. Less than half (44%) of the lowest skilled manual workers thought that they would be able to do their current job when they were 60, while more than two-thirds (72%) of the most highly skilled non-manual workers thought so (Eurofound 2012).

South-east European countries

Albania, Turkey, and the countries emerging from the Socialist Federal Republic of Yugoslavia have also harmonized their national laws with the EU *acquis communautaire*. The Socialist Federal Republic of Yugoslavia had strong occupational health and safety services, but these have been weakened in the years of transition, partly due to the extensive privatization of the public sector and the collapse of the big state-owned industrial combines, as well as the growth in the number of self-employed people and of the informal sector.

Although many national strategies and action plans have been drawn up, their implementation lags behind that in western Europe, due to a lack of capacity and, in some countries, lack of political will. The total number of specialized occupational health physicians in south-east Europe is under 500, whereas more than 2000–2500 are needed. Occupational health surveillance and disease registry systems are also insufficient, leading to serious under-reporting.

Countries of the former Soviet Union

In the Soviet Union, occupational health services were delivered through centrally planned and managed networks of sanitary-epidemiological (san-epid) facilities. The transition period has generally undermined occupational health and safety programmes and structures. The reasons are similar to those in the countries of south-east Europe and include a lack of transparency and accountability, lack of genuine social dialogue, and indiscriminate privatization of public services.

The scale of occupational fatalities and injuries is so extensive that they cost Russian employers on average 10–15% of their payroll (Fudge and Owens 2006). However, the under-reporting of accidents is huge, especially among SMEs and in the informal economy. The situation is further aggravated in those countries that have retained the outdated system of compensation for work in hazardous working conditions ("hazard pay"), which does not encourage employers to improve working conditions.

There have, however, also been some positive developments. With the support of ILO, most countries in the region have prepared national profiles analysing their national occupational safety and health systems and prepared programmes for improvement.

Kazakhstan has adopted an occupational safety and health programme, while Kyrgyzstan and Tajikistan have signed tripartite general agreements that include consideration of occupational safety and health issues. In Azerbaijan, the government has pledged to modernize labour inspection and occupational safety and health. Kyrgyzstan has become the lead country in the sub-region introducing ILO's Work Improvement in Neighbourhood Development (WIND) programme for the improvement of working conditions in farms and rural enterprises.

In Georgia, the situation was very different, as the former government terminated all occupational safety and health-related inspection services and minimum safety requirements. After a number of serious workplace accidents, employers and trade unions voluntarily set up an occupational safety and health centre and agreed to start implementing ILO recommendations for occupational safety and health management systems without involvement of the government. The new government faces the task of rebuilding the national occupational safety and health system.

One of the lessons to emerge from the experience of the former Soviet countries is that major advances can be achieved when ministries of labour and health (and in some cases environment and emergency response) cooperate to provide safe and healthy workplaces. This helps to foster collaboration between multiple inspectorates (such as for labour, the environment, technical issues, mining), saving resources and decreasing duplication of inspections. Furthermore, the introduction of modern occupational safety and health management systems, based on an open social dialogue at enterprises, helps to achieve a shift of occupational health and safety systems towards a prevention-oriented risk assessment and management approach.

Current challenges

The globalization of capital and labour markets, coupled with rapid population growth in low-income countries, results in an almost endless supply of cheap labour, encouraging limited attention to hazard control and occupational health and safety (Gochfeld 2005). Many countries have seen a trend to deregulate, privatize, and outsource public services, including for occupational health and safety. As mentioned above, this is especially common in many former Soviet countries leading to the deterioration of both working conditions and occupational health services. Profit-oriented providers of occupational health services are compelled to satisfy the needs of their clients, often without participation of trade unions or workers' representatives and at a cost to professional and ethical standards.

The occupational health and safety of migrant workers in Europe is another major concern (Rechel, Mladovsky et al. 2013). The vulnerability of most migrants leaves them exposed to hazardous working environments, labour exploitation, and inadequate access to health services, with higher rates of occupational accidents (Agudelo-Suárez, Ronda-Pérez et al. 2011). Those most at risk are migrants working in precariously irregular conditions, and in mining, construction, heavy manufacturing, and agriculture.

The financial crisis, which began in 2007, has placed extra strain on the occupational health and safety of European workplaces. It has led to the deregulation of labour laws, affecting occupational safety and health policies and increasing the incidence of occupational diseases. The experience in other parts of the world (Min, Min et al. 2010) suggests that cutting back on occupational safety and health during an economic crisis is likely to have a sustained negative effect. The findings of a recent survey carried out on behalf of Germany's major health insurers indicate that companies in manufacturing industries with between 50 and 499 employees are showing less interest in implementing occupational health and safety management than they used to before the economic crisis (Bechmann, Jäckle et al. 2010).

New technologies (such as nanotechnology), atypical work organizations, and demographic changes at the workplace are associated with new and re-emerging risks. Work-related stress and psychosocial problems are among the leading causes of sick leave and early retirement. Unemployment, job insecurity, discrimination, and exclusion from work also increase the risk of physical and mental disorders. Child labour still exists in several countries of the WHO European Region, such as during the cotton harvest in central Asia (ILO 2006). Another global phenomenon is that production is being moved to emerging economies where occupational health standards are lower.

The ageing of working populations is another challenge for policy-makers of many European countries (Rechel, Grundy et al. 2013). For both biological and social reasons, older workers are particularly vulnerable in the workplace. It is crucial to improve working conditions and manage non-communicable diseases (NCDs) through workplace health promotion programmes to enable workers to remain in the workforce (WHO 2012c). Workplaces provide an important entry point for NCD prevention and health promotion programmes aimed at tackling NCD risk factors in the working population.

Strategic directions for the future

To strengthen occupational health across the WHO European Region, three strategic directions will be crucial: to mainstream occupational health and safety into essential public health operations, achieve universal coverage of occupational health services for all workers, and provide NCD prevention and health promotion in healthy workplaces.

Mainstreaming occupational health and safety into essential public health operations

The protection and promotion of workers' health is an essential public health function (WHO 2003, 2012b). Mainstreaming occupational health and safety into essential public health operations implies an improved integration of occupational health professions and other specialists into multidisciplinary preventive services capable of detecting, assessing, and advising on the management of occupational, environmental, social, and lifestyle hazards affecting the working ability, health, and well-being of employees.

National action plans on workers' health between relevant ministries (e.g. for health and labour), social partners, and other major national stakeholders need to be elaborated taking into account the international instruments mentioned above. Such plans should include national profiles, priorities for action, objectives and targets, actions and mechanisms for implementation, monitoring and evaluation. Local alliances of health and labour authorities, large enterprises, external occupational and environmental health services, and primary health care services can help to work towards full coverage of all workers, including those in SMEs and the informal sector (WHO 2002).

There are solid theoretical and practical grounds for mainstreaming occupational health and safety into public health. Four conceptual frameworks are of relevance. The first is eco-social theory, which integrates social and biological analyses of disease distribution using a multilevel, dynamic, and historical approach to explain health inequalities. The second is integrated workplace intervention models that address both individual risk-taking behaviours and environmental risk factors. Third is the life-course approach, in which the effects on health of cumulative life experiences, including occupational exposures, are evaluated. Finally, sustainable production seeks integrated solutions to occupational and environmental hazards through primary prevention. The health of workers may be most effectively advanced by expanding the scope of occupational safety and health beyond the constraints of the workplace to embrace the lives of workers, including in their homes and communities and over the life course (Quinn 2003).

There are also compelling economic arguments for mainstreaming occupational health and safety in public health services. While a very high proportion of the economic costs of occupational injury and disease fall on parties external to the employer in question (Kankaanpää, van Tulder et al. 2008), investing in workplace prevention still yields substantial benefits for employers. An international study quantified the return on prevention by calculating the costs and benefits of investments in occupational safety and health in companies in Australia, Austria, Azerbaijan, Canada, the Czech Republic, Germany, Hong Kong (China), Romania, the Russian Federation, Singapore, Sweden, Switzerland, Turkey, the United States, and Vietnam (International Social Security Association 2011). Figure 5.3 shows how the

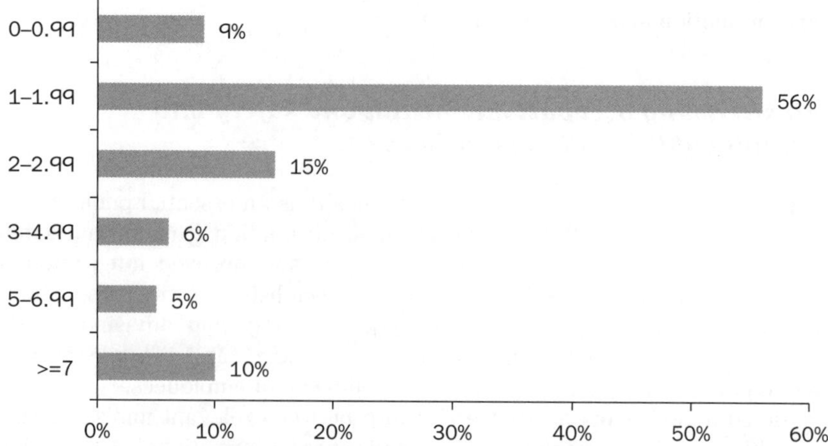

Figure 5.3 Return on workplace prevention expected by employers in 15 countries

Source: Authors' compilation, based on the International Social Security Association (2011)

companies rated the return on prevention, i.e. the expected economic return for investing in workplace prevention. Across all countries, the average return on prevention was 2.2, so that for every €1 invested per employee per year, companies on average expected an economic benefit of €2.2 (International Social Security Association 2011).

Universal coverage of occupational health services for all workers

In addition to mainstreaming occupational health and safety, another strategy for the future should be scaling up the coverage of occupational health services for all workers. Due to ethical, legal, and economic reasons, large enterprises striving for sustainable business tend to invest in comprehensive occupational health services, except in countries where the enforcement of labour and health standards is weak. However, as mentioned above, occupational health services are rarely provided to workers in small enterprises and the informal sector.

When considering strategic priorities for developing occupational health services in the WHO European Region, it is important to take account of the widely varying needs, capacities, and trajectories of individual countries. Conceptually, four stages of development can be distinguished (Figure 5.4).

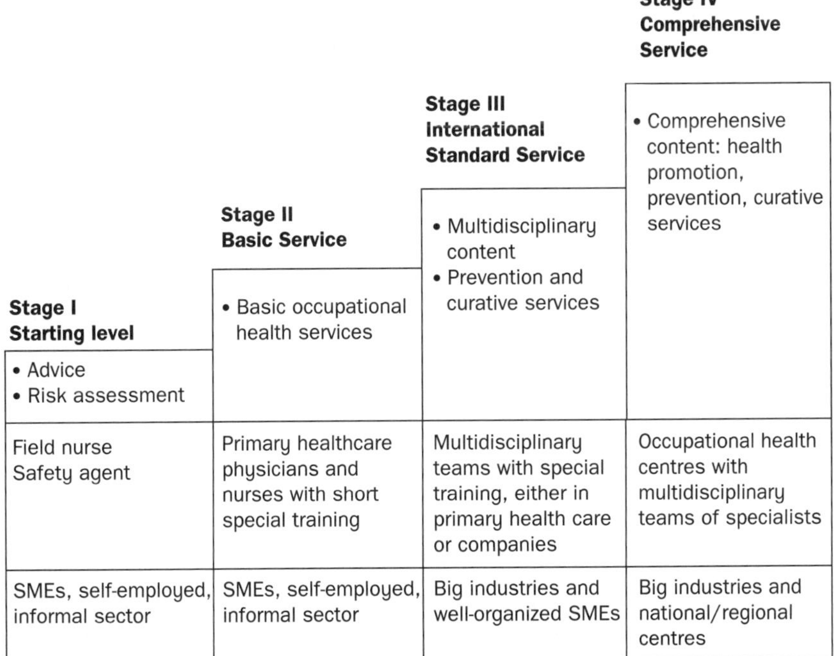

Figure 5.4   Stages of developing occupational health services

Note: SMEs = small and medium-sized enterprises
Source: Authors' compilation, based on Rantanen (2007)

Stages I and II primarily apply to the smallest enterprises, the self-employed and the informal sector. Large companies and well-organized SMEs should, however, always start by establishing Stage III services. This is also the level that should be the minimum objective for each country and workplace in the long term, as stipulated by ILO Conventions Nos. 161 and 155.

Stage I: Starting level

This is a reasonable starting point for workplaces or workers that do not have any occupational health services. The aim is to lower the threshold for initiation, but still ensure basic occupational health services. It relies on field occupational health service workers (if possible, a nurse and safety agent) who have a short training in occupational health and safety and work for a primary health-care unit or another grassroots level facility. The service focuses on risks of accidents, heavy physical work, basic sanitation and hygiene, and the most hazardous chemical, physical, and biological factors (including HIV/AIDS). Advising clients to seek help from specialized services constitutes an important part of the service.

Stage II: Basic occupational health services

This service works as closely as possible with workplaces and communities. Service provision may vary, depending on local circumstances and needs. The personnel, usually a physician and a nurse, have a short training (lasting approximately 10 weeks) in occupational health. They sometimes benefit from the support of a safety expert who is competent in accident prevention and basic safety.

Stage III: Services meeting international standards

This level should be the minimum objective for each country and workplace, as stipulated in ILO conventions. The service infrastructure can take several different forms and the service is primarily preventive, although curative services may also be provided. The staff should be multidisciplinary and led by a specially trained expert (usually an occupational health physician or nurse). However, the multidisciplinary content of the service can also be ensured through appropriate support services from occupational hygienists and specialized units, such as institutes of occupational health.

Stage IV: Comprehensive occupational health services

This level is usually found in large companies in industrialized countries or may be provided by large occupational health centres that provide services for a large number of companies. The staff work as a multidisciplinary team and often include several specialists, such as specialist physicians, occupational health nurses, occupational hygienists, ergonomists, psychologists or safety engineers. The services are comprehensive and include prevention, curative services, health promotion and promotion of work ability.

Providing basic occupational health services in primary health care

Integration of occupational health services into primary health care is a key component of Stage II, with the aim of achieving comprehensive coverage of occupational health services for all workers. Close collaboration between occupational health and primary care can help to enhance productivity and extend working lives much more than a fragmented approach (WHO 2011). Key guiding principles for an integrated approach to occupational health in primary health care emerged from a global conference on the topic in 2011 (Box 5.3).

Prevention of non-communicable diseases and health promotion in healthy workplaces

As mentioned above, workplaces are recognized as an important entry point for NCD prevention programmes. Most of the 300,000 lives lost in the WHO European Region from work-related diseases (not including deaths from injury) are due to NCDs. Risk factors for these diseases can be mitigated by the organized efforts of society. An excellent example is elimination of asbestos-related cancers and lung diseases through the elimination of asbestos exposure at the workplace.

NCD prevention programmes at the workplace should not only target occupational or work-related NCD hazards, but also other NCD risk factors, such as physical inactivity, unhealthy dietary habits, tobacco and alcohol consumption, job-related stress, and work–life imbalance. When designed and

Box 5.3 Guiding principles for an integrated approach to occupational health and primary care

- Workers' health is part of general health and life.
- Health systems should facilitate local strategies to meet workers' health needs.
- In moving towards universal coverage, those at greatest risk or having the greatest needs should be targeted first. This will require attention to essential interventions, financing, and human and technical capacities.
- When developing policies about workers' health, all relevant stakeholders should be involved (although national and local governments have a leading role to play).
- Training in health and work should be part of the professional training of all health workers.
- The empowerment of workers and encouragement of decision-makers is critical for the promotion of the health and safety of workers.

Source: Adapted from WHO (2012a)

executed as a comprehensive initiative for healthy workplaces, workplace health promotion is effective in reducing NCD risk factors (WHO 2011). However, workplace health promotion activities at the level of individual companies are more likely to be effective when implemented as an integral part of occupational health services and other activities at the workplace and in the health sector in general (Rantanen and Kim 2012). The conceptual framework for healthy workplaces shown in Figure 5.5 clarifies the four major avenues of influence that employers, with the participation of workers, can take.

The model provides guidance for a holistic approach to healthy workplaces, particularly when employers, workers, and their representatives work together in a collaborative manner. Workplace health promotion, while primarily addressing personal health behaviour and the psychosocial work environment for NCD prevention, should be linked with a healthier physical work environment and active community involvement of the enterprise. Workplaces are situated

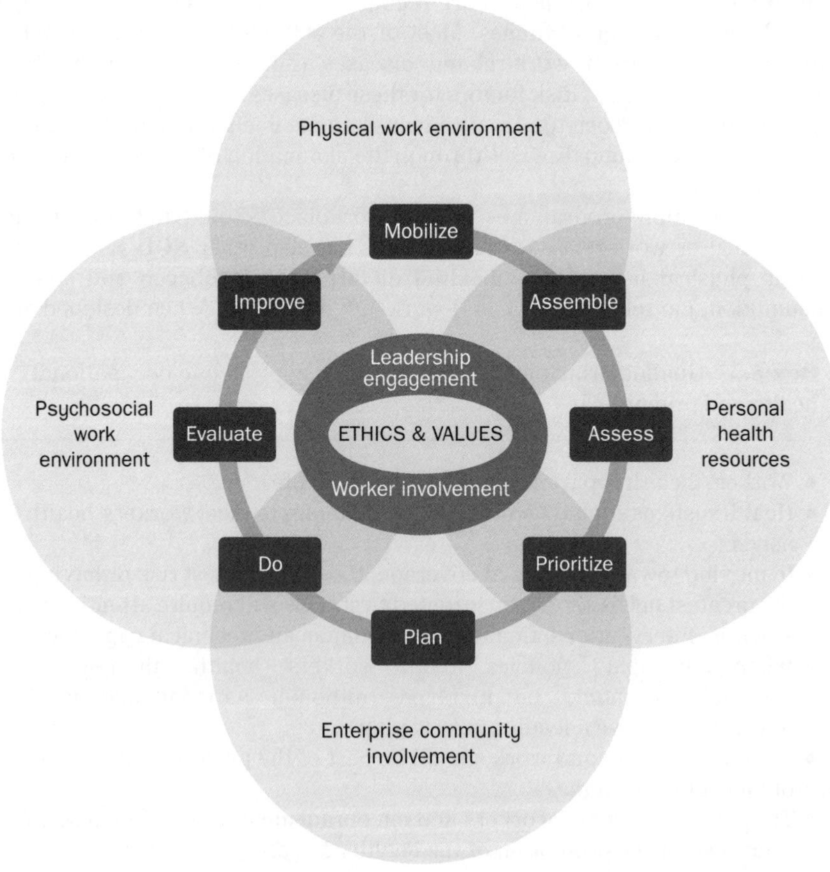

Figure 5.5 Healthy workplace model

Source: WHO (2009)

within a much larger context. Governments, legislation, civil society, market conditions, and health systems, all have a tremendous impact on workplaces and on what can be achieved by the various groups engaged in the workplace. It is crucial to engage these diverse actors and to recognize that different countries in Europe have very different needs and challenges, as do smaller and larger enterprises. Whatever the circumstances, worker involvement and leadership engagement should be at the core of healthy workplace initiatives (Burton 2010).

Conclusion

Work plays a central role in society: it provides the means of acquiring income, prestige and a sense of worth, and offers a way of participating and being included as a full member in the life of the community (WHO 2012d). Being unemployed effectively excludes people from such participation and the benefits that employment brings. Worryingly, the current economic crisis has seen levels of unemployment rise dramatically in some European countries, particularly among younger workers. This is likely to have negative effects on health, but also has implications for the provision of occupational health services, as these tend to ignore people outside of employment.

In addition to improving employment prospects, countries in Europe should aspire to reduce exposure to unhealthy or unsafe work and strengthen measures to secure healthy workplaces. This includes improving psychosocial conditions through measures to promote greater job control, job security, flexible hours and other family-friendly practices, adequate social protection, and rewards and status commensurate with effort. A good-quality job with a high level of job control and a correct balance between effort and reward is an important prerequisite for health and its determinants (such as a good standard of living, self-esteem, and social participation). This can also contribute to a healthy and productive workforce, with secondary benefits for families and communities (WHO 2012d).

While this chapter has provided a broad overview of the status of occupational health and safety in the WHO European Region, more research is needed to measure the performance of occupational health services between and within countries. Internationally standardized approaches would be a major step towards allowing a more objective comparison of the scope and effectiveness of occupational health and safety programmes in different parts of Europe (WHO 2002).

Modern public health services need to include a strong programme for health and safety in the workplace, particularly targeting vulnerable workers and high-risk sectors. Intersectoral cooperation between health, labour, and other sectors at the local, national, and international level is particularly important, in line with "whole-of-government" and "Health in All" policy approaches. Government leadership, in collaboration with social partners, is necessary, as well as a combination of vertical sector-specific and horizontal intersectoral policies (Finnish Ministry of Social Affairs and Health 2013).

In addition to mainstreaming occupational health and safety, scaling up basic occupational health services through the integration of occupational health services into primary health care, and strengthening NCD prevention and health promotion in healthy workplaces are the major strategic developments for the future. Improved conditions of work, with mechanisms that enable people to influence the design and improvement of their work, will create a healthier, happier, and more productive workforce.

Policies will also need to address: promoting sustainable green economic growth; transferring knowledge and skills; increasing employability, especially among young people; achieving greater job stability among the most vulnerable people; reducing exposure to unhealthy work and the associated risks of disease and injury; managing health risks by enforcing national regulations and providing good occupational health services; developing standardized tools for monitoring and risk management; and implementing methods known to improve safe and healthy work, with priority given to high-risk groups, including unemployed people (WHO 2012d).

In achieving a better work–life balance, a number of supportive measures can be put in place, including: granting family-related leave; improving the provision of child care; organizing working time to include flexible arrangements; abolishing conditions that lead to wage differences between men and women; harmonizing school and working hours; and reviewing the opening hours of shops. Employment policies should also provide measures that encourage a more equitable division of leave for child care and care of older people between men and women. There are still large differences between countries in terms of such supportive social policies.

One of the main negative impacts of the deregulation of occupational health and safety policies in a number of European countries is the lack of effective enforcement by public authorities. Ascertaining the quality, effectiveness, and efficiency of occupational health services should be a shared responsibility of national and local health authorities, associations of health professionals, and organizations of employers and employees. It would make it possible to move closer to the implementation of relevant international and European commitments. Various networks and resources in occupational health and safety, such as the network of WHO Collaborating Centres, the Baltic Sea Network on Occupational Health and Safety, the South East European Network on Workers' Health, and the International Commission on Occupational Health, can help to realize the vision of occupational health and safety for all workers in Europe.

References

Agudelo-Suárez, A. A., E. Ronda-Pérez and F. G. Benavides (2011). "Occupational health." In *Migration and Health in the European Union*. B. Rechel, P. Mladovsky, W. Deville, B. Rijks, R. Petrova-Benedict and M. McKee, Eds. Maidenhead, Open University Press: 155–168.

Bechmann, S., R. Jäckle, P. Lück and R. Herdegen (2010). *Motive und Hemmnisse für Betriebliches Gesundheitsmanagement (BGM)*, IGA-Report 20. Berlin, AOK-Bundesverband.

Burton, J. (2010). *WHO Healthy Workplace Framework and Model: Background and supporting literature and practices* [http://www.who.int/occupational_health/healthy_workplace_framework.pdf, accessed 19 September 2013].

Commission on the Social Determinants of Health (CSDH) (2008). *Closing the Gap in a Generation: Health equity through action on the social determinants of health.* Final Report of the Commission on Social Determinants of Health. Geneva, WHO.

Concha-Barrientos, M., D. Imel Nelson, T. Driscoll, L. Punnett, K. Steenland and M. Fingerhut (2004). "The global burden of selected occupational disease and injury risks." In *Comparative Quantification of Health Risks: Global and regional burden of disease attributable to selected major risk factors.* M. Ezzati, A. D. Lopez, A. Rodgers and C. J. L. Murray, Eds. Geneva, WHO: 1651–1802.

Council of the European Communities (1989). Council Directive 89/391/EEC of 12 June 1989 on the introduction of measures to encourage improvements in the safety and health of workers at work [http://eur-lex.europa.eu/LexUriServ/LexUriServ.do?uri=CELEX:31989L0391:en:HTML, accessed 26 February 2013]. Brussels, Council of the European Communities.

Eurofound (2012). *Fifth European Working Conditions Survey.* Luxembourg, Publications Office of the European Union.

European Agency for Safety and Health at Work (2013). *European Directives* [http://osha.europa.eu/en/legislation/directives/directives-intro, accessed 26 February 2013].

European Commission (2004). Communication from the Commission to the European Parliament, the Council, the European Economic and Social Committee and the Committee of Regions on the practical implementation of the provisions of the Health and Safety at Work Directives 89/391 (Framework), 89/654 (Workplaces), 89/655 (Work Equipment, 89/656 (Personal Protective Equipment), 90/269 (Manual Handling of Loads and 90/270 (Display Screen Equipment). Brussels, European Commission.

European Commission (2007). Communication from the Commission to the European Parliament, the Council, the European Economic and Social Committee and the Committee of the Regions on improving quality and productivity at work: Community strategy 2007–2012 on health and safety at work [http://eur-lex.europa.eu/LexUriServ/LexUriServ.do?uri=COM:2007:0062:FIN:EN:PDF]. Brussels, European Commission.

European Commission (2013). *Evaluation of the European Strategy on Safety and Health at Work 2007–2012* [http://ec.europa.eu/social/BlobServlet?docId=10016&langId=en, accessed 15 September 2013].

European Network for Workplace Health Promotion (ENWHP) (2013). [http://www.enwhp.org/, accessed 25 February 2013].

Fidler, D. P. (2003). *Developments involving SARS, International Law, and Infectious Disease Control at the Fifty-Sixth Meeting of the World Health Assembly* [http://www.asil.org/insigh108.cfm, accessed 25 February 2013]. Washington, DC, ASIL Insights.

Finnish Ministry of Social Affairs and Health (2013). *Health in All Policies: Seizing opportunities, implementing policies.* K. Leppo, E. Ollila, S. Pena, M. Wismar, S. Cook, Eds. [http://www.euro.who.int/__data/assets/pdf_file/0007/188809/Health-in-All-Policies-final.pdf, accessed 29 September 2013]. Helsinki, Ministry of Social Affairs and Health.

Fudge, J. and R. Owens (2006). "Precarious work, women and the new economy: the challenge to legal norms." In *Precarious Work, Women and the New Economy: The Challenge to Legal Norms.* J. Fudge and R. Owens, Eds. Oxford, Hart: 3–28.

Gochfeld, M. (2005). "Occupational medicine practice in the United States since the industrial revolution." *Journal of Occupational and Environmental Medicine* **47**(2): 115–131.

International Labour Organization (ILO) (1985). *Convention on Occupational Health Services* (No. 161). Geneva, ILO.

International Labour Organization (ILO) (2006). *Global Report on Child Labour*. Geneva, ILO.

International Labour Organization (ILO) (2009). *Facts on Safety and Health at Work* [http://www.ilo.org/wcmsp5/groups/public/—-dgreports/—-dcomm/documents/publication/wcms_105146.pdf, accessed 25 February 2013]. Geneva, ILO.

International Social Security Association (ISSA) (2011). *The Return on Prevention: Calculating the costs and benefits of investments in occupational safety and health in companies*. Geneva, ISSA.

Joint ILO/WHO Committee on Occupational Health (1995). *Working Document of the Twelfth Session of the Joint ILO/WHO Committee on Occupational Health*, 5–7 April 1995. Geneva, ILO/WHO.

Kankaanpää, E., M. van Tulder, M. Aaltonen and M. De Greef (2008). "Economics for occupational safety and health." *Scandinavian Journal of Work, Environment and Health* Suppl **5**: 9–13.

László, K., H. Pikhart, M. Kopp, M. Bobak, A. Pajak, S. Malyutina, G. Salavecz and M. Marmot (2010). "Job insecurity and health: a study of 16 European countries." *Social Science and Medicine* **70**(6): 867–874.

Min, K., J. Min, J. Park, S. Park and K. Lee (2010). "Changes in occupational safety and health indices after the Korean economic crisis: analysis of a national sample, 1991–2007." *American Journal of Public Health* **100**(11): 2165–2167.

Quinn, M. M. (2003). "Occupational health, public health, worker health." *American Journal of Public Health* **93**(4): 526.

Rachiotis, G., C. Alexopoulos and S. Drivas (2010). "Occupational morbidity and the state of occupational health in Greece." *Occupational Medicine (London)* **60**(4): 315–316.

Rantanen, J. (2005). "Basic occupational health services – their structure, content and objectives." *Scandinavian Journal of Work, Environment and Health* **1**: 5–15.

Rantanen, J. (2007). *Basic Occupational Health Services*. Helsinki, Finnish Institute of Occupational Health.

Rantanen, J. and R. Kim (2012). *Situation Analysis and Recommendations for Stewardship on Workplace Health Promotion in Poland*. [http://www.euro.who.int/__data/assets/pdf_file/0011/181856/e96758-Eng.pdf, accessed 20 September 2013]. Copenhagen, WHO Regional Office for Europe.

Rechel, B., E. Grundy, J.-M. Robine, J. Cylus, J. P. Mackenbach, C. Knai and M. McKee (2013). "Ageing in the European Union." *The Lancet* 381(9874): 1312–1322.

Rechel, B., P. Mladovsky, D. Ingleby, J. P. Mackenbach and M. McKee (2013). "Migration and health in an increasingly diverse Europe." *The Lancet* 381(9873): 1235–1245.

Takala, J., P. Hämäläinen and K. Saarela (2009). "Roles of occupational safety and health organisations in global and regional prevention strategies." *Occupational Health Southern Africa Journal* **15**(2a): 17–23.

World Health Organization (WHO) (1996). *WHO Global Strategy for Occupational Health for All*, WHA49.12. Geneva, WHO.

World Health Organization (WHO) (2002). *Good Practice in Occupational Health Services: A contribution to workplace health*. Copenhagen, WHO Regional Office for Europe.

World Health Organization (WHO) (2003). *Essential Public Health Functions: A three-country study in the Western Pacific Region*. Manila, WHO Regional Office for the Western Pacific.

World Health Organization (WHO) (2007). *Workers' Health: Global plan of action*. Geneva, WHO.

World Health Organization (WHO) (2009). *Healthy Workplaces: A WHO global model for action*. Geneva, WHO.

World Health Organization (WHO) (2011). *Action Plan for Implementation of the European Strategy for the Prevention and Control of Noncommunicable Diseases 2012–2016*. Copenhagen, WHO Regional Office for Europe.

World Health Organization (WHO) (2012a). *Connecting Health and Labour: Bringing together occupational health and primary care to improve the health of working people*. Executive Summary. Global Conference "Connecting Health and Labour: What Role for Occupational Health in Primary Health Care," The Hague, Netherlands, 29 November–1 December 2011. Copenhagen, WHO Regional Office for Europe.

World Health Organization (WHO) (2012b). *European Action Plan for Strengthening Public Health Capacities and Services*. Copenhagen, WHO Regional Office for Europe.

World Health Organization (WHO) (2012c). *Strategy and Action Plan for Healthy Ageing in Europe, 2012–2020*. Copenhagen, WHO Regional Office for Europe.

World Health Organization (WHO) (2012d). *Health 2020 Policy Framework and Strategy* [http://www.euro.who.int/en/who-we-are/governance/regional-committee-for-europe/sixty-second-session/working-documents/eurrc628-health-2020-policy-framework-and-strategy, accessed 15 September 2013]. Copenhagen, WHO Regional Office for Europe.

World Health Organization (WHO) (2013). *European Health for All Database*, July 2013 edition. Copenhagen, WHO Regional Office for Europe.

chapter six

Environmental health

Giovanni Leonardi, Bernd Rechel

Introduction

Environmental health comprises those aspects of human health that are determined by factors in the environment. It also refers to the theory and practice of assessing, correcting, and preventing those factors in the environment that can potentially have an adverse effect on the health of present and future generations (WHO 1994). Environmental *public* health can be defined as the science and art of preventing disease, prolonging life, and promoting health where environmental hazards are the key factor, through the organized efforts of society (Spiby 2006). Environmental health services are those services that implement environmental health policies through monitoring and control activities, promote the improvement of environmental parameters, and encourage the use of environmentally friendly and healthy technologies and behaviours. They also have a leading role in developing and suggesting new areas for environmental health policies (WHO 1994). However, it is important to stress that understandings of environmental health differ widely across the countries of Europe (Public Health Services Gelderland Midden 2011).

Environmental health is shaped by all those responsible for the environment, including housing, transport, agriculture, and employment, going far beyond health systems. As a consequence, environmental health has often been neglected by public health services and actions. Furthermore, although environmental influences on human health, well-being, and development have become increasingly clear, consensus on the urgency and means of addressing them is still lacking.

The environment has both direct and indirect effects on health. While traditional concerns of environmental health, such as the prevention of the toxic effects of chemicals, remain relevant globally (Prüss-Üstun, Vickers et al. 2011), the breakdown of ecosystems is becoming ever more important. Major global concerns include climate change, the loss of biodiversity, the depletion of stratospheric ozone, ocean acidification, the availability of fresh water, and changes in land use (Rockstrom, Steffen et al. 2009). It is becoming increasingly evident that sustainable population health depends on the successful transition to an economy that maintains the ecosphere (Meadows, Meadows et al. 1972; Daly 2005; Czech 2008; Jackson 2009; Max-Neef 2010). Ecosystems include air, water, soil, and vegetation and are necessary to enable life, including human life, but are being eroded as a result of human interventions (Rees 2002). Understanding these impacts is a new task for environmental health, requiring new approaches, methods, and tools that allow human development and prosperity that is not associated with ecological destruction and that can be used at the local level and beyond (Costanza, Kubiszewski et al. 2011).

This chapter begins by giving a brief overview of major environmental health hazards and the burden of disease that can be attributed to them. It then describes the main elements of environmental health services and the disciplines involved in this area. This is followed by a brief description of the varying training systems in place in Europe. The chapter then discusses what actions can be undertaken at international, national, and local level. The concluding section identifies steps to strengthen environmental health in Europe.

Environmental health hazards

Recognition of environmental health hazards varies across disease groups and conditions. Injuries are an area in which preventable environmental factors are well recognized, including those arising from road traffic injuries, falls, unintentional poisonings, fires, drowning, and natural hazards (e.g. floods, storms, periods of excessively hot or cold weather, and earthquakes).

It is also well established that exposure to certain environmental risk factors causes cancer at several sites of the body. One of the main environmental risk factors is smoking, responsible for about 70% of lung cancer cases globally. Other environmental risk factors for lung cancer include exposure to radon, ionizing radiation, asbestos, and other chemicals (e.g. chromium, nickel, cadmium, arsenic), and carcinogens that have also been linked to a range of other cancers, as detailed, for example, in reports by the International Agency for Research on Cancer.

The effects of carcinogens have been particularly well documented in occupational settings, with 28 chemical or biological agents considered, in a 2004 report, to be definite, 27 probable, and 113 possible occupational carcinogens (Siemiatycki, Richardson et al. 2004). Knowledge of occupational carcinogens is also relevant to the general population, where carcinogens are present outside the workplace and the distribution of exposures is known. Many other disease groups already have a confirmed or strongly suspected link to chemicals (Lippmann 2009; Prüss-Üstun, Vickers et al. 2011). For example, exposure to lead, methylmercury, polychlorinated biphenyls (PCBs), arsenic, toluene, and other chemicals has been confirmed or strongly suspected to cause cognitive development delays, Parkinson's disease, and attention-deficit disorder. There is also increasing recognition of endocrine disruptors – chemicals that interfere with the hormone system of mammals, causing tumours, birth defects, and other developmental disorders.

A comprehensive consideration of environmental factors can help to capture their overall impact on health, and identify the policy options available to national or local government bodies outside the health sector (Nriagu 2011). With this aim, the World Health Organization has coordinated overviews of the burden of disease attributable to specific environmental hazards, including climate change, outdoor air pollution (Ostro 2004), water (Prüss-Üstun, Bos et al. 2008), sanitation and hygiene, lead (Fewtrell, Kaufmann et al. 2003), mercury (Poulin and Gibb 2008), second-hand smoke (Oberg, Jaakkola et al. 2011), noise (WHO 2011a), and solar ultraviolet radiation (Lucas 2010).

It is also important to recognize that poorer countries and the most disadvantaged population groups are at an increased risk of poor environmental health. An assessment in 2012 found that there are major inequalities in environmental health in the WHO European Region, both within and across countries (WHO 2012). Whereas almost all countries in the EU have, for example, an adequate water supply, a sizeable share of the population in several former Soviet countries does not, with almost 40% of the rural population in Tajikistan lacking adequate access to water (WHO 2012). However, major differences in environmental health indicators also exist within the EU, with important differences across old and new member states; overcrowding is suffered by about 10% of the population in 15 "old" EU member states, but by an estimated 47% in the 12 "new" EU member states that joined in 2004 and 2007 (WHO 2012). Levels of air pollution also differ greatly, with countries in western Europe having been much more successful in reducing emissions than those in central and eastern Europe. For example, the average passenger car in central and eastern Europe has up to ten times higher nitrogen oxides emissions than its equivalent in western Europe (Mackenbach, Henschel et al. 2013).

Burden of disease attributable to environmental health hazards

Estimates of the burden of disease attributable to preventable factors tend to focus on direct effects that are readily quantifiable (Ezzati, Hoorn et al. 2003), and this is also true for estimates concerning the effects of environmental factors. In the 2004 round of the Global Burden of Disease, an estimated 24% of the global disease burden (healthy life years lost) and 23% of all deaths (premature mortality) were attributed to preventable environmental factors (Prüss-Üstün and Corvalán 2006). In the 2010 round, the number of disability-adjusted life years (DALYs) attributable to all of the environmental determinants studied, except exposure to lead, was estimated to have fallen, in some cases quite substantially, leading to a drop in the rankings of health determinants for most (Lim, Vos et al. 2013). However, in many cases the burden of disease was not quantifiable, although the health impacts were readily apparent. For instance, the disease burden associated with changed, damaged or depleted ecosystems was not quantified. Consequently, the estimated burden of disease attributable to environmental factors is almost certainly an underestimate.

While quantifiable evidence on the effects of environmental factors is crucial to motivate public health workers and to make a case for environmental health action in other sectors, it is an insufficient basis for developing effective environmental health services. In addition to estimates of the current burden of disease, approaches are needed that enable estimation of the impact of future trends. Mathematical modelling and its application to the development of decision support tools, for example, is an increasingly important tool for environmental health services. Others are provided by social sciences such as anthropology.

Main elements of environmental health services

Environmental health services typically include the following activities (Fitzpatrick and Bonnefoy 1998):

- risk assessment;
- risk management;
- risk communication;
- intersectoral cooperation and consultation;
- education and training;
- research.

These areas of environmental health services are constantly evolving. One of the latest European policy documents, the Parma Declaration on Environment and Health, adopted at the Fifth Ministerial Conference on Environment and Health in 2010, identified the following key environmental and health challenges:

- the health and environmental impacts of climate change and related policies;
- the health risks to children and other vulnerable groups posed by poor environmental, working, and living conditions (especially the lack of water and sanitation);
- socio-economic and gender inequalities in the human environment and health, amplified by the financial crisis;
- the burden of non-communicable diseases (NCDs), in particular to the extent that it can be reduced through adequate policies in areas such as urban development, transport, food safety and nutrition, and living and working environments;
- concerns raised by persistent, endocrine-disrupting, and bio-accumulating harmful chemicals and (nano)particles; and by novel and emerging issues; and
- insufficient resources in parts of the WHO European Region.

In addition to these new and emerging challenges, some traditional concerns of environmental health continue to require attention. One of them is housing. During the twentieth century, marked health improvements were achieved in Europe by improving the quality of housing and urban settlements. In the nineteenth century, local governments in many European countries had established campaigns for housing improvement in response to inadequate living conditions, characterized by overcrowding, lack of hygiene, and inadequate sanitation. These traditional risks are still prevalent in some countries, but new hazards related to housing have also been recognized. In the EU, injuries at home and during leisure activities and sport kill more than twice as many people than do road traffic injuries (EuroSafe 2013), while indoor pollutants or mould cause asthma, allergies, and respiratory diseases. There is growing evidence of the potential harmful effect that unsatisfactory housing can have on the health of occupiers. Four interrelated elements of housing can be distinguished: the house (or dwelling), the home (the social, cultural, and economic structure created by the household), the neighbourhood (or immediate housing environment), and the community (the population and services within the neighbourhood). Each of these individual elements has the potential to have a direct or indirect impact on physical, social, and mental health (WHO 2011b).

One area of intervention relates to falls within houses. In the Russian Federation, Kyrgyzstan, and Belarus, children are 22 times more likely to die from a fall than children in the European countries with the lowest mortality rates, Sweden, Netherlands, and the United Kingdom. One major reason for these differences is housing, with improved stair design and safe window design in the countries with lower mortality rates (WHO 2008b). Interventions effective in reducing housing-related health burdens are often among the most cost-efficient available (DiGuiseppi, Jacobs et al. 2010). Smoke alarms are an effective measure to reduce mortality from home fires, with mortality twice as high in homes without functioning smoke alarms (WHO 2011b). Yet overall, the evidence on the health impact of improvements in housing is still limited (WHO 2011b).

Waste management is becoming an increasingly complex matter in many European countries. Of concern are the effects on health of exposure to waste materials and the products of waste management (WHO 2007). In view of the limited ability to characterize all health risks, consideration should be given to application of a precautionary approach, with respect to the creation of new facilities and the mitigation of exposure to emissions and leachates of existing sites.

The sound management of chemicals is another area of environmental health. Chemical safety requires that all activities involving chemicals are undertaken in such a way as to ensure the safety of human health and the environment. It covers all chemicals, natural and manufactured, and the full range of exposure situations from the natural presence of chemicals in the environment to their extraction or synthesis, industrial production, transport, use, and disposal.

The health impacts of environmental noise are a growing concern among both the general public and policy-makers in Europe. Specific health effects include cardiovascular disease, cognitive impairment, sleep disturbance, tinnitus, and annoyance. It has been estimated that environmental noise in western European countries results annually in 61,000 DALYs lost due to ischaemic heart disease, 45,000 DALYs lost due to cognitive impairment of children, 903,000 DALYs lost due to sleep disturbance, 22,000 DALYs lost due to tinnitus, and 587,000 DALYs lost due to annoyance (WHO 2011a).

The establishment of disease registries in several countries provides a resource that could be used to gain a better understanding of the effects of environmental factors. There is also considerable scope to integrate toxicological knowledge in the design and interpretation of population-based epidemiological studies.

Man-made climate change will affect human health in many ways, mostly adversely (McMichael, Woodruff et al. 2006). Epidemiological evidence on how climatic trends affect health outcomes is accumulating. Public health services need to take account of the projected future health effects of climate change, in order to plan their policies and strategies for the next decades. Research to date has mostly focused on thermal stress, extreme weather events, infectious diseases, and to a lesser degree, projected future regional food yields and hunger prevalence. A broader approach will need to address a wider spectrum of health risks, due to the possibility of social, demographic, and economic disruptions resulting from climate change. Evidence on adverse health effects and better anticipation of future trends will strengthen the case for pre-emptive policies, and inform priorities for the planning of adaptive strategies (Leonardi 2010).

The central challenge is to leave future generations a biosphere that is intact. This requires the adoption of policies and practices that ensure sustainability, and moving to an economy that only consumes as much as the natural environment can produce (McMichael, Smith et al. 2000). The challenge is a political one (i.e. to make the necessary transition happen in practice) and requires not only action at the local and national level, but also – despite all the challenges in moving to a binding international framework for reducing greenhouse gas emissions (Vidal 2011) – by the international community.

Both the climate and human health are likely to benefit from a transition to an ecologically and socially sustainable model of social and economic development. Climate change threatens health, while many unhealthy activities are carbon-intensive (NHS Sustainable Development Unit 2010). Some of the causes of the growing burden of obesity, for example, such as the consumption of meat and other energy-dense foods, also have a range of negative consequences for the environment (Neff, Parker et al. 2011). Reducing greenhouse gas emissions through reductions in private car use and increased active travel (walking and cycling), on the other hand, benefits both the climate and population health. Low carbon technologies, strategies, and lifestyles have ancillary or collateral benefits for health, the so-called "health co-benefits". In some cases, the health benefits partly or fully offset the costs of implementing these policies (Haines 2012). The need to embrace more sustainable policies also applies to the health sector, which is a major source of greenhouse gas emissions (NHS Sustainable Development Unit 2008). Healthcare public health can play an important role in drawing attention to helping improve environmental awareness (see Chapter 8, "Healthcare public health").

Disciplines involved in environmental health

As in other areas of public health, professionals play a key role (see Chapter 15, "Developing the public health workforce"). Over 70 professional categories relevant to environmental health in Europe were identified in a review published in 1998, which included academics, medical specialists, environmental scientists (e.g. epidemiologists, natural scientists, social scientists, and experts in occupational hygiene), and practitioners (such as environmental health officers, technicians, and architects) (Fitzpatrick and Bonnefoy 1998). Yet, in the 15 years since then, few of these professions have increased their involvement in environmental health; on the contrary, the pressure of tight budgets seems to have reduced the number of professionals involved. Nevertheless, a wide range of disciplines and fields of knowledge continues to be required in environmental health services (Table 6.1).

Table 6.1 Fields of knowledge relevant to the core areas of environmental health

Core area	*Field of knowledge*
Accident and injury prevention and control	Predictive modelling of accident scenarios Contingency and logistical management Accident perception and psychology Accident and risk economics
Water quality	Water and wastewater chemistry Applied hydrology Hydrogeology Marine sciences Hydromechanics Water supply and water treatment technologies Agriculture, industrial and energy management
Air quality	Climatology Industrial and energy management Meteorology Atmospheric chemistry Atmospheric and climatological modelling
Food quality and safety	Agricultural management economics Veterinary science Soil science Food production technology Hazard analysis systems Health promotion Biotechnology and genetic modification technology
Waste management and soil pollution	Solid and liquid waste management Soil science Contaminated land management and rehabilitation Waste avoidance management
Human ecology and housing	Construction management Rural management Architecture Urban planning Building and housing science
Health of people at work	Ergonomics Occupational safety Environmental protection Engineering technology Occupational hygiene Bioengineering technology
Energy	Energy consumption modelling and prediction Long-distance monitoring and remote sensing techniques Geographical information systems
Transport management	Transport and logistics economics Transport modelling Motor engineering Transport behavioural studies Road safety studies

(Continued)

Table 6.1 Fields of knowledge relevant to the core areas of environmental health (*continued*)

Core area	*Field of knowledge*
Land use planning	Town and country planning Open space management Nature conservancy and wildlife protection Contaminated land management Agricultural management Natural resource and energy management
Agriculture	Plant and crop science Animal husbandry Veterinary science Chemical and pesticide safety Marine and fisheries sciences
Ionizing and non-ionizing radiation	Natural background radiation monitoring and protection techniques Nuclear power plant safety auditing Nuclear waste management Radiation monitoring Predictive modelling techniques Rehabilitation techniques for contaminated sites Applied epidemiological techniques for investigating exposure to non-ionizing radiation sources
Noise control	Noise exposure assessment techniques Noise-induced annoyance study skills Community noise assessment
Tourism and recreational activities	Bathing water quality Leisure facility control Applied ecology Littoral and estuarine sciences
Vector control	Entomology Parasitology Applied zoology Infectious disease control techniques

Source: Authors' compilation, adapted from Fitzpatrick and Bonnefoy (1998)

In view of the great diversity of professional categories involved in environmental health, the need for close collaboration across a wide range of topic areas and disciplines is apparent. There is also a clear need for intersectoral collaboration (see Chapter 12, "Intersectoral working"). Where partnerships have been developed between public health and practitioners in other sectors, these have facilitated the design and implementation of interventions that can reduce the environmentally induced disease burden. A number of policy instruments have been used to address environmental issues across sectors (Box 6.1).

Box 6.1   Policy instruments for intersectoral action in environmental health

Intersectoral action and health in all policies can be achieved in the area of environmental health through a number of policy instruments:

- **High-level political declarations:** these allow for shared agenda-setting and cooperation between health and environment sectors. Examples include ministerial conferences in the WHO European Region.
- **Long-term cooperative action programmes:** these result from high-level political declarations and can lead to networking and the exchange of good practice. Examples include the Transport, Health and Environment Pan-European Programme (THE PEP).
- **Norms and standards:** national and international norms, standards, and legislation are often based on evidence developed by the health sector. Examples include WHO guidelines on drinking-water quality, air quality, and noise, which have formed the basis for relevant EU directives.
- **Multilateral environment agreements:** these are often developed and implemented with the help of environmental health. Examples include the Convention on the Protection and Use of Transboundary Watercourses and the Convention on Long-Range Transboundary Air Pollution.
- **International Health Regulations:** these now include chemical and radiological events of international public health concern (see Chapter 4, "The health security framework in Europe").
- **Litigation over environmental contamination:** this is often used by NGOs to draw attention to environmental health concerns. Examples include the classification of global warming emissions as "pollutants" in the United States following a court case brought by the Natural Resources Defense Council.

Source: Dora, Pfeiffer et al. (2013)

Training in environmental health

A review of the training structures in 15 EU member states found that there is no common definition of environmental health and that there is no agreement as to the number of professionals trained or needed across Europe (Public Health Services Gelderland Midden 2011). This mirrors the findings related to public health in general (see Chapter 15, "Developing the public health workforce").

The training of professionals working in environmental health differs substantially across European countries and no common curriculum exists. In Finland, for example, physicians are not trained specifically in the environment and health, only in occupational health, and other professionals cover the environment and health field. In the Netherlands, a speciality in environmental health for physicians was established in the late 1980s and other professionals trained in environmental health or biomedical sciences were added in the 1990s. In Belgium, a mix of professionals, ranging from psychologists to biologists, are working in environmental health. In Poland, an Environmental Health Training Centre has been established, but there was a perceived need to institutionalize training on the environment and health for general practitioners and paediatricians (Public Health Services Gelderland Midden 2011).

Training objectives, as well as the competencies covered, also differ greatly across countries. In one European country, professionals may receive training in toxicology but not in risk communication, while the reverse may be true in the neighbouring country, with negative implications for cross-border collaboration and exchange (Public Health Services Gelderland Midden 2011). This indicates that there is substantial scope for increased collaboration and harmonization in Europe, both with regard to the training curricula of professionals in environmental health, and the definitions, job titles and roles, and the registration of professionals (Public Health Services Gelderland Midden 2011).

Action at the international level

A number of international organizations are active in the area of environmental health and a range of international guidelines, norms, and standards have been developed. The United Nations Environment Programme (UNEP), established as a result of the 1972 UN Conference on the Human Environment, coordinates UN environmental activities, many of which have an impact on human health. Together with the World Meteorological Organization, it set up the Intergovernmental Panel on Climate Change in 1988. Following the UN Conference on Sustainable Development in Brazil in 2012 (marking the twentieth anniversary of the 1992 United Nations Conference on Environment and Development in Rio de Janeiro), the UN General Assembly decided to strengthen and upgrade UNEP. Other UN agencies responsible for aspects of environmental health include the United Nations Development Programme (UNDP), the Food and Agriculture Organization (FAO), the International Maritime Organization (IMO), and the International Labour Organization (ILO). An example of a relevant multilateral agreement is the United Nations Framework Convention on Climate Change. The Kyoto Protocol to this convention set binding obligations on industrialized countries to reduce emissions of greenhouse gases. Although the protocol was criticized for being not effective enough to reduce worldwide emissions, it may still pave the way to a more effective successor document.

The WHO Regional Office for Europe has organized several Ministerial Environment and Health conferences as part of a process that also involves UN agencies and the EU. In the Parma Declaration on Environment and Health, adopted at the Fifth Ministerial Conference on Environment and Health in 2010, the ministers of health and environment in the European Region of WHO pledged to step up their efforts to address environmental and health challenges and set clear targets for the next decade.

The EU adopted a European Environment and Health Strategy in 2003, also referred to as the SCALE (Science, Children, Awareness, Legal instrument, Evaluation) initiative, followed by the Environment and Health Action Plan for 2004–2010. The Action Plan is currently being implemented. It aims to provide national governments with scientifically sound information to reduce the adverse health impacts of certain environmental factors. Examples of EU-wide hazard surveillance include the monitoring of air and water quality, undertaken by all local authorities, as well as the activities instituted by the EU Directives on Integrated Pollution Prevention and Control and on the Control of Major-Accident Hazards.

Ensuring the safety of drinking water is an essential activity of environmental health services in all European countries and international agencies have been instrumental in setting standards and norms. The WHO Water Quality Guidelines provide a framework based on a preventive, risk-based approach (WHO 2011c). The framework comprises three key components: health-based targets established by a competent health authority, adequate and properly managed systems (adequate infrastructure, proper monitoring, and effective planning and management), and a system of independent surveillance. Such a framework is usually enshrined in national standards, regulations or guidelines, in line with relevant policies and programmes as well as local circumstances, taking into consideration environmental, social, economic, and cultural issues and political priority-setting. However, it is important to stress that water contamination and its effects on the health of humans and whole ecosystems is just one aspect of the wider challenge of sustainable water management. The real issue that needs to be considered when examining what strategies and policies may alleviate the consequences of water contamination is the scarcity of water relative to human pressures, arising from the growing use of water for the production of food, goods, and to absorb waste (Leonardi 2006).

Air quality standards are another important component of environmental health policies that has been driven by international institutions. Although a minimum level of air quality standards has been legislated for EU member states, national standards both within the EU and across the WHO European Region vary, as countries adopt different approaches for balancing health risks, technological feasibility, economic considerations, and various other political and social factors, which in turn depend on, inter alia, the level of economic development and national capability in air quality management. WHO has published guidelines for air quality both outdoors (WHO, 1987, 2000, 2006) and indoors (WHO 2010). These guidelines are intended to support actions on air quality that protect public health in different contexts. They stress that, when formulating policy targets, governments should consider their own local circumstances before adopting the guidelines as legally binding standards. While there has been a decline in air pollution in Europe in recent years, this is not primarily due to stricter regulations, but reflects an underlying shift of polluting industries to countries outside Europe, as well as the impact of the global economic crisis.

Action at national and sub-national level

Stakeholders from within and outside the health sector need to take action to address environmentally mediated causes of disease (Prüss-Üstün and Corvalán 2006). The approaches needed for effective environmental health services comprise many methods familiar to practitioners in other domains of public health, but also methods that are more typical of natural scientists. These include not only basic environmental sciences, such as chemistry, physics, and geology (applied to identify the source and distribution of potentially hazardous substances), but also branches of engineering concerned with the whole range of human activities affecting air, water, and soil, such as agriculture, building, manufacturing, and transport.

The institutions at the local, regional, and national level that deliver environmental health services in the countries of the WHO European Region are extremely diverse, and involve both the public and private sector (Fitzpatrick and Bonnefoy 1998). A broad range of stakeholders is involved, at local and national level (MacArthur 2002). However, no recent overview seems to have been conducted on how environmental health services are organized across the WHO European Region. In addition to state institutions, there is also a range of other stakeholders in environmental health, including citizens' groups (such as activists who have been injured, e.g. CO Awareness, a charity that supports victims of carbon monoxide poisoning and other products of combustion), non-governmental organizations (NGOs), corporations, and independent professionals. Intergovernmental organizations also play an important role.

The local level is particularly important for the development and implementation of action on the environment and health, such as involving communities in decision-making processes, as in initiatives such as Healthy Cities. A number of requirements for successful action on the environment and health have been identified, including a multisectoral approach, community participation, and municipal action, supported by national commitment and leadership (MacArthur 2002).

Environmental health policies should be realistic and enforceable and take into account government structures, market forces, availability of public sector financing, the scope of legislation, and lobbying activities. Policies and instruments that can be used by national governments in Europe to strengthen or reform environmental health services in this sense include (MacArthur and Bonnefoy 1998):

- applying principles of environmental management to the objectives of environmental health services;
- developing strategies on policy formulation, situation assessment, priority setting, planning, public participation, and management;
- institutional development, including the location of environmental health services at the most appropriate level of government;
- reviewing the functions of environmental health services in relation to the overall objectives of the public health service (this includes options for legal remedies, for licenses and pre-development controls, and for economic sanctions and penalties);

- using mechanisms for environmental health services that are part of the broader economic and financial system, and the different mixtures of national and local sources of funding in Europe;
- evaluating the effectiveness of environmental health services.

Policy-makers are increasingly required to justify their decisions on economic grounds. However, the costs and benefits of environmental interventions are often surrounded by a degree of uncertainty and political controversy. Recognizing this, in 2013 the WHO Regional Office for Europe initiated an Environmental Health Economics Network (EHEN), with the aim of making better use of available economic evidence for decisions on the environment and health. While the benefits of interventions are often difficult to quantify, there is accumulating evidence on the costs of inaction. The costs caused by air pollution from traffic in the EU, for example has been estimated to amount to €25 billion per year, while noise pollution from traffic in the EU results in costs estimated as €7 billion per year (WHO 2013a). There is also increasing evidence of the benefits of action. Providing affordable warm housing through insulation and heating in the United Kingdom, for example, can give a return on investment after less than a year (WHO 2013a). Within urban settings, it is often possible to identify a cluster of cost-saving interventions and approaches, such as safe green spaces, safer driving, and encouraging walking and cycling, that can be delivered as part of a service package, creating multiple efficiencies and "win–win" solutions for health, society, the economy, and the environment (WHO 2013a).

Decision-makers in non-health departments also often prefer evidence on policies beneficial to health to be presented in terms of the competencies of their department. For example, rather than evidence that is focused on disease or exposure, a review summarizing all disease outcomes that would benefit from interventions within the housing sector at national or local level is much closer to the agenda of decision-makers in government departments that focus on housing (Braubach, Jacobs et al. 2011). This approach has the advantage of providing evidence on interventions in the framework of a single setting (Keall, Ormandy et al. 2011).

Environmental impact assessments are another important way of taking account of the impact of the environment on health (see Chapter 13, "Health impact assessment"). They have been used increasingly since the 1960s and have become mandatory in many European countries. In EU member states, a first directive on environmental impact assessments was adopted in 1985, with several amendments since.

While action at local and national level is crucial, it is becoming increasingly important to consider the global dimension of environmental health policies, in particular their ecological implications. Local environmental health services need to prioritize actions in line with local policies and needs, but also take account of the global context. The scope of environmental health services has thus expanded beyond the environment of the immediate "human setting" to include the more distant environment of "ecosystem services".

In view of the finite nature of fossil fuel reserves, it will become increasingly important to consider the energy requirements of various sectors (energy, transport, housing, but also health services). World production of oil is likely to peak in the near future, while demand continues to rise, resulting in a growing supply–demand gap that will increase the cost of energy in the long term.

One of the important roles of public health leaders and experts will be to anticipate potential consequences for the health of the population, such as through rising healthcare costs, and communicate them in consistent, transparent, and understandable ways to policy-makers and the public, including the careful communication of uncertainty where insufficient evidence exists (Nisbet, Maibach et al. 2011). Local (public) health departments face particular challenges in adapting to this new situation, as they are likely to face budget constraints as well as increasing public health needs and rely in many essential public health operations on fossil fuel consumption (Barnett, Parker et al. 2011). However, action will be needed in all sectors to prepare for a post-carbon future (Schwartz, Parker et al. 2011). This will require appropriate political and financial arrangements and incentives (Greer 2011).

A plethora of public health techniques and approaches have been applied to environmental factors affecting health, from case reports (following incidents) to individual and community trials (evaluating interventions). The accumulated evidence makes it possible to distinguish three basic scenarios underlying prevention activities (Box 6.2).

Box 6.2 Scenarios underlying prevention activities in environmental health

- The available information is sufficient to justify prevention, prevention activities exist, and they are effective, acceptable, and affordable.
- The available information is sufficient to justify prevention, as health effects are probable and prevention appears possible, but no prevention activities are available that are sufficiently effective, acceptable, and affordable.
- The available information is confined to a concern that an environmental component of causation exists for a given disease, but no further environmental, clinical, toxicological, or other data support this assumption; overall, such information is insufficient to justify prevention.

In the first of these scenarios, prevention activities seem well justified to prevent adverse effects on human health. Examples that illustrate the range of potential interventions include:

- access to improved sources of drinking water;
- pedestrian- and bicycle-friendly land use and transport;
- leisure and workplace facilities and policies that support active transport and more active lifestyles in general;
- phasing out leaded gasoline;
- access to cleaner household energy.

Once the interventions to be taken forward in a given geographical area are agreed, public health services are in a position to design information systems that make it possible to monitor progress. Environmental factors can be monitored by stand-alone information systems or mechanisms that supplement existing surveillance systems (see Chapter 3, "Monitoring the health of the population"). For example, surveillance activities that focus on the hazard (hazard surveillance) are typically not undertaken within a local public health service, but can inform public health actions by local and national authorities or other agencies. Only a limited number of chemicals fall into this category, including several "classical" air pollutants, such as SO_2, NO_x, particulate matter, and carbon monoxide, as well as several carcinogens. For these chemicals, the aim of surveillance should be to minimize exposure, as there is a confirmed association with human morbidity and mortality. Surveillance programmes for these chemical hazards focus largely on their emissions, enabling interventions to reduce such emissions, sometimes through a legal duty to do so. Examples of national or local initiatives are pollen monitoring networks and the activities by national and local environment agencies related to waste management.

Many environmental health interventions are as cost-effective as health-sector interventions (Prüss-Üstün and Corvalán 2006). The effectiveness of controlling environmental determinants of disease has, for example, been assessed with regard to air quality, in terms of both the reduced burden of disease and the economic costs and benefits. The introduction of air quality controls in industrialized countries has reduced the burden of cardiovascular and respiratory morbidity for such a small cost per DALY that these controls have been described as one of the most cost-effective regulations ever introduced. The replacement of lead in petrol with an alternative anti-knocking agent is another example of an action to reduce exposure to a hazard known to cause adverse health effects. It has since become apparent, however, that replacing lead with benzene may lead to other adverse health effects, making it difficult to evaluate the effect of this intervention on the overall disease burden.

Conclusion

In general, the functions of environmental health are not disputed, but far too often they are only provided as general statements or policies, without effective intergovernmental steering and implementation. Environmental health requires strong governance and political leadership (see Chapter 16, "Developing public health leadership"), as it spans governmental departments of health, environment, housing, transport, energy, and trade, and also involves the general population and private companies.

To strengthen environmental health in Europe, it is also essential to enhance the resilience of environmental health services and the communities they serve to respond to threats to the environment and to health (WHO 2013b). In line with the maxim that "all disasters begin locally", addressing environmental health hazards such as climate change will require local public health systems to become more resilient (Barnett, Parker et al. 2011). This will require investments in local capacities in the areas of communication, learning, risk awareness, and "social capital" (Castleden, McKee et al. 2011; Schwartz, Parker et al. 2011).

Preparing for a post-carbon future is another major challenge (Greer 2011). While there is growing awareness of the expected health effects of climate change and of possible policies and strategies to address these (WHO 2003), not enough is known about how, or if, these policies and strategies can be implemented. This gap between policies and implementation has been noted with regard to the United Kingdom, but it is also likely the case for many other European countries (Nichols, Maynard et al. 2009). Often, environmental targets are set too far into the future, and the promises and aspirations of politicians prove unachievable.

National and local public health services can take a number of actions to advance the environmental health agenda. They can decrease energy use in public health services and the wider health system, reconfigure health infrastructure and personnel, educate local communities about sustainable environmental action and its health benefits, and increase intersectoral collaboration (Barnett, Parker et al. 2011). Prioritization mechanisms are needed that can guide the allocation of scarce resources, with an increased focus on prevention and considerations of cost-effectiveness (Barnett, Parker et al. 2011).

In the area of preventing non-communicable diseases, a number of policies and strategies have been identified (WHO 2008a), but these are often poorly integrated with the management of environmental hazards to health (Ritsatakis and Makara 2009). While the role of environmental factors is often fairly clear, they have received far less attention than interventions that aim to modify individual behaviour. Obesity, for example, cannot only be addressed through changing individual diets, but also, and much more effectively, through the provision of healthy urban landscapes that include green spaces that encourage physical exercise, with proven benefits in terms of cardiovascular and mental health (Chow, Lock et al. 2009). Most actions that reduce greenhouse gas emissions, including in the areas of transport, household energy, food and agriculture, and electricity generation, also have public health benefits. The task for public health is to advocate for the implementation of these interventions as a win–win solution capable of addressing both climate change and health, that will be more effective and socially acceptable than when addressing these dimensions separately (Haines, McMichael et al. 2009).

It is becoming increasingly apparent that the future of environmental health services in Europe will require a synergy of traditional environmental health concerns (related to the immediate environment of human settings) with new needs (related to whole ecosystems and the biosphere). This may not be such a daunting task. What is needed is the development and implementation of appropriate policies, based on political support, better training of environmental health professionals, intersectoral cooperation, involvement of civil society, a clear distribution of responsibilities, and a strong system of monitoring and evaluation.

References

Barnett, D. J., C. L. Parker, V. A. Caine, M. McKee, L. M. Shirley and J. M. Links (2011). "Petroleum scarcity and public health: considerations for local health departments." *American Journal of Public Health* **101**(9): 1580–1586.

Braubach, M., D. E. Jacobs and D. Ormandy (2011). *Environmental Burden of Disease Associated with Inadequate Housing: Methods for quantifying health impacts of selected housing risks in the WHO European Region.* Bonn, WHO European Centre for Environment and Health, WHO Regional Office for Europe.

Castleden, M., M. McKee, V. Murray and G. Leonardi (2011). "Resilience thinking in health protection." *Journal of Public Health (Oxford)* **33**(3): 369–377.

Chow, C., K. Lock, K. Teo, S. Subramanian, M. McKee and S. Yusuf (2009). "Environmental and societal influences acting on cardiovascular risk factors and disease at a population level: a review." *International Journal of Epidemiology* **38**: 1580–1594.

Costanza, R., I. Kubiszewski, D. Ervin, R. Bluffstone, J. Boyd, D. Brown, H. Chang, V. Dujon, E. Granek, S. Polasky, V. Shandas and A. Yeakley (2011). "Valuing ecological systems and services." *F1000 Biology Reports* **3**: 14.

Czech, B. (2008). "Prospects for reconciling the conflict between economic growth and biodiversity conservation with technological progress." *Conservation Biology* **22**(6): 1389–1398.

Daly, H. E. (2005). "Economics in a full world." *Scientific American* **293**(3): 100–107.

DiGuiseppi, C., D. E. Jacobs, K. J. Phelan, A. D. Mickalide and D. Ormandy (2010). "Housing interventions and control of injury-related structural deficiencies: a review of the evidence." *Journal of Public Health Management and Practice* **16**(5 Suppl.): S34–S43.

Dora, C., M. Pfeiffer and F. Racioppi (2013). "Lessons from environment and health for HiAP." *Health in All Policies: Seizing opportunities, implementing policies.* K. Leppo, E. Olilla, S. Pena, M. Wismar and S. Cook, Eds. Helsinki, Finnish Ministry of Social Affairs and Health: 255–285.

EuroSafe (2013). *Injuries in the European Union: Report on injury statistics 2008–2010.* Amsterdam, EuroSafe.

Ezzati, M., S. V. Hoorn, A. Rodgers, A. D. Lopez, C. D. Mathers and C. J. Murray (2003). "Estimates of global and regional potential health gains from reducing multiple major risk factors." *The Lancet* **362**(9380): 271–280.

Fewtrell, L., R. Kaufmann and A. Prüss-Üstün (2003). *Lead: Assessing the environmental burden of disease at national and local level.* WHO Environmental Burden of Disease Series, No. 2. Geneva, WHO.

Fitzpatrick, M. and X. Bonnefoy (1998). *Environmental Health Services in Europe 3: Professional profiles.* WHO Regional Publications, European Series, No. 82. Copenhagen, WHO Regional Office for Europe.

Foster, J. (2008). *The Sustainability Mirage.* London, Earthscan.

Greer, J. (2011). *The Wealth of Nature: Economics as if survival mattered.* Gabriola Island, BC, New Society Publishers.

Haines, A. (2012). "Sustainable policies to improve health and prevent climate change." *Social Science and Medicine* **74**(5): 680–683.

Haines, A., A. McMichael, K. Smith, I. Roberts, J. Woodcock, A. Markandya, B. Armstrong, D. Campbell-Lendrum, A. Dangour, M. Davies, N. Bruce, C. Tonne, M. Barrett and P. Wilkinson (2009). "Public health benefits of strategies to reduce greenhouse-gas emissions: overview and implications for policy makers." *The Lancet* **374**(9707): 2104–2114.

Jackson, T. (2009). *Prosperity without Growth: Economics for a finite planet.* London, Earthscan.

Keall, M. D., D. Ormandy and M. G. Baker (2011). "Injuries associated with housing conditions in Europe: a burden of disease study based on 2004 injury data." *Environmental Health* **10**: 98.

Leonardi, G. (2006). "Water contamination: a question of sustainability." *Eurohealth* **12**(2): 14–17.

Leonardi, G. (2010). "Adaptation to climate change." In *Environmental Medicine*. J. G. Ayres, R. M. Harrison, G. L. Nichols and R. L. Maynard, Eds. London, Hodder Arnold.

Lim, S., T. Vos, A. Flaxman, G. Danaei, K. Shibuya, H. Adair-Rohani, M. Amann, H. Anderson, K. Andrews, M. Aryee and C. Atkinson (2013). "A comparative risk assessment of burden of disease and injury attributable to 67 risk factors and risk factor clusters in 21 regions, 1990–2010: a systematic analysis for the Global Burden of Disease Study 2010." *The Lancet* **380**(9859): 2224–2260.

Lippmann, M. (2009). *Environmental Toxicants: Human exposures and their health effects*, 3rd edition. New York, Wiley.

Lucas, R. (2010). *Solar Ultraviolet Radiation: Assessing the environmental burden of disease at national and local levels*. Environmental Burden of Disease Series, No. 17. Geneva, WHO.

MacArthur, I. and X. Bonnefoy (1998). *Environmental Health Services in Europe 2: Policy options*. WHO Regional Publications, European Series, No. 77. Copenhagen, WHO Regional Office for Europe.

MacArthur, I. D. (2002). *Local Environmental Health Planning: Guidance for local and national authorities*. WHO Regional Publications, European Series, No. 95. Copenhagen, WHO Regional Office for Europe.

Mackenbach, J., S. Henschel, P. Goodman, S. Medina and M. McKee (2013). "Air pollution." *Successes and Failures of Health Policy in Europe: Four decades of divergent trends and converging challenges*. J. Mackenbach and M. McKee, Eds. Maidenhead, Open University Press: 239–254.

Max-Neef, M. (2010). "The world on a collision course and the need for a new economy." *Ambio* **39**(3): 200–210.

McMichael, A. J., K. R. Smith and C. F. Corvalan (2000). "The sustainability transition: a new challenge." *Bulletin of the World Health Organization* **78**(9): 1067.

McMichael, A. J., R. E. Woodruff and S. Hales (2006). "Climate change and human health: present and future risks." *The Lancet* **367**(9513): 859–869.

Meadows, D. H., D. L. Meadows, J. Randers and W. W. Behrens (1972). *The Limits of Growth*. New York, Universe Books.

Neff, R. A., C. L. Parker, F. L. Kirschenmann, J. Tinch and R. S. Lawrence (2011). "Peak oil, food systems, and public health." *American Journal of Public Health* **101**(9): 1587–1597.

NHS Sustainable Development Unit (2008). *NHS England Carbon Emissions: Carbon footprinting report*. London, NHS Sustainable Development Unit.

NHS Sustainable Development Unit (2010). *Saving Lives, Saving Money, Securing the Future*. Sustainability, Health and the NHS Factsheet. London, NHS Sustainable Development Unit.

Nichols, A., V. Maynard, B. Goodman and J. Richardson (2009). "Health, climate change and sustainability: a systematic review and thematic analysis of the literature." *Environmental Health Insights* **3**: 63.

Nisbet, M. C., E. Maibach and A. Leiserowitz (2011). "Framing peak petroleum as a public health problem: audience research and participatory engagement in the United States." *American Journal of Public Health* **101**(9): 1620–1626.

Nriagu, J. (2011). *Encyclopedia of Environmental Health*, 5 volume set. Burlington, MA, Elsevier.

Oberg, M., M. S. Jaakkola, A. Woodward, A. Peruga and A. Prüss-Üstün (2011). "Worldwide burden of disease from exposure to second-hand smoke: a retrospective analysis of data from 192 countries." *The Lancet* **377**(9760): 139–146.

Ostro, B. (2004). *Outdoor Air Pollution: Assessing the environmental burden of disease at national and local level.* Environmental Burden of Disease Series, No 5. Geneva, WHO.

Poulin, J. and H. Gibb (2008). *Mercury: Assessing the environmental burden of disease at national and local levels.* Environmental Burden of Disease Series, No. 16. Geneva, WHO.

Prüss-Üstün, A. and C. Corvalán (2006). *Preventing Disease through Healthy Environments: Towards an estimate of the environmental burden of disease.* Geneva, WHO.

Prüss-Üstün, A., R. Bos, F. Gore and J. Bartram (2008). *Safer Water, Better Health: Costs, benefits and sustainability of interventions to protect and promote health.* Geneva, WHO.

Prüss-Üstün, A., C. Vickers, P. Haefliger and R. Bertollini (2011). "Knowns and unknowns on burden of disease due to chemicals: a systematic review." *Environmental Health* **10**: 9.

Public Health Services Gelderland Midden (2011). *Training of Professionals in Environment and Health.* Luxembourg, European Commission Directorate General for Health and Consumers.

Rees, W. E. (2002). "Footprint: our impact on Earth is getting heavier." *Nature* **420**(6913): 267–268.

Ritsatakis, A. and P. Makara (2009). "Gaining health." In *Analysis of Policy Development in European Countries for Tackling Noncommunicable Diseases.* J. L. Farrington, R. Geneau and B. Pettersson, Eds. Copenhagen, WHO Regional Office for Europe.

Rockstrom, J., W. Steffen, K. Noone, A. Persson, F. S. Chapin, III, E. F. Lambin, T. M. Lenton, M. Scheffer, C. Folke, H. J. Schellnhuber, B. Nykvist, C. A. de Wit, T. Hughes, S. van der Leeuw, H. Rodhe, S. Sorlin, P. K. Snyder, R. Costanza, U. Svedin, M. Falkenmark, L. Karlberg, R. W. Corell, V. J. Fabry, J. Hansen, B. Walker, D. Liverman, K. Richardson, P. Crutzen and J. A. Foley (2009). "A safe operating space for humanity." *Nature* **461**(7263): 472–475.

Schwartz, B. S., C. L. Parker, J. Hess and H. Frumkin (2011). "Public health and medicine in an age of energy scarcity: the case of petroleum." *American Journal of Public Health* **101**(9): 1560–1567.

Siemiatycki, J., L. Richardson, K. Straif, B. Latreille, R. Lakhani, S. Campbell, M.-C. Rousseau and P. Boffetta (2004). "Listing occupational carcinogens." *Environmental Health Perspectives* **112**(15): 1447–1459.

Spiby, J. (2006). *Developing Competencies in Environmental Public Health: Chemical hazards & poisons report* [http://www.hpa.org.uk/web/HPAwebFile/ HPAweb_C/1194947321801, accessed 26 February 2012].

Vidal, J. (2011). "Brokering a deal to replace Kyoto will take years, EU ministers say." *British Medical Journal* **343**: d7963.

World Health Organization (WHO) (1987). *Air Quality Guidelines for Europe.* WHO Regional Publications, European Series, No. 23. Copenhagen, WHO Regional Office for Europe.

World Health Organization (WHO) (1994). *Action Plan for Environmental Health Services in Eastern and Central Europe and the Newly Independent States.* Report on a WHO Consultation, Sofia, Bulgaria, 19–22 October 1993. Copenhagen, WHO Regional Office for Europe.

World Health Organization (WHO) (2000). *Air Quality Guidelines for Europe,* 2nd edition. WHO Regional Publications, European Series, No. 91. Copenhagen, WHO Regional Office for Europe.

World Health Organization (WHO) (2003). *Climate Change and Human Health: Risks and responses. Summary.* Geneva, WHO.

World Health Organization (WHO) (2006). *Air Quality Guidelines: Global update 2005. Particulate matter, ozone, nitrogen dioxide and sulfur dioxide.* Copenhagen, WHO Regional Office for Europe.

World Health Organization (WHO) (2007). *Population Health and Waste Management: Scientific data and policy options.* Report of a WHO Workshop. Rome, WHO.

World Health Organization (WHO) (2008a). *2008–2013 Action Plan for the Global Strategy for the Prevention and Control of Noncommunicable Diseases.* Geneva, WHO.

World Health Organization (WHO) (2008b). *European Report on Child Injury Prevention.* Copenhagen, WHO Regional Office for Europe.

World Health Organization (WHO) (2010). *WHO Guidelines for Indoor Air Quality: Selected pollutants.* Copenhagen, WHO European Centre for Environment and Health, WHO Regional Office for Europe.

World Health Organization (WHO) (2011a). *Burden of Disease from Environmental Noise: Quantification of healthy life years lost in Europe.* Geneva, WHO.

World Health Organization (WHO) (2011b). *Environmental Burden of Disease Associated with Inadequate Housing: Methods for quantifying health impacts of selected housing risks in the WHO European Region.* M. Braubach, D. E. Jacobs and D. Ormandy, Eds. Bonn, WHO Regional Office for Europe.

World Health Organization (WHO) (2011c). *Guidelines for Drinking-water Quality,* 4th edition [http://www.who.int/water_sanitation_health/publications/2011/dwq_chapters/en/index.html, accessed 4 January 2012]. Geneva, WHO.

World Health Organization (WHO) (2012). *Environmental Health Inequalities in Europe: Assessment report.* Copenhagen, WHO Regional Office for Europe.

World Health Organization (WHO) (2013a). *The Case for Investing in Public Health.* A public health summary report for EPHO 8. Copenhagen, WHO Regional Office for Europe.

World Health Organization (WHO) (2013b). *Health and the Environment in the WHO European Region: Creating resilient communities and supportive environments.* Copenhagen, WHO Regional Office for Europe.

chapter seven

Food security and healthier food choices

João Breda, Trudy Wijnhoven,
Mojca Gabrijelčič, Louise Sigfrid

Introduction

Food, nutrition, and obesity have gained increasing political attention in recent years, with the realization that the global obesity epidemic coexists, in many countries, with widespread under-nutrition, and food shortages. While at the beginning of the twentieth century the main goal of nutrition policies in Europe was to prevent hunger, with policy focused on agriculture, today the focus is on tackling obesity and under-nutrition, while ensuring the environmental and economic sustainability of food production and consumption. This links with other global issues, such as climate change, population growth, and the growing demand for energy and water (Global Food Security 2011). In the WHO European Region, obesity is rising steeply in many countries, although decreasing in some, while at the same time the number of malnourished people (including micronutrient deficiencies) is stubbornly high in many countries and social groups. These developments have negative implications for population health, health systems, and the wider economy and are accentuated through the current economic crisis, with more people facing unemployment and poverty and an increase in health inequalities in parts of the WHO European Region.

To address these challenges, it will be crucial to create environments that support healthy food choices throughout the life-course and make these choices easy, accessible, and cheap. It will also be necessary to meet the rising demand for food in ways that are equitable as well as environmentally, socially, and economically sustainable. There is also a need to ensure that food is contributing to balanced, healthy, and safe diets, and to reduce over-consumption and food waste. Meeting these challenges requires effective policies and regulations, as well as multidisciplinary partnerships working across sectors and borders. This chapter outlines the current situation and the challenges ahead, as well as providing examples of existing networks and partnerships and good practice from across Europe. It begins by setting out key challenges for food and nutrition in Europe today, including food security, diet and malnutrition, obesity, foodborne diseases, and sustainability and wastage. The chapter then turns to a discussion of international initiatives and policies, which is followed by an overview of national policy actions. A concluding section brings together the key findings of the chapter.

Food security

The 1996 World Food Summit defined food security as follows: "when all people at all times have access to sufficient, safe, nutritious food to maintain a healthy and active life" (WHO 2013b). Importantly, it is not only the amount of food available, or the purchasing power to buy it, but also its nutritional quality and safety.

Food security is built on three pillars (Figure 7.1):

- Availability: sufficient quantities of food are available on a consistent basis.
- Access: sufficient resources are available to obtain appropriate food for a nutritious diet.
- Utilization: appropriate use, based on knowledge of nutrition and care, as well as adequate water and sanitation.

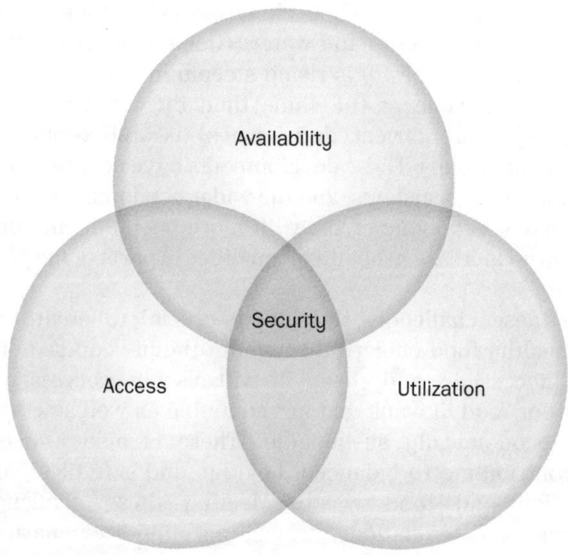

Figure 7.1 The three pillars of food security

Source: Global Climate Change and Human Health (2013)

Some of the challenges in providing food security across Europe are as follows (Global Food Security 2011):

- demographic changes and urbanization;
- climate change – increasing carbon dioxide, greenhouse gases, temperature, and extreme weather events;
- environmental impacts of farming – increasing water and land use, pollution, and decreasing biodiversity;
- limited resources for agriculture – in terms of land, fresh water, and energy;
- social and cultural drivers – urbanization, changing consumer needs, preferences and habits;
- economic drivers – trade, land, and food markets.

In the poorer countries in Europe, poverty affects more than half of the population, which can lead to food insecurity and the consumption of unsafe foods of poor nutritional quality (WHO 2008a). The current economic crisis has reduced food security in several European countries, with Greece recording the steepest decline (Global Food Security 2013).

Food security, however, is clearly a much more pressing problem in other parts of the world. Over 900 million people globally are estimated to be under-nourished, most of them in Sub-Saharan Africa and in South Asia (European Commission 2013d). In some developing countries, food prices are very high and subject to volatility, affecting in particular access to food by people on low incomes. Other factors affecting food security include civil war, natural disasters, political instability, and urbanization, and how well a country is prepared to respond to these (Global Food Security 2013). In 1996, leaders at the World Food Summit in Rome set the goal of halving the number of food-insecure people in the world to 400 million by 2015. This target is likely to be missed. Yet, gains have been made, largely through poverty alleviation and innovations that improve market access, increase households' ability to purchase food and boost the availability of more nutritious crops. This indicates that food security can be achieved, provided there are appropriate international and national policies on agriculture and economic development in place (Global Food Security 2013).

Malnutrition

Public health nutrition can be defined as "promotion and maintenance of nutrition-related health and wellbeing of populations, through the organised efforts and informed choices of society" (Gibney, Margetts et al. 2004). Malnutrition develops when the body does not get the right amount of energy, protein, vitamins, and other nutrients needed to maintain health and normal organ function. Malnutrition is not only confined to people who are obviously undernourished – overweight and obese people can suffer from it too. In Europe, an estimated 33 million people are at risk of malnutrition, including pregnant women, older people, those with chronic diseases, and socially isolated and poorer people (WHO/UNICEF 2006).

Many children in the WHO European Region, in particular in some central Asian countries, suffer from deficiencies in micronutrients, such as iodine, iron, and vitamin A. This has been attributed to a lack of access to balanced and appropriate diets (including fresh fruit and vegetables), poor implementation of food fortification programmes (such as salt iodization), and low levels of awareness, particularly with regard to nutrition for infants and young children (Rokx, Galloway et al. 2002). Iron deficiency is the most common nutritional deficiency in children worldwide and an estimated 11 million children below 5 years of age in Europe (22% of the total) are anaemic (WHO 2008b). Another challenge in many European countries are low rates of exclusive breastfeeding at 6 months (Rokx, Galloway et al. 2002; Cattaneo, Yngve et al. 2005). There are also growing concerns across Europe about malnutrition in hospitals and care homes, with calls to raise awareness and train health professionals in recognizing the signs of malnutrition. In the European Union (EU), 10% of individuals over the age of 65 and almost one-third of patients in hospitals and nursing homes were found to be at risk of malnutrition (Stratton, Green et al. 2003; Ljungqvist, van Gossum et al. 2010).

Malnourishment is a serious issue with long-term consequences, including poor educational achievement by children and young people (WHO/UNICEF 2006). It can result in compromised immune responses, leading to an increased risk of infections, poor wound healing, delayed recovery from illness, and longer hospitalization (Kondrup, Johansen et al. 2002). The European Nutrition for Health Alliance reported that hospital stays of malnourished patients are on average three days longer than for those with adequate nutrition, while those diagnosed with nutrition problems in the community consumed an additional €1128 in healthcare resources over six months per person compared with similar well-nourished individuals (European Nutrition for Health Alliance 2013). It has been estimated that the cost of malnutrition in the EU alone totals €120 billion per year (Ljungqvist, van Gossum et al. 2010).

Obesity

Europe is also seeing an increased burden of obesity. Across the WHO European Region, the growing intake of foods rich in salt, sugars, saturated and trans-fatty acids leads to unbalanced diets with a high energy density, resulting in diet-related non-communicable diseases, such as cardiovascular disease, diabetes, some forms of cancer, as well as mental health issues (WHO 2003; McElroy, Kotwal et al. 2004; Solfrizzi, Frisardi et al. 2011). These not only shorten life expectancy (mortality increases sharply once the overweight threshold is crossed), but also reduce the quality of life. Furthermore, the costs of overweight and obesity are staggering, not only to individuals but also to society and the overall economy (IOTF/EASO 2002).

In 46 of the 53 countries of the WHO European Region, the adult prevalence of overweight and obesity is over 50% (WHO 2007, 2012a). Similar levels can be found throughout the EU, where more than half of the adult population are overweight or obese and an average of almost 1 in 5 (17%) is obese. The prevalence among adults ranges from around 1 in 12 in Romania and Switzerland to over 1 in 4 in Hungary and the United Kingdom, although some of these variations may be due to different methodologies in data collection. While there is little difference in average obesity rates between men and women, there is variation within individual countries, with more men than women being obese in Malta, Iceland, and Norway, while a higher proportion of women are obese in Latvia, Turkey, and Hungary (OECD 2012a). The prevalence of obesity among children is also rising in many countries (see below for information on WHO's Childhood Obesity Surveillance Initiative, COSI).

Current trends suggest that the average body mass index among both adults and children will continue to increase in the coming years across Europe. In some countries, obesity- and overweight-related diseases are concentrated among the poor and less educated, thus contributing to increasing health inequalities (OECD 2012b).

Obesity is to a large extent driven by low levels of physical activity and poor dietary choices, owing to social, cultural, technological, economic, and political factors, such as the global food system (see Chapter 6, "Environmental health") and its increasing reliance on processed and energy-rich foods (Bock, Atzel et al. 2012). Obesity-generating ("obesogenic") environments (Swinburn, Egger et al. 1999) have emerged, driven by questionable urban planning, as well as economic drivers and technological developments. To decrease the burden of obesity, it is crucial to create environments that support healthy food choices throughout the life-course (WHO 1986, 2004, 2013d). Prevention in early life can target several risk factors at once and amplify benefits and cost-effectiveness as, for example, in the case of promoting breastfeeding and appropriate complementary feeding. The problem of overweight and obesity is not only complicated, but also complex (Rutter 2011); it thus needs complex societal and political solutions. As the causal factors range from environmental, educational, technological to cultural and behavioural issues, the solutions require multidisciplinary and intersectoral partnerships (see Chapter 12, "Intersectoral working"), including a whole-of-government approach and health impact assessments of policies outside the health sector (see Chapter 13, "Health impact assessment"). In particular, it needs a strong regulatory framework, including effective measures to properly monitor obesity, improve school nutrition and reduce the exposure of children to the marketing of foods that are high in fat, sugar, and salt, coupled with local interventions that include planning solutions to change environments that do not favour physical activity and the adoption of healthier diets. Preventing obesity is a win–win–win solution, and should be at the forefront of national and international health policies.

Foodborne diseases and other hazards

Foodborne diseases represent a considerable public health burden and pose a major challenge to the public health system. Salmonellosis and campylobacteriosis are the most commonly reported foodborne diseases in Europe. Foodborne illnesses can also result from pesticides or medicines in food and naturally toxic substances (see Chapter 6, "Environmental health"). With the globalization of food markets, climate change, and increasing international travel, there is a risk of new outbreaks of foodborne diseases in

Europe. Antimicrobial resistance is a related challenge, partly related to the non-human use of antimicrobial agents. The growth of global trade and travel allows resistant microorganisms to be spread rapidly through humans and food (WHO 2013a). Various chemical hazards also represent a public health risk, while food allergies are another concern that is increasingly recognized (WHO 2008a).

The bovine spongiform encephalopathy (BSE) outbreak in the 1980s and 1990s highlighted the impact of decisions made in other sectors on human health, but also demonstrated the importance of retaining public confidence in policy-makers. Poor agricultural practices and policies and difficulties regulating the agricultural sector led to BSE being transmitted from cows to humans as a new fatal disease (the new variant Creutzfeld–Jakob disease) (McKee, Lang et al. 1996). This illustrated the role public health and public health nutrition should play in ensuring a whole-of-government approach during the development of agriculture, food, and other policies (Lock, Gabrijelcic Blenkus et al. 2003).

Sustainability and wastage

Another problem is that the current global food system may generate inequalities that pose enormous environmental challenges, such as coping with a growing population and the increasing demand for food, energy, and water. In this context, the problem of food waste is becoming ever more evident (FAO 2013b). Around one-third of the food produced globally is lost or wasted, while at the same time more than one billion people around the world are undernourished. Food waste not only serves as a reminder of gross social injustice, it also represents a substantial loss of resources such as land, water, energy, and labour. In the EU alone, an estimated 90 million tonnes of food, or 180 kg per person, are wasted every year, with much of this food still suitable for human consumption (European Commission 2011b). Food waste occurs at every stage of the production and supply chain, as well as at the consumption stage. Some of it is caused by legislation and trade markets, some by consumer preferences and habits. The European Environment Agency aims to halve the disposal of edible food in the EU by 2020 through the combined efforts of farmers, the food industry, retailers, and consumers, including more resource-efficient production techniques and more sustainable food choices (European Environment Agency 2012).

International policies and initiatives

Several international organizations are supporting actions in Europe that aim to improve food security and ensure safe, healthy, and nutritious diets in sustainable and equitable ways. These include in particular the WHO Regional Office for Europe and the EU with its services (DG SANCO) and specialized bodies, the European Food Safety Authority, and the European Centre for

Disease Prevention and Control (ECDC). All of these agencies are leading on a range of policies and partnerships with stakeholders from across Europe. Public health has an important role to play in informing these policies and actions in terms of providing intelligence, research, advocacy, surveillance, monitoring, and evaluation.

The World Health Organization

The World Health Organization has developed several policy frameworks and action plans to address diet-related non-communicable diseases (NCDs), nutrition, food safety, and food security. Following on from a first European Action Plan for Food and Nutrition Policy for 2000–2005, WHO adopted a second action plan for 2007–2012 (WHO 2008a), with the goals of reducing the prevalence of diet-related NCDs, reversing the obesity trend among children and adolescents, reducing the prevalence of micronutrient deficiencies, and reducing the incidence of foodborne diseases. The envisaged measures to achieve these goals include (WHO 2008a):

- supporting a healthy start;
- ensuring a safe, healthy, and sustainable food supply;
- providing comprehensive information and education to consumers;
- taking integrated action to address related determinants (e.g. physical activity, alcohol consumption, safe drinking water, and other environmental factors);
- strengthening nutrition and food safety in the health sector;
- monitoring, evaluation, and research.

The action plan further recommended adoption of population nutrition goals in line with recommendations by WHO and the Food and Agriculture Organization of the United Nations (FAO) (Box 7.1).

In 2012, WHO also published a guide on prevention strategies for reducing childhood obesity, highlighting best practice examples of population-based approaches (Figure 7.2) (WHO 2012b).

Box 7.1 Population nutrition goals based on WHO and FAO recommendations

- < 10% of daily energy intake from saturated fatty acids;
- < 1% of daily energy intake from trans-fatty acids;
- < 10% of daily energy intake from free sugars;
- ≥ 400 g of fruits and vegetables a day;
- < 5 g a day of salt.

Source: Paris and Polton (2008)

Structures to support policies and interventions	Population-wide policies and initiatives	Community-based interventions
• Leadership • 'Health-in-All' policies • Dedicated funding for health promotion • NCD monitoring systems • Workforce capacity • Networks and partnerships • Standards and guidelines	• Restrictions on marketing of unhealthy foods and beverages to children • Nutrition labelling • Food taxes and subsidies • Fruit and vegetable initiatives • Physical activity policies • Social marketing campaigns	• Multi-component community-based interventions • Early childcare settings • Primary and secondary schools • Other community settings

Figure 7.2   Population-based approaches to childhood obesity prevention

Source: WHO (2012b)

At the Ministerial Conference on Nutrition and Noncommunicable Diseases in the Context of Health 2020, in Vienna in July 2013, ministers of health and representatives of member states of the WHO European Region reaffirmed their commitment to existing European and global frameworks to address important NCD risk factors, notably unhealthy diet and physical inactivity. Ministers recognized that a healthy diet can contribute to achieving the global targets on NCDs adopted by the 66th World Health Assembly, including achieving a 25% relative reduction in premature mortality from NCDs by 2025. They also acknowledged the importance of multisectoral action and health system capacity, universal health coverage, and evidence-based methods in preventing and treating NCDs within comprehensive and integrated national strategies.

Building on the new European policy framework Health 2020, countries agreed to facilitate decisive action to prevent and tackle overweight, obesity, and under-nutrition. This includes supporting food systems that encourage healthy eating, are sustainable, and ensure equity. Policy options for governments to consider include production, consumption, marketing, availability, access, economic measures, and education-based interventions, taking into account the cultural dimensions of nutrition. Member states agreed to prioritize five action areas (WHO 2013d):

- create healthy food and drink environments and encourage physical activity for all population groups;
- promote the health gains of a healthy diet throughout the life-course, especially for the most vulnerable;
- reinforce health systems to promote health and to provide services for NCDs;
- support surveillance, monitoring, evaluation, and research of the population's nutritional status and behaviours;
- strengthen governance, alliances, and networks and empower communities to engage in health promotion and prevention efforts.

At the Vienna Ministerial Conference, high salt intake was identified as one of the main risk factors for high blood pressure, which increases the risk of stroke, cardiovascular disease, and kidney disease. Research has shown that reducing salt intake to less than 5 g per day reduces the risk of stroke by 23%

and cardiovascular disease by 17% (WHO 2013c). Yet, the average intake of salt across Europe is estimated to be about 8–11g, far exceeding the recommended levels. In view of the clear association between salt intake and hypertension, WHO has developed a target as part of a more comprehensive set of nine voluntary global targets and 25 indicators to monitor and assess progress in the implementation of strategies to reduce the burden of NCDs. The goal is to reduce dietary salt intake by 30% by 2025 (WHO 2013c).

The WHO European Childhood Obesity Surveillance Initiative

There is a need to ensure robust data collection, monitoring, and surveillance systems to enable comparisons over time, between countries, and to detect new trends (see Chapter 3, "Monitoring the health of the population"). In the area of obesity, a comprehensive European surveillance system has been set up in the form of the European Childhood Obesity Surveillance Initiative (COSI), led by the WHO Regional Office for Europe. This initiative aims to measure routinely trends in overweight and obesity in primary school children (6–9 years) to gain a better understanding of the scope of the problem in this population group and permit intercountry comparisons within the WHO European Region. Data from countries that have taken part in COSI so far show a high prevalence of overweight and obesity among 6–9-year-olds, but also variation between countries, with the highest prevalence in southern Europe (Box 7.2).

Between 2008 and 2011, the WHO Regional Office for Europe and the European Commission also ran a collaborative project entitled "Monitoring progress

Box 7.2   Selected findings from WHO's European Childhood Obesity Surveillance Initiative

The first round of data collection took place during the school year 2007/2008 with 13 countries participating: Belgium (the Flemish region), Bulgaria, Cyprus, Czech Republic, Ireland, Italy, Latvia, Lithuania, Malta, Norway, Portugal, Slovenia, and Sweden. The prevalence of overweight ranged from 19% to 49% among boys and from 18% to 43% among girls, while the prevalence of obesity ranged from 6% to 27% among boys and from 5% to 17% among girls (based on the 2007 WHO growth reference).

The second round of data collection was undertaken in 2009/2010 in 15 countries. It found that the prevalence of obesity among children is rising in many countries, while levelling off in a very few. The prevalence of overweight (including obesity) ranged from 18% to 57% among boys and from 18% to 50% among girls; 6–31% of boys and 5–21% of girls were obese.

Source: Wijnhoven, van Raaij et al. (2013)

on improving nutrition and physical activity and preventing obesity in the European Union" (WHO 2008–2011), which highlighted the need for monitoring and surveillance, as well as for the implementation of policies and action plans and the sharing of good practice. The project identified four priority areas:

Surveillance

- nutritional status, dietary habits, physical activity or inactivity
- awareness, knowledge, attitudes, and other behaviours

National policies and action plans

- policy documents on food and nutrition, physical activity, and obesity
- actions to implement the policies: programmes, legislation, public–private partnerships, and voluntary actions

Flagging of successful initiatives

- national, regional, and local programmes
- preventative interventions in different settings (e.g. schools, workplaces, communities, primary health care, and hospitals)

Status of implementation

- including progress in key commitments contained within the European Charter on Counteracting Obesity, the WHO European Food and Nutrition Action Plan, and the Vienna Declaration on Nutrition and Noncommunicable Diseases in the context of Health 2020.

The European Union

In 2010, the EU took a significant step towards cooperating with developing countries to address food and nutrition security challenges by adopting an EU policy framework for food security (European Commission 2013a). The framework highlights priorities for the EU and its member states, including the implementation of an action plan around six policy priorities by 2020:

- supporting effective governance;
- supporting regional agriculture and food and nutrition security policies;
- improving smallholder resilience and rural livelihoods;
- strengthening social protection mechanisms for food and nutrition security, particularly for vulnerable population groups;
- enhancing nutrition, particularly for mothers, infants, and children;
- enhancing coordination between development and humanitarian actors to build resilience and promote sustainable food and nutrition security.

Aiming to step up its efforts to fight against world hunger, food insecurity, and malnutrition, the EU also adopted in 2013 a new policy, "Enhancing Maternal and Child Nutrition", which aims to improve the nutrition of mothers and children in order to reduce disease, mortality, and the growth impediments caused by under-nutrition. The new policy also provides for more vigorous collaboration with the private sector, which is expected to contribute to activities such as product safety control, the fortification of food with minerals and vitamins, and awareness-raising through social marketing (European Commission 2013c).

The European Common Agricultural Policy (CAP), implemented since 1962, includes a system of agricultural subsidies and other programmes. While this policy has protected European farming and helped to ensure that populations in the EU have access to safe and relatively affordable food and are protected against famine, it has been criticized on the grounds of its cost, inequities in the allocation of subsidies, and its environmental and humanitarian impact. It has also been argued that EU subsidies to European farmers amount to unfair competition on a global scale, preventing developing countries from competing equitably on European markets. Public health professionals have also criticized the CAP for not considering health, even though agricultural products have a major influence on diets. In light of these criticisms, the CAP was reformed in 2013, with changes including a fairer distribution of the CAP budget between member states, strengthened crisis management and reserves, and a focus on green farming with payments linked to environmentally friendly farming practices, such as crop diversification, maintaining permanent grassland, conserving areas of ecological interest, and support for organic farming (European Commission 2013b).

In 2007, the European Commission published a strategy on nutrition, overweight, and obesity (European Commission 2007). The strategy established partnership groups between member states, the private sector, and civil society to exchange ideas and enter into voluntary commitments. However, an evaluation of the strategy found that, while it had delivered progress on objectives, its approach was too soft and there was a need for more intrusive measures, such as stricter regulation, which would be more effective in combating overweight and obesity (PHEIAC 2013). In February 2014 the EU adopted an Action Plan on Childhood Obesity for 2014–2020.

In 2008, the EU also developed a common EU framework for salt reduction. The overall goal of this framework is to help reduce salt intake at population level in order to achieve national or WHO recommendations.

Other international agencies

FAO and the World Trade Organization (WTO) are examples of other large, international agencies that play a role in food security and nutrition globally and in Europe. FAO is an intergovernmental organization with 194 member states and one member organization, the EU. Its main aim is to make sure people have regular access to enough high-quality food to lead active, healthy lives. FAO states that growth in the agriculture sector is one of the most effective means of reducing poverty and achieving food security. There is sufficient capacity in the world to produce enough food to feed everyone adequately, but, despite progress made over the last decades, 870 million people still suffer from chronic hunger (FAO 2013a). FAO creates and shares critical information about food, agriculture, and natural resources and plays a connector role by identifying and working with different expert partners and facilitating a dialogue between those who have the knowledge and those who need it (FAO 2013a).

The WTO with its 159 member states is a worldwide organization for trade and a forum for governments to negotiate trade agreements and settle disputes. WTO oversees the global system of trade agreements and negotiated an agriculture agreement in 1994, a significant step towards fairer competition and a less distorted sector. Member governments have agreed to work towards improving market access and reducing trade-distorting subsidies in agriculture (WTO 2013). However, the WTO has been heavily criticized for placing trade interests above health and for the secrecy and power imbalances in its disputes procedures.

National policy actions

Ministries of health play a leading role in developing food security, healthy diets, and obesity policies, as well as in engaging other partners and sectors, such as agriculture, social affairs, consumer affairs, and education. At national level, nutrition policies are at different stages of development across Europe. Some countries are still at the beginning of the process, while others take a more comprehensive approach, include obesity prevention in their public health strategies, and adopt a whole-of-government and "Health in All Policy" approach. Important ministries outside the health sector include those responsible for education, welfare, social services, transport and planning, agriculture, the environment, and finance.

Governments can help people to change their lifestyle by making healthy options more widely available, or by making existing ones more accessible and affordable, and unhealthy options less accessible and more expensive. They must balance those measures that seek to inform the public with those that regulate the food environment, including the use of price policies and marketing restrictions. The latter are generally more effective but give rise to opposition from powerful corporate interests (OECD 2012b). No matter what approach is taken (or what combination thereof), there is increased recognition of the importance of governance, clear leadership and roles, communication, education, and workforce capacity for effective multidisciplinary public health actions in the area of nutrition and obesity. There are also increasing efforts to interact with, rather than oppose, industry in policies and action plans at the implementation level.

A number of initiatives on food and nutrition are under way in Europe that can be implemented at national level and are good examples of working in intersectoral partnerships. The EU-wide School Fruit Scheme aims to facilitate healthy food choices in schools and involves intersectoral working between the health, education, and agriculture sectors. The primary objective is to increase children's consumption of fruit and vegetables by making them available in schools (European Commission 2012). Evaluations indicate a positive impact, as the example of Slovenia illustrates (Box 7.3). In some countries, the scheme has been complemented by other initiatives. In Slovenia, these included the

Box 7.3 Evaluation of the School Fruit Scheme in Slovenia

Owing to effective cooperation between the agriculture, education, and health sectors, the School Fruit Scheme was successfully implemented in Slovenia. A short-term evaluation showed not only a positive impact on changes in attitudes and behaviour (particularly among boys, younger children, and children from less well-off families), but also an increased consumption of fruit and vegetables.

traditional breakfast initiative (Ministry of Agriculture and the Environment 2011) and the Slovene food day initiative (Ministry of Agriculture and the Environment 2012). These schemes represent win–win–win situations for all three sectors involved (health, education, and agriculture).

Food taxes and subsidies

There is good evidence that price has an effect on consumption choices and that changes in price can be used to improve population health. There is also evidence to indicate that monetary incentives to encourage the purchase of healthier items may be effective, such as discounted low-fat snacks from vending machines and discount coupons for fruit and vegetables. Taxes on unhealthy foods have been shown to be extremely cost-effective measures and several countries have explored fiscal measures to reduce consumption of unhealthy foods. France, for example, has introduced a tax on sugary drinks, with the proceeds earmarked for programmes to help combat obesity (WHO 2012b). Finland has implemented a tax on soft drinks, as well as on confectionary products (OECD 2012b). Hungary has introduced a tax on selected manufactured foods with high sugar, salt or caffeine content, such as carbonated sugary drinks. The tax only affects products that have healthier alternatives (OECD 2012b). Another example is the salt tax in Hungary, which is part of a wider initiative (Box 7.4).

Box 7.4 The national salt initiative in Hungary

Hungary is part of the EU framework for salt reduction. Its national salt initiative is part of the National Public Health Programme 2003–2013. In February 2010, the national salt reduction programme "STOP SALT!" was launched. The programme included:

- a situation assessment;
- identification of the main food products to be included in the programme;
- reformulation of products by the industry and public catering establishments;
- an awareness-raising campaign for the public;
- a monitoring and evaluation component;

> - food products such as salty snacks, soup, and other powders and artificial seasonings fall under the Public Health Product Tax Act of 2011, popularly called the 'chips tax', based on their salt content;
> - the involvement of industry: the Hungarian Bakers' Association, for example, assembled more than 1500 bakers to sign a contract in which they undertook voluntarily to decrease the salt content of their bread by 2017.
>
> *Source*: WHO (2013c)

There has been some scepticism around the effectiveness of taxes on unhealthy foods (see Chapter 14, "Organization and financing of public health"), with some arguing that an increase in price does not necessarily lead to the purchase of a healthy product instead. It has also been argued that price increases will hit the poorest the hardest and are therefore unfair. The argument for such taxes emphasizes their effectiveness in changing the behaviour of those who are most at risk – low-income populations (Chaufan, Hee Hong et al. 2009). However, it is necessary to get the level of taxation right, given their primary role of changing behaviour rather than revenue generation. A study in the United States found that a relatively low tax (1% per dollar or 1% of overall value) would not appreciably alter consumption, but generate $40–$100 million in tax revenues (Kuchler, Tegene et al. 2004); these resources could be used for obesity prevention initiatives. In France and Hungary, at least part of the revenues from the new taxes will contribute to the financing of health and social security expenditures (OECD 2012b). It is also important to ensure public buy-in and support. Denmark introduced a saturated fat tax, which, according to early reports, achieved a 6% reduction in the consumption of saturated fats. However, due to the resistance the initiative encountered, the government scrapped the tax.

Restricting trans-fatty acids

Denmark was the first country in Europe to implement stringent laws restricting the trans-fat content of foods. In 2003, the Danish Nutrition Council affirmed that there were substantial harmful effects on health from trans-fats, with no positive effects, and that they could be eliminated from food without any adverse effect on taste, price or the availability of foods. Legislation was enacted, limiting trans-fats to 2% of the fat and oil content in foods. Other countries, such as Switzerland, Iceland, Austria, Norway, and Sweden, followed the same model. Still others aimed to reduce trans-fats using self-regulatory methods. While this approach has resulted in a reduction in trans-fats in countries such as the Netherlands and the United Kingdom, some specialists argue that self-regulatory approaches are more likely than regulatory approaches to increase inequities. Private sector companies have also implemented voluntary changes to their food compositions and preparation techniques in order to reduce the amount of trans-fats. However, these changes will need to be monitored carefully, as it has transpired that the trans-fat content of food products such as fries or industrial popcorn differs across Europe, with multinational corporations allowing a higher content of trans-fats in eastern than in western European countries (WHO 2013c).

Labelling

In most European countries, it is mandatory for processed foods to display nutrition information on the product packaging, including levels of energy, protein, fat, saturated fat, carbohydrates, sugars, and sodium. Front-of-pack nutrition signposting systems, such as the "traffic-light" system, where nutrient contents such as fat, sugar, and salt are colour-coded into high, moderate, and low levels have been implemented by some countries (Box 7.5) (WHO 2012b). Nutrition labelling has been shown to encourage healthier diets among those who read the labels. Traffic-light labelling may also encourage food producers to improve product formulation. However, their effectiveness has led some major food corporations to oppose them on spurious grounds. Some local public health departments in the United Kingdom have launched a similar system targeting restaurants and workplace canteens. Where caterers have been encouraged and advised on how to prepare and provide healthier food options and market healthy options on their menus, consumers choose healthier options when eating away from home (Brighton and Hove City Council 2009). While efforts to ensure EU-wide implementation of traffic-light systems have so far been unsuccessful, EU legislation on the labelling of food prevents presentation and advertising that is designed to mislead consumers about products' characteristics or effects (WHO 2013c).

Integrating obesity prevention and nutrition into primary care

In many European countries, primary care physicians are increasingly involved in delivering preventive services, including: health checks and advice on healthy lifestyles (see Chapter 8, "Healthcare public health"; Chapter 10,

Box 7.5   "Keyhole" labelling

Denmark, Norway, and Sweden have agreed on a common Nordic food-labelling symbol, known as the "keyhole", implemented in 2009. Labelling is on a voluntary basis. Foods labelled with the keyhole symbol contain less fat, sugars, and salt and more fibre than food products of the same type not carrying the symbol. The aim is to make it easier and less time-consuming to find healthier products in food stores. It is also hoped that the keyhole system will stimulate manufacturers to reformulate products and develop healthier alternatives.

Source: WHO (2013c)

"Health promotion"; Chapter 14, "Organization and financing of public health"). However, the extent to which they provide health promotion and advice on healthy lifestyles varies between and within countries. Barriers to integrating obesity prevention into primary health care can be structural, organizational or relate to the skills and attitudes of health workers. Public health services and governments have a role in ensuring that primary care is supported to deliver preventative public health services, such as through the training of health workers in nutrition, weight management, advice on diets and healthy lifestyles, as well as recognizing malnutrition.

Community programmes

There is a need to identify best practices and innovative models for providing preventative support in the community. Many obesity prevention interventions have focused on single settings and been designed without community involvement. In addition, many interventions have only been for the short term, limiting benefits and sustainability. Evidence shows that the most successful obesity interventions have multiple components and are adapted to the local context. An example of a sustainable, comprehensive community initiative is the EPODE Network (Box 7.6).

Box 7.6 EPODE (*Ensemble Prévenons l'Obésité Des Enfants*; Together Let's Prevent Childhood Obesity)

EPODE is a capacity-building approach for communities to implement effective and sustainable strategies to promote healthier lifestyles and prevent childhood obesity. The aim is to reduce childhood obesity through a societal process in which local environments, childhood settings, and family norms become more supportive and facilitate the adoption of healthy lifestyles in children aged 0–12 years, their families, and local stakeholders. It was launched in 2004 in ten French communities and is based on national guidelines on diet and physical activity. The methodology promotes the involvement of multiple stakeholders at national level (ministries, health groups, NGOs, and private partners) and at local level (political leaders, health professionals, families, teachers, and business communities). Funding comes from public and private partnerships at national and local level. Private sponsors are mainly from the food industry, health insurance companies, and the food distribution sector. Five years after the launch, 90% of the original pilot communities were still active. The initiative has now been expanded to other countries and more than 500 communities across the world are now part of an EPODE programme, including in Belgium, Spain, and Greece. The Netherlands, Portugal, and Scotland have launched similar programmes.

Source: WHO (2012b)

Industry involvement

Industry involvement includes collaborative action involving the food and catering industries, food retailers, and restaurants, as well as other types of industry associated with a sedentary lifestyle, such as the automobile, TV, film, and electronic games industries. There is growing recognition in Europe that more needs to be done to halt the obesity epidemic, and that the private sector needs to be involved. Industry clearly plays an important role in food reformulation, such as in reducing the salt and sugar content of its products. It can also expand the marketing of healthy food options, restrict the marketing of unhealthy options (especially to children), and provide better information to consumers.

Industry involvement, however, is not without considerable risk. To prevent obesity, there is a need to shift eating habits and cultures to reduce calorie intake as well as create opportunities for more active lifestyles. Increased physical activity alone cannot stop the obesity epidemic. The leading food corporations are aware of this, but some still argue that the main driver of rising levels of obesity is inadequate physical activity, whereas it is well accepted by the international scientific community that both diet and physical activity play a role. Often, multinational corporations are eager to associate themselves with sports events and physical activity. Two of the major food multinationals, for example, were "gold" sponsors of the 2012 Olympic Games in London, illustrating the influence industry can have on public health policies.

Conclusion

This chapter has reviewed some of the key challenges for food and nutrition in Europe today, including food security, malnutrition, and obesity. It has argued that one of the key challenges for the future will be to ensure sustainable food resources for a growing population with increased demand on energy and water. Food security is not just a European but a global challenge (Global Food Security 2011). The global food system is unsustainable (see Chapter 6, "Environmental health"). It consumes resources faster than they are replenished and renewed, accounting for 70% of total global water withdrawals and 10–12% of greenhouse gas emissions (FAO 2013a). To ensure food security, the global food system has to be redesigned to bring sustainability centre stage. This requires concerted global and national action across several policy domains (European Commission 2011a).

Malnutrition is another concern, in particular for pregnant women, children, older people, those with chronic diseases, and socially isolated and poorer people. Challenges are particularly acute in the countries of the Caucasus and Central Asia, but malnutrition also occurs in western Europe, in particular among older and hospitalized people. It will be necessary to address these problems through multisectoral approaches (see Chapter 12, "Intersectoral working"), but also through the training of health professionals. Furthermore, there is a clear need to tackle socio-economic inequalities and translate political commitments into practice (see Chapter 11, "Tackling the social determinants of health").

Finally, the obesity epidemic is another major public health challenge and both governments and societies as a whole need to act to curb the epidemic. Addressing obesity requires approaches that strike a balance between individual and population-wide approaches and between education-based and multisectoral, regulatory, and environmental interventions.

This chapter has presented some examples of the action that can be taken at international and national level. What permeates these examples is the need to involve other sectors to prevent ill health and promote better health and well-being (Schäffer Elinder, Lock et al. 2006; Gillespie, Egal et al. 2013). Public health has a clear role to play in these efforts, not just in providing advocacy, expertise and leadership, and facilitating intersectoral working, but also in monitoring, surveillance, research, and evaluation.

References

Bock, A., B. Atzel, et al. (2012). *Tomorrow's Health Society: Research priorities for foods and diets*. Brussels, The European Commission, Joint Research Centre.

Brighton and Hove City Council. (2009). *Healthy Choice Award* [www.brighton-hove.gov.uk/content/business-and-trade/food-safety/healthy-choice-award-0, accessed 15 October 2013].

Cattaneo, A., A. Yngve. B. Koletzko and L. R. Guzman (2005). "Protection, promotion and support of breast-feeding in Europe: current situation." *Public Health Nutrition* **8**: 39–46.

Chaufan, C., G. Hee Hong and P. Fox (2009). "Taxing 'sin foods' – obesity prevention and public health policy." *New England Journal of Medicine* **361**: e113.

European Commission (2007). *White Paper on a Strategy for Europe on Nutrition, Overweight and Obesity Related Health Issues* [http://ec.europa.eu/health/ph_determinants/life_style/nutrition/documents/nutrition_wp_en.pdf]. Brussels, European Commission.

European Commission (2011a). *Future of Global Food and Farming: How can science support food security?* [http://ec.europa.eu/dgs/jrc/downloads/jrc_20110330_seminar_programme.pdf]. Brussels, European Commission.

European Commission (2011b). Roadmap to a Resource Efficient Europe: Communication from the Commission to the European Parliament, the Council, the European Economic and Social Committee and the Committee of the Regions, COM(2011)571/final. Brussels, European Commission.

European Commission (2012). Report from the Commission to the European Parliament and the Council in accordance with Article 184(5) of Council Regulation (EC) No. 1234/2007 on the implementation of the European School Fruit Scheme [http://ec.europa.eu/agriculture/sfs/documents/documents/com2012-768_en.pdf]. Brussels, European Commission.

European Commission (2013a). *Boosting Food and Nutrition Security through EU Action: Implementing our commitments* [http://ec.europa.eu/europeaid/what/food-security/documents/boosting_food_and_nutrition_security_through_eu_action_ec_swd.pdf]. Brussels, European Commission.

European Commission (2013b). *The Common Agricultural Policy (CAP) and Agriculture in Europe* [http://ec.europa.eu/agriculture/faq/, accessed 15 October 2013]. Brussels, European Commission.

European Commission (2013c). *Enhancing Maternal and Child Nutrition in External Assistance: An EU policy framework* [http://ec.europa.eu/europeaid/documents/

enhancing_maternal-child_nutrition_in_external_assistance_en.pdf].	Brussels, European Commission.

European Commission (2013d). *Fighting Hunger* [http://ec.europa.eu/europeaid/what/food-security/]. Brussels, European Commission.

European Environment Agency (EEA) (2012). *Food Waste* [http://www.eea.europa.eu/signals/signals-2012/close-ups/food-waste, accessed 17 October 2013]. Copenhagen, EEA.

European Nutrition for Health Alliance (ENHA) (2013). *European Nutrition for Health Alliance* [www.european-nutrition.org/index, accessed 15 October 2013]. London, ENHA.

Food and Agriculture Organization (FAO) (2013a). *Food and Agriculture Organization of the United Nations* [http://www.fao.org/about/what-we-do/en/, accessed 15 October 2013]. Rome, FAO.

Food and Agriculture Organization (FAO) (2013b). *Save Food: Global initiative on food losses and waste reduction* [http://www.fao.org/save-food/en/, accessed 15 October 2013]. Rome, FAO.

Gibney, M. J., B. M. Margetts, J. M. Kearney and L. Arab, Eds. (2004). *Public Health Nutrition*. Oxford, Blackwell Science.

Gillespie, S., F. Egal and M. Park (2013). "Agriculture, food and nutrition." In *Health in All Policies: Seizing opportunities, implementing policies*. K. Leppo, E. Ollila, S. Peña, M. Wismar and S. Cook, Eds. Helsinki, Ministry of Social Affairs and Health of Finland.

Global Climate Change and Human Health (2013). *Food Security* [http://climatechangehumanhealth.org/activities/food-security/].

Global Food Security (GFS) (2011). *GFS Strategic Plan 2011–2016* [http://www.foodsecurity.ac.uk/assets/pdfs/gfs-strategic-plan.pdf]. Global Food Security, UK. London: GFS.

Global Food Security (GFS) (2013). *Global Food Security Index 2013* [http://foodsecurityindex.eiu.com/]. London, The Economist Intelligence Unit.

International Obesity Taskforce/European Association for the Study of Obesity (IOTF/EASO) (2002). *Obesity in Europe* [http://www.iaso.org/site_media/uploads/Sep_2002_Obesity_in_Europe_Case_for_Action_2002.pdf]. London, IOTF.

Kondrup, J., N. Johansen, L. M. Plum, L. Bak, I. H. Larsen, A. Martinsen, J. R. Andersen, H. Baemthsen, E. Bunch and N. Lauesen (2002). "Incidence of nutritional risk and causes of inadequate nutritional care in hospitals." *Clinical Nutrition* **21**(6): 461–468.

Kuchler, F., A. Tegene and J. M. Harris (2004). "Taxing snack foods: what to expect for diet and tax revenues." *Current Issues in Economics of Food Markets* No. 747-08 [http://www.ers.usda.gov/media/306707/aib74708_1_.pdf].

Ljungqvist, O., A. van Gossum, M. Sanz and F. de Man (2010). "The European fight against malnutrition." *Clinical Nutrition* **29**(2): 149–150.

Lock, K., M. Gabrijelcic-Blenkus, M. Martuzzi, P. Otorepec, P. Wallace, C. Dora A. Robertson and J. M. Zakotnic (2003). "Health impact assessment (HIA) of agriculture and food policies: lessons learnt from HIA development in the Republic of Slovenia." *Bulletin of the World Health Organization* **81**(6).

McElroy, S. L., R. Kotwal, S. Malhotra, E. B. Nelson, P. E. Keck and C. B. Nemeroff (2004). "Are mood disorders and obesity related? A review for the mental health professional." *Journal of Clinical Psychiatry* **65**(5): 634–651.

McKee, M., T. Lang and J. Roberts (1996). "Deregulating health: policy lessons of the BSE affair." *Journal of the Royal Society of Medicine* **89**: 424–426.

Ministry of Agriculture and the Environment (MAE) (2011). *Traditional Slovenian Breakfast* [http://tradicionalni-zajtrk.si/, accessed 10 May 2013]. Ljubljana, MAE.

Ministry of Agriculture and the Environment (MAE) (2012). *Dan slovenske hrane* [http://tradicionalni-zajtrk.si/media/uploads/public/document/54-plakat_dan_slo_hrane_sl.pdf, accessed 10 May 2013]. Ljubljana, MAE.

OECD (2012a). *Health at a Glance: Europe 2012* [http://www.oecd.org/health/health-systems/HealthAtAGlanceEurope2012.pdf]. OECD Publishing.

OECD (2012b). *Obesity Update 2012* [http://www.oecd.org/health/49716427.pdf]. Paris, OECD.

Paris, V. and D. Polton (2008). "France: targeting investment in health." In *Health Targets in Europe: Learning from experience.* M. Wismar, M. McKee, K. Ernst, D. Srivastava and R. Busse, Eds. Copenhagen, WHO Regional Office for Europe on behalf of the European Observatory on Health Systems and Policies: 101–122.

Public Health Evaluation and Impact Assessment Consortium (PHEIAC) (2013). *Evaluation of the Implementation of the Strategy for Europe on Nutrition, Overweight and Obesity Related Health Issues.* Brussels, PHEIAC.

Rokx, C., R. Galloway and L. Brown (2002). *Prospects for Improving Nutrition in Eastern Europe and Central Asia.* Washington, DC, World Bank.

Rutter, H. (2011). "Where next for obesity?" *The Lancet* **378**: 746–747.

Schäffer Elinder, L., K. Lock and M. Gabrijelcic-Blenkus (2006). "Public health, food and agriculture policy in the European Union." In *Health in All Policies: Prospects and potentials.* T. Ståhl, M. Wismar, E. Ollila, E. Lahtinen and K. Leppo, Eds. Helsinki, Ministry of Social Affairs and Health of Finland: 93–110.

Solfrizzi, V., V. Frisardi, D. Seripa, G. Logroscino, B. P. Imbimbo, G. D'Onofrio, F. Addante, D. Sancarlo, L. Cascavilla, A. Pilotto and F. Panza (2011). "Mediterranean diet in predementia and dementia syndromes." *Current Alzheimer Research* **8**(5): 520–542.

Stratton, R. J., C. J. Green and M. Elia, Eds. (2003). *Disease-Related Malnutrition: An evidence-based approach to treatment.* Wallingford, UK, CABI Publishing.

Swinburn, B., G. Egger and F. Raza (1999). "Dissecting obesogenic environments: the development and application of a framework for identifying and prioritizing environmental interventions for obesity." *Preventive Medicine* **29**(6): 563–570.

Wijnhoven, T. M., J. M. van Raaij, A. Spinelli, A. I. Rito, R. Hovengen, M. Kunesova, G. Starc, H. Rutter, A. Sjöberg, A. Petrauskiene, U. O'Dwyer, S. Petrova, V. Farrugia Sant'angelo, M. Wauters, A. Yngve, I. M. Rubana and J. Breda (2013). "WHO European Childhood Obesity Surveillance Initiative 2008: weight, height and body mass index in 6–9-year-old children." *Pediatric Obesity* **8**(2): 79–97.

World Health Organization (WHO) (1986). *The Ottawa Charter for Health Promotion* [www.who.int/healthpromotion/conferences/previous/ottawa/en/print.html]. Geneva, WHO.

World Health Organization (WHO) (2003). *Diet, Nutrition and the Prevention of Chronic Diseases* [http://whqlibdoc.who.int/trs/who_trs_916.pdf]. Geneva, WHO.

World Health Organization (WHO) (2004). *Food and Health in Europe: A new basis for action.* Copenhagen, WHO Regional Office for Europe.

World Health Organization (WHO) (2007). *The Challenge of Obesity in the WHO European Region and Strategies for Response.* Copenhagen, WHO Regional Office for Europe.

World Health Organization (WHO) (2008a). *WHO European Action Plan for Food and Nutrition Policy 2007–2012* [http://www.euro.who.int/__data/assets/pdf_file/0017/74402/E91153.pdf]. Copenhagen, WHO Regional Office for Europe.

World Health Organization (WHO) (2008b). *Worldwide Prevalence of Anaemia 1993–2005* [http://whqlibdoc.who.int/publications/2008/9789241596657_eng.pdf]. Geneva, WHO.

World Health Organization (WHO) (2008–2011). Joint WHO/European Commission project to monitor progress in improving nutrition and physical activity and preventing obesity in the European Union. [http://www.euro.who.int/en/

health-topics/disease-prevention/nutrition/activities/monitoring-and-surveillance/ joint-whoec-project-to-monitor-progress, accessed 15 October 2013]. Copenhagen, WHO Regional Office for Europe.

World Health Organization (WHO) (2012a). *The World Health Statistics 2011* (http:// apps.who.int/ghodata/, accessed 2 November 2013). Geneva, WHO.

World Health Organization (WHO) (2012b). *Population-based Approaches to Childhood Obesity Prevention* [http://apps.who.int/iris/bitstream/10665/80149/1/9789241504782_ eng.pdf]. Geneva, WHO.

World Health Organization (WHO) (2013a). *Antimicrobial Resistance* [http://www.who. int/mediacentre/factsheets/fs194/en/]. Geneva, WHO.

World Health Organization (WHO) (2013b). *Trade, Foreign Policy, Diplomacy and Health: Food Security* [www.who.int/trade/glossary/story028/en/]. Geneva, WHO.

World Health Organization (WHO) (2013c). *Mapping Salt Reduction Initiatives in the WHO European Region* [www.euro.who.int/_data/assets/pdf_file/0009/186462/ Mapping-salt-reduction-initiatives-in-the-WHO-European-Region.pdf]. Copenhagen, WHO Regional Office for Europe.

World Health Organization (WHO) (2013d). *Vienna Declaration on Nutrition and Noncommunicable Diseases in the Context of Health 2020* [http://www.euro.who. int/_data/assets/pdf_file/0009/193878/Vienna-Declaration.pdf, accessed 4 November 2013]. Copenhagen, WHO Regional Office for Europe.

World Health Organization/UNICEF (WHO/UNICEF) (2006). *WHO, UNICEF, and SCN Informal Consultation on Community-based Management of Severe Malnutrition in Children* [http://www.who.int/child_adolescent_health/documents/fnb_v27n3_ suppl/en/index.html]. Geneva, WHO/UNICEF/UN System Standing Committee on Nutrition.

World Trade Organization (WTO) (2013). World Trade Organization homepage [http:// www.wto.org/english/thewto_e/whatis_e/who_we_are_e.htm, accessed 15 October 2013]. Geneva, WTO.

chapter eight

Healthcare public health

*Martin McKee, Bernd Rechel,
Reinhard Busse*

Introduction

The set of activities referred to in some countries as healthcare public health is the least well understood aspect of public health in Europe. It refers to the roles played by those with public health skills (in areas such as epidemiology, statistics, economic evaluation, health service research, and sociology) to maximize the health gain achieved by the delivery of health care both to individuals and populations. Thus, for example, such public health professionals would be involved in developing the terms for a contract between a health authority or an insurance fund and a hospital to deliver a care pathway, ensuring it is effective, as shown by clinical trials, appropriate, in relation to the population it is aimed at, efficient, based on evidence from cost-effectiveness studies, and equitable, which may require the provision of written material in ethnic minority languages or in formats that are accessible to those with partial sight, and which incorporate evidence on the most appropriate ways to communicate with patients who are more or less literate. These individuals might work on either side of this relationship, for the purchaser of care or the provider. However, in many countries such roles do not exist, or are confined to the organization of specific areas of delivery, such as screening programmes. Elsewhere, these roles are filled by individuals who do not see themselves as public health professionals, such as health economists, but who do use, to varying degrees, skills that fall within the boundaries of what is elsewhere termed "healthcare public health". Examples include many of the professional staff working in organizations such as the National Institute for Health and Care Excellence in England, the Haute Autorité de Santé in France, and the Institute for Quality and Efficiency in Health Care (IQWiG) in Germany.

The development of healthcare public health has been slow in many countries. In some, this reflects the view of medicine as a liberal profession, whose practitioners should be free to decide how they provide care, while expecting a third party funder to pay them for doing what they feel is most appropriate for the individual patient. In others, it reflects a somewhat restrictive view of public health from its practitioners, who see public health as involved primarily in policies and interventions that affect entire populations, such as ensuring clean water supplies or campaigns to reduce smoking. Yet public health has an important, if frequently poorly appreciated role to play in the organization and delivery of health care so that it serves the needs not only of those patients who seek the services of health professionals, but also for the entire population.

The rationale for healthcare public health

A population perspective on health care is important for several reasons. First, individuals who need health care may not be aware that they do so. They may develop symptoms that they dismiss as normal, trivial, or perhaps part of the ageing process, and consequently fail to seek timely care (Oliver, Pearson et al. 2005). If symptoms are the initial sign of something serious, the delay may lead to more complex and expensive treatment, such as when someone with diabetic foot disease ends up having an amputation, or even dies, when the symptoms were the first manifestation of what was then a treatable cancer (Maringe, Walters et al. 2012). Crucially, such a failure to convert a need for health care into a demand may be socially patterned. Thus, some groups in the population may be prone to greater delays than others, whether because of inadequate knowledge, expectations, or real or perceived barriers to care (Petherick, Cullum et al. 2013). Public health professionals, drawing on epidemiological, sociological, and anthropological insights, can help to ensure that health services are designed in ways that meet the needs of all groups of the population (Healy and McKee 2004).

Second, the resources available to any health system are limited. It may, for example, not be possible to recruit sufficient health professionals, especially where the need is for those with highly specialized skills. In some cases, pharmaceuticals may be in short supply, such as in the early stages of an influenza pandemic before vaccine manufacturing capacity has been scaled up. The available funding is also finite and choices have to be made. This can be, and usually is, done through a process of negotiation, in which those with the most power and the loudest voices win, regardless of the impact on the overall health of the population. However, it can also be done through a public health approach, where the number of people who need a particular intervention is quantified, the effectiveness of the intervention in achieving a given amount of health gain is determined, and the cost of providing the intervention is assessed. The information so generated can then inform the choices that must be made. This will inevitably mean trade-offs, such as between investment in services for cancer or mental health (Abel-Smith, Figueras et al. 1995). These issues cannot be addressed adequately without taking a population perspective.

Third, as the complexity of health care increases, in parallel with technological advances, increasing specialization, and the complexity of health problems in ageing populations (Doyle, McKee et al. 2009; Barnett, Mercer et al. 2012), a public health perspective can inform the design of services, achieving the linkages necessary to provide a seamless service for the patient who may require inputs from many different healthcare providers.

Fourth, it is not sufficient to design and implement health services; they must be monitored and evaluated continuously to ensure that they are achieving optimal health outcomes. Again, a public health perspective is necessary to determine whether these outcomes are being achieved and whether they are being achieved for the entire population.

Fifth, it is now well established that timely and effective care can be a significant contributor to improved population health. This has been demonstrated by research over several decades on the concept of mortality amenable to health care (Nolte and McKee 2004). Conditions have been identified where death should not occur in the presence of timely and effective care. Examples include diabetes at young ages, bacterial infections, vaccine-preventable diseases, and common surgical emergencies such as appendicitis. Mortality rates for such avoidable causes have fallen much more rapidly than for other causes of death: between 1997/98 and 2006/07, amenable mortality in 16 OECD countries fell on average by 31.7%, versus only 14.0% for other causes of death (Table 8.1). That the indicator "amenable mortality" is not only

Table 8.1 Levels of mortality amenable to health care versus other causes of death in 16 OECD countries, 1997/98 and 2006/07 (age-standardized death rates, age 0–74 per 100,000 population)

	"Avoidable" mortality amenable to health care			*Other causes of death*		
	1997/98	*2006/07*	*Change (%)*	*1997/98*	*2006/07*	*Change (%)*
Australia	87.95	56.92	–35.2	203.70	164.57	–19.0
Austria	108.92	67.31	–38.2	232.23	201.70	–13.1
Denmark	113.01	80.13	–29.1	307.22	265.66	–13.5
Finland	116.22	73.78	–36.5	239.26	223.36	–6.7
France	75.62	55.00	–27.3	267.68	223.75	–16.4
Germany	106.18	76.42	–28.0	245.84	209.49	–14.8
Greece	97.27	76.65	–21.2	213.53	186.77	–12.5
Ireland	134.36	77.82	–42.1	248.45	196.81	–21.8
Italy	88.77	59.88	–37.1	224.46	174.62	–22.2
Japan	81.42	61.17	–24.9	192.97	166.11	–13.9
Netherlands	96.89	65.55	–32.2	239.42	200.85	–16.1
New Zealand	114.54	78.64	–31.3	225.82	189.65	–16.0
Norway	98.64	63.63	–35.5	215.92	188.97	–12.5
Sweden	88.44	61.25	–31.7	190.94	173.33	–9.2
United Kingdom	126.45	82.54	–34.7	224.80	202.85	–9.8
United States	120.22	95.54	–21.5	278.06	258.85	–6.9
Average			**–31.7**			**–14.0**

Note: Deaths from ischaemic heart disease not included.
Source: Nolte and McKee (2011)

theoretically convincing but actually related to the availability of health care has been shown by Sundmacher and Busse (2011) for avoidable cancer deaths: mortality was significantly lower in German districts with a higher physician-to-population ratio.

Finally, the potential of health care to improve population health cannot be taken as given, but depends on the availability of effective, affordable, and accessible health care for the entire population. For example, there has been less progress regarding "avoidable mortality" in the United States than in most other OECD countries, as a substantial proportion of the population there lacks access to routine care (Nolte and McKee 2012). Even in health systems with near-universal population coverage, which in theory should provide easy access to all, there may be considerable disparities in utilization, with some population groups, such as migrants, ethnic minorities, and the poor, at a particular disadvantage (Healy and McKee 2004). It is thus not enough to look only at those who use services – it is also important to consider those who do not. However, utilization is only one aspect of the provision of health care, and quality of care and adherence to treatment also matter. The effectiveness of health care thus depends on population coverage, entitlements to services, accessibility, treatment adherence, and quality of care. The combination of these factors has been termed "community effectiveness" (Tugwell, Bennett et al. 1984) and the major task of healthcare public health is to improve this effectiveness.

Where health care can be informed by public health

Assessment of need

Assessing the healthcare needs of a population should be the first step to public health professionals' involvement in the organization and delivery of health care, in order to create a benchmark for any measures to improve "community effectiveness". While this sounds straightforward, it is in fact quite complicated – the first question to ask, namely "need for what?", is not easy to answer. It is not sufficient to show that the health of the population, or a group within the population, is poor. It is also necessary to show that there is an intervention that could improve that population's health. Need may thus be defined as the ability to benefit.

Approaches to health needs assessment are often divided into three broad groupings (Stevens and Gabbay 1991). The first is *epidemiologically based needs assessment*, which seeks to determine the number of people with a certain condition for which there is an intervention available that will treat or improve it, and who are not otherwise unsuitable to receive it. This requires knowledge of the prevalence of the condition in the population, the criteria for using the intervention, and the benefit it can produce. This approach is both technically challenging, as it requires that there is a simple means of assessing ability to benefit, and too expensive for routine use. Nonetheless, where it can be done it can provide valuable evidence to feed into other types of needs assessment (Box 8.1).

Box 8.1 Assessing the need for prostatectomy in an English district

Enlargement of the prostate is a common condition in older men, which results in difficulty in passing urine and can, on occasions, lead to complete obstruction. However, surgery can result in a number of unpleasant side-effects. An epidemiologically based health needs assessment was undertaken in an English district (Sanderson, Hunter et al. 1997). First, a standardized symptom questionnaire was selected, allowing the severity of symptoms to be measured on a scale. Next, a formal consensus development exercise was undertaken with a panel of urologists and general practitioners, informed by a systematic review of the literature, to agree the point on the scale at which surgery might be appropriate (Hunter, McKee et al. 1994). A survey was then undertaken among men in the population in the age group most at risk for prostate problems. In addition to asking about symptoms and severity, and presenting them with information about the operation, including its benefits and risks, they were also asked about other aspects of their general health, so as to identify those who had other problems that might preclude surgery. In this way, it was possible to ascertain both the prevalence of men who might benefit from surgery and, among them, those who would wish to receive it (Hunter, McKee et al. 1995). The resulting data, broken down by age band, could then be applied to other settings.

The second approach is *comparative needs assessment*, such as between geographical areas or population groups, which can help to identify gross disparities in the extent to which existing services meet need. This makes two major assumptions. First, that the optimal treatment rate in a population can be determined from data on utilization. Second, it assumes that the need in a population can be estimated by comparing utilization with that in the reference population, after adjusting for known characteristics, such as the age distribution.

The third approach is termed *corporate needs assessment*. This involves building consensus about what is needed among health professionals, patients, patient representatives, and other interested parties. This approach involves gathering information from a wide range of sources.

In practice, these different approaches are often combined in an iterative process that brings together information from many different sources:

1. It will begin by identifying a particular health problem. The problem may have been brought to the attention of the authorities as a result of a health survey, concerns by patients or healthcare providers, new findings from research, or political imperatives.
2. The health problem in question must then be defined. This involves agreeing case definitions, obtaining estimates of disease incidence and prevalence, and reviewing information on services, as well as the extent to which they meet existing demand. In some cases, this initial search will identify existing systematic needs assessments that can be applied without significant

additional work. If this is not the case, the next step will be to determine the size and nature of the problem. This may require a population survey.

3. The third step is to determine existing levels of provision. Unfortunately, in many countries, this is more difficult than it might seem because of the existence of multiple providers in both the public and private sector. For example, some facilities might only provide care for groups defined by their employment, for example the military, or for those with private medical insurance. Thus, in a study undertaken in London, England, the utilization of coronary revascularization in different local government areas differed substantially when the procedures undertaken in private healthcare facilities were included (Mindell, Klodawski et al. 2008).

A fourth step involves seeking the views of patients, professionals, and other stakeholders. A range of methods can be used, including standard market research techniques (involving interviews and focus groups), formal consultative mechanisms with patient and provider representatives, and citizen juries (Tempfer and Nowak 2011). However, all of these suffer from the challenge of achieving representativeness (McKee 2010). In particular, it is not always clear who should be asked. Those who are appointed representatives of patients or providers are rarely typical of those whom they are supposed to represent. It has been especially difficult to involve those whose need is greatest and who face the largest barriers to obtaining care, such as people from ethnic minority communities, undocumented migrants, those who are homeless, and those who have mental disabilities or illness (Box 8.2).

Box 8.2   Meeting the needs of marginalized populations

A survey of major European cities identified many services supporting provision of mental health services for homeless people, asylum seekers and refugees, and street sex workers, although there were few initiatives targeting irregular migrants or travelling communities, perhaps because the former have limited entitlement to care in many European countries while there may be little awareness of the needs of the latter. Other than for asylum seekers/refugees and for irregular migrants, the availability of professional interpreters was low, even though all of these groups often face language barriers. Payment of "out-of-pocket" fees was common, especially in services for homeless people, even though it is known that even a small up-front charge can deter people from accessing health care. Only few services made data publicly available on patient characteristics and experiences, consistent with the weak tradition of evaluation in public health in most European countries. There were few outreach activities and most services had exclusion criteria and did not operate outside office hours, while many had waiting lists. The authors concluded that there is a need for new ways of providing services for marginalized groups with mental disorders that are flexible and appropriate to their needs.

Source: Priebe, Matanov et al. (2013)

A fifth step is to identify the range of interventions that can most appropriately meet the needs that have been identified. This will draw on evidence from health technology assessment and organizational research, both of which are discussed further below.

The final step is to agree priorities for action, taking account of resource implications and proposals for interventions to meet other healthcare needs in the population.

Health technology assessment

Healthcare public health involves ensuring that the care that is provided to patients is effective. Given the competing demands on resources, new interventions should be assessed to ensure that they really work. Health technology assessment (HTA), which determines whether new interventions do indeed work, besides relying on a systematic evaluation of the "efficacy" of an intervention as measured in (randomized) clinical trials, draws extensively on the traditional skills of public health, including epidemiology, economic evaluation, and outcome measurement (e.g. patient-reported outcomes).

Since the establishment of the first national health technology agency in Sweden in the 1980s, similar agencies have been set up in many other European countries. They include the National Institute for Health and Care Excellence (NICE) in England, the Haute Autorité de Santé in France, and the Institute for Quality and Efficiency in Health Care (IQWiG) in Germany (Velasco Garrido, Kristensen et al. 2008). These agencies cover a variable range of interventions. Some take a narrow view of technology, focusing on pharmaceuticals and medical equipment, while others also consider models of care. Moreover, in many countries, agencies for health technology assessment are complemented by organizations with more specific foci on specialized areas, such as vaccines, or on areas where particular ethical or other issues arise, such as fertility-related technology. The extent to which their advice is binding, and on whom, varies greatly according to the governance arrangements in the health system in question. With the support of a succession of European Commission funded projects, such as EUR-ASSSESS and EUnetHTA, extensive collaborations between agencies for health technology assessment have been established that serve as a basis for exchanging knowledge and experience and developing shared methodologies (Velasco Garrido, Kristensen et al. 2008). Based on the requirement to foster such collaborations in the "EU Directive on the application of patients' rights in cross-border health care", EUnetHTA has been established with EU funding as a so-called Joint Action, which includes members officially nominated by member states.

The importance of HTA is growing. First, it is increasingly recognized that advances in technology are the major upward pressure on healthcare expenditure in Europe, much more so than ageing populations (Busse, van Ginneken et al. 2012). Second, previous successes in areas such as pharmaceuticals mean that many new products offer at best marginal benefits, often at great cost. Third, a series of scandals has demonstrated serious flaws in the European regulatory system for medicines, such as the refusal by some major companies to disclose full data on clinical trials. There is a clear need for systems that go beyond the narrow perspective of the main regulatory body, the European Medicines Agency, which has gone to great lengths to avoid disclosure of information on drug effectiveness and safety (Goldacre 2013). Fourth, the increasing commercialization of health care in some European countries creates incentives for companies (both equipment manufacturers and healthcare delivery companies) to aggressively market products that offer no benefit, and which may be harmful (McCartney 2012).

Setting priorities

Faced with scarce financial resources, those responsible for funding and delivering health care must make difficult choices. Ideally, such choices should be informed by objective assessments of benefit, but this cannot be a mechanistic process. It is also necessary to take account of societal values. In England, NICE has developed a system of prioritization that uses cost-utility analysis, whereby both the cost of an intervention and its benefits, expressed as quality-adjusted life years (QALYs), are measured and compared with those associated with other interventions. However, decisions are also informed by citizens' panels, whose members contribute to an understanding of societal values and how they impact on actual clinical decisions (Rawlins 2012). Furthermore, despite the aim to depoliticize decisions, the government, the media, and pharmaceutical companies continue to wield influence (Teutsch and Rechel 2012).

Allocating resources

Assuming that health technology assessment has identified efficacious and cost-effective technologies and that priority-setting has helped to identify those which are socially valued and offer the greatest benefits, the necessary financial, human, and technological resources have to be made available across a country to provide equal, ideally needs-based, access. In most European countries, the allocation of financial resources to geographical entities (or health insurers) is separated from "needs-based planning" of physicians, hospitals or technologies. Both activities are highly political, because even small changes in any formula can mean significant differences, both negative and positive, for a given area or insurer. However, the actual discussions – and decisions – often take place behind closed curtains, and public health expertise, even if highly relevant, is not necessarily involved.

Essentially, the underlying question is the same for both activities – which factors should be taken into account? While the majority of resource allocation formulae in use internationally concentrate on allocating resources primarily according to the size of the problem (i.e. health need), Mooney and Houston (2004) outline an alternative approach that incorporates "capacity to benefit" (i.e. the extent to which one population's health problems may be more amenable to health intervention than others) and management, economic, and social infrastructure (i.e. the ability of an area to deliver health benefits to its population). With regard to the factors related to need, there is consensus that easily available demographic parameters, such as age and gender, are insufficient; however, there is debate about the extent, and the ways, to include socio-economic area factors, such as the percentage of single households, levels of education, or average disposable income (Rice and Smith 2002). Others advocate measures of morbidity, which are often favoured by countries using competitive health insurers (van de Ven, Beck et al. 2007). In theory, such measures are desirable, but all existing indicators (e.g. documented diagnoses, prescriptions, hospitalizations) tend to be higher in areas with higher levels of health care (e.g. in urban versus rural areas), while persons in need without adequate utilization are not captured by these measures or are under-represented.

Designing models of care

The design of healthcare delivery systems can make a major difference to population health outcomes. This was illustrated in a comparison of infant mortality in an English region, where neonatal care was decentralized, with mortality in the state of Victoria in Australia, where it was centralized. After adjustment for birth weight and other factors, the decentralized model of care was associated with double the mortality rate (Pearson, Shann et al. 1997) – an association that has also been shown within Germany (Heller, Schnell et al. 2003). In the United States, Birkmeyer and colleagues (Birkmeyer, Siewers et al. 2002) reported a volume–outcome relationship (i.e. better outcomes in hospitals with higher numbers of procedures) for many types of procedures, with the largest difference in mortality in the case of pancreatic resection, ranging from 16.3% to 3.8%. Data from a series of cohorts of patients with diabetes and from comparisons of incidence and mortality data indicate that more integrated models of care achieve better outcomes (Nolte, Bain et al. 2006). A public health perspective will aim to build on the growing body of research on the organization and delivery of health care and in particular the development of integrated models that address the spectrum of patient needs.

Improving the process of care (process quality)

For health interventions to improve population health, health professionals play two important roles: they have to select the "appropriate" intervention for the patient at the right time, and they have to provide the intervention at a high level of quality (see next section). That health services are often provided inappropriately (i.e. to patients who cannot sufficiently benefit from them at the time they get them) has long been established. This "appropriateness research" (Brook 2009) has shown, for example, high rates of inappropriate coronary angiography, bypass surgery, and carotid endarterecomy, not only in the United States, but also in several European countries.

Activities to improve the process of care – in regard to appropriateness, timeliness, responsiveness, etc. – are therefore receiving increasing attention. Among them are clinical guidelines and disease management programmes. Although guideline development has often been led by clinicians, in a number of European countries healthcare public health has played a role in developing, disseminating, and evaluating clinical guidelines, drawing on the core public health skills of critically assessing evidence and evaluating interventions (Legido-Quigley, Panteli et al. 2012). Many countries in western Europe now have programmes to develop guidelines at national, regional or local level. However, the processes vary in terms of their transparency and explicit use of scientific evidence. The European AGREE collaboration has done much to enhance the methodological robustness of guidelines (AGREE Collaboration 2003).

Monitoring results (outcome quality)

Although most health care is provided by dedicated professionals, not all of them are as highly trained – and occasionally things go wrong. There have been a number of well-documented scandals where care fell far short of acceptable standards (Carter and Jarman 2013). Healthcare public health involves putting in place systems that can identify such failings and intervene where necessary. By looking across health facilities, healthcare public health has the potential to identify differences in outcome that require further investigation (Berta, Seghieri et al. 2013). However, this is not straightforward.

The simplest approach, at least in theory, is to compare mortality rates in different hospitals. However, the experience of doing so in England offers a cautionary tale. Even after addressing some of the more obvious problems, such as adjusting for age, diagnosis, and co-morbidities, many problems remain (Mohammed, Deeks et al. 2009; Girling, Hofer et al. 2012). First, dying in hospital may not be an adverse outcome for some, such as when a patient has been admitted for palliative care. This may be particularly common where there are no alternative facilities nearby. It is, of course, possible to flag the records of those admitted for this purpose, but this practice, just like diagnostic coding, is highly susceptible to gaming. A second problem relates to the random variation associated with relatively small numbers. While monitoring outcomes may thus have some value, considerable caution is required, as there may be many false positives, as well as false negatives, where hospitals with real problems are overlooked.

Health facilities in which there are serious quality problems are often recognized as such by those who work in them or come into contact with them in other ways. Putting in place systems that make it as easy as possible for individuals to draw attention to such failings without fear of punishment can help to identify health facilities that offer sub-standard levels of care (Jarman 2012).

This does not mean that comparative data are of no value. In some countries, there has been considerable investment in registers of patients receiving particular procedures, such as that maintained by cardiac surgeons in the United

Kingdom. These more specialized databases enable the adoption of much more sophisticated case-mix adjustment tools and explicit and clearly agreed case definitions (Black and Tan 2013). In some cases, they also incorporate patient-reported outcome measures (PROMS) (Black 2013). Crucially, by ensuring that the physicians involved have ownership of the system, the risk of gaming is significantly reduced.

Data for healthcare public health

Healthcare public health requires data on the burden of disease in the population and on outcomes that can be linked to the delivery of health care (see Chapter 3, "Monitoring the health of the population"). One approach, mentioned above, is mortality amenable to health care, using data from existing vital registration systems. Where deaths from a particular condition are unexpectedly high in a population, they should be investigated. This will typically involve gathering data from a range of sources, for example a review of case notes of those who have died, or a multi-method assessment of those with the condition to understand their experiences of seeking and obtaining health care.

An example of the former was a retrospective review of clinical data on 1000 people dying after major trauma in England (Anderson, Woodford et al. 1988). This review identified a number of failings in the immediate response and subsequent management and led to significant changes in practice. Subsequent research has shown how death rates from major trauma have steadily fallen in England and Wales, not as a result of any one particular change, but rather from a combination of different practices (Lecky, Woodford et al. 2000).

An example of the latter is the structured evaluation of the experience of patients with diabetes and their healthcare providers as a means to identify failings in the health system (Box 8.3).

Box 8.3 Diabetes as a lens through which to understand health system performance

Insulin-dependent diabetes is an ideal tracer condition to evaluate the organization and delivery of health care, as people with diabetes can easily be identified and, where the health system fails, the results are apparent – including serious complications, such as amputations or blindness, and premature death. Studies undertaken in Georgia (Balabanova, McKee et al. 2009) and Kyrgyzstan (Beran, Abdraimova et al. 2012) have looked at how these health systems function through the eyes of those with diabetes and their healthcare providers. Both identified failings in human resources (with health professionals lacking necessary skills), physical resources (such as a lack of functioning systems to procure and distribute insulin, unaffordability of glucose monitors, and the lack of equipment to provide foot care), and the overall management of resources (with limited follow-up of patients and high private, out-of-pocket payments).

In some countries, there are additional data sources that offer important insights into the extent to which health care meets population health needs. The most widely available are cancer registers. However, these cover the entire population in only a few countries, such as the United Kingdom, Estonia, Slovenia, and the Nordic countries. Elsewhere, they are limited to small and not necessarily representative regions. They provide information on many different aspects of cancer care. First, they identify those cancers which are only discovered when persons die, the so-called "death certificate only" cases. If these represent an unduly high proportion of overall cases in the register, this suggests problems in access to care. Similar information can be obtained from data on stage at diagnosis. Ideally, cancer should be identified as early as possible, given the often significantly better prognosis of early-stage disease. Cancer registry data also provide information on quality of care, making it possible to compare survival in different populations and different settings. However, caution is required in interpreting these data, due to the phenomenon of lead-time bias, whereby improvements in early detection may prolong recorded survival, although the time when death occurs remains unchanged. Data from cancer registries have been extremely influential in identifying differences in performance and leading to changes in policy and practice (Abdel-Rahman, Stockton et al. 2009), with major benefits arising from collaboration among European registries within the framework of successive EUROCARE projects (Sant, Allemani et al. 2009).

Although cancer registers are the most widely available sources of data on health outcomes at the population level, a similar approach has been adopted on a smaller scale for other conditions. Stroke registers have been established in a number of European countries and comparative analyses have highlighted improved outcomes associated with better organized care (Ayis, Coker et al. 2013).

There are also a number of Europe-wide registers of rare diseases, although coverage is variable, and many suffer from uncertain funding streams, being maintained purely by the enthusiasm of a few individuals (Rare Diseases Task Force 2011). Nonetheless, these have once again identified significant variations in management and outcomes, such as for cystic fibrosis, in different European countries (Colombo and Littlewood 2011).

Health care as an opportunity to promote health

The encounter between the patient and a health professional is more than simply a mechanism to reach a diagnosis or prescribe treatment. It is also a valuable opportunity to prevent disease and promote health (see Chapter 10, "Health promotion"). Healthcare public health includes policies that maximize these opportunities (McKee 2002).

It is axiomatic that a healthcare facility should be designed and operated in a way that is health promoting, not only for the patients that use it, but also for the staff that work in it. There is now an extensive body of experience that has been accumulated by the Health Promoting Hospitals network in Europe, although progress in expanding the concept beyond the pioneers has been limited (Whitehead 2004). Measures include the external environment of hospitals, to encourage active transport, such as through the construction of cycle lanes and storage facilities, banning smoking near health facilities (in those cases where there is not already a nationwide ban), serving healthy food, and reducing the carbon footprint of the facility's operations (Rechel, Wright et al. 2009). Unfortunately, such health facilities are still limited in number.

The design of health facilities can itself promote or impede recovery. Thus, patients with an attractive view recover more quickly and require less pain relief. One problem that is often overlooked in hospital design is the high noise level, which may lead to sleep deprivation among patients. Much can be done by using appropriate noise-reducing materials (Rechel, Erskine et al. 2009).

Health facilities should also be designed in ways that make them accessible to the entire population. This includes architectural features that place no barriers in the way of people with disabilities, including those in wheelchairs and those with impaired vision or hearing. It also includes ensuring that signs indicating directions are easily visible, understandable, and where appropriate, in a range of languages (Rechel, Erskine et al. 2009).

Finally, the clinical consultation is an ideal setting for conveying health-promoting messages (see Chapter 10, "Health promotion"; Chapter 14, "Organization and financing of public health"). When meeting health professionals, patients are often receptive to advice on how to change their lifestyle. A planned admission to hospital is another good opportunity to review a patient's lifestyle. Smokers undergoing non-urgent surgery are at greater risk of a range of complications, including chest infections and impaired wound healing. Consequently, there is a strong case for preadmission referral to a smoking cessation service, where patients may be given advice on the risks involved and, where necessary, prescribed nicotine replacement therapy (McKee, Gilmore et al. 2003). There is a growing body of evidence of the effectiveness of brief interventions combined with pharmacotherapy in helping patients to stop smoking (Stead and Lancaster 2012) or avoid hazardous alcohol consumption (Spanou, Simpson et al. 2010).

In summary, healthcare public health includes input into the design and operation of health facilities and measures to ensure that every clinical encounter is seen as an opportunity to promote health. However, there is also a need for much more rigorous evaluative research in this area (McHugh, Robinson et al. 2010).

Collaborative working

The activities described in this chapter will, in some countries, represent a major departure from the traditional role of public health, which has tended to become separated from the delivery of health care. However, this division is increasingly recognized as artificial. Change, however, will require much more than new organizational models. It will require the creation of a culture based on mutual respect, in which clinicians recognize the value of the epidemiological, statistical, and evaluative skills that some public health professionals have to offer, but also a culture in which public health professionals develop a much better understanding of the rapidly changing scientific basis of medicine, as well as the complexity that clinicians wrestle with on a day-to-day basis. This, in turn, has implications for the selection, training, and remuneration of the public health workforce, which, in some countries, is still seen as a refuge for those unable to succeed in the clinical setting.

Conclusion

Health care has been recognized as an important determinant of population health. Yet, in many countries in Europe, public health has failed to engage seriously with it. Instead, healthcare provision has been left to those who provide it. The type of health care they provide, and the quantity of it, is most commonly determined by demand. In other words, where large numbers of patients are queuing up to obtain services, those services will be expanded, as long as there is a funding system in place to ensure that it is affordable, or in some cases profitable. Little, if any, attention is given to those who do not translate their need for care into demand. The result is that those who are already disadvantaged, such as the poor, those from ethnic minorities, and undocumented migrants, will remain excluded from the system. In contrast, a public health perspective involves looking at how the health system is responding to the needs of the entire population, including those whose voices would not otherwise be heard.

Although a comprehensive public health perspective such as that described in this chapter can improve the delivery of health care for the entire population, in practice it is rarely adopted. This is in part because it presupposes several things. The first is that there is some entity with responsibility for the health care delivered to a population defined in some way, typically by geography, but potentially by employment or some other characteristic. Without a population denominator and, moreover, without sources of information on the characteristics of that denominator in terms of age, gender, socio-economic status, and ethnicity, among others, it is not possible to assess the extent of differential utilization of services and thus, by inference, potential unmet need. This inevitably means that the healthcare public health function has more hurdles to overcome in countries where health care is predominantly paid for by social insurance funds than in those where it is predominantly funded by taxes (McKee, Delnoij et al. 2004). However, progress is also being achieved in social insurance systems, such as the French Agences Régionales de Santé, which, since 2010, have coordinated care delivered by a diverse array of providers within geographically defined regions.

The second presumption is that there is an acceptance that the organization and delivery of health care should not simply be left to emerge from either a market or a planning process that is largely devoid of evidence. This is increasingly being recognized in several European countries, for example by the creation of regional agencies to plan networks to care for people with complex disorders, such as cancer. An example is the very successful regional cancer networks in England, although these are now in jeopardy, as a result of the government's 2013 health reforms (Hawkes 2012).

The third presumption is that there are public health professionals with the expertise to implement such a perspective. In many European countries, one or all of these presumptions does not hold true. Yet, even there, as noted above, some elements may be in place – such as assessment of effectiveness (e.g. through health technology assessment), monitoring and evaluation (in the form of quality assurance), or the incorporation of health promotion or public health into healthcare delivery – although the extent to which those undertaking these activities see themselves as fulfilling public health roles may vary.

Crucially, a public health perspective will involve looking at the ways in which the health system responds to need. This includes ensuring that effective care is being provided and ineffective care withdrawn. It also involves asking whether services are used by everyone able to benefit and not just a selected few. In particular, a public health perspective will provide a voice for those who, for whatever reason, may not otherwise be heard. Finally, a public health perspective will ensure that health promotion and prevention is an intrinsic part of the clinical encounter.

References

Abdel-Rahman, M., D. Stockton, B. Rachet, T. Hakulinen and M. P. Coleman (2009). "What if cancer survival in Britain were the same as in Europe: how many deaths are avoidable?" *British Journal of Cancer* **101**(Suppl. 2): S115–S124.

Abel-Smith, B., J. Figueras, W. Holland, M. McKee and E. Mossialos (1995). *Choices in Health Policy: An agenda for the European Union*. Luxembourg, Dartmouth.

AGREE Collaboration (2003). "Development and validation of an international appraisal instrument for assessing the quality of clinical practice guidelines: the AGREE project." *Quality and Safety in Health Care* **12**(1): 18–23.

Anderson, I. D., M. Woodford, F. T. de Dombal and M. Irving (1988). "Retrospective study of 1000 deaths from injury in England and Wales." *British Medical Journal* **296**(6632): 1305–1308.

Ayis, S. A., B. Coker, A. Bhalla, I. Wellwood, A. G. Rudd, A. Di Carlo, Y. Bejot, D. Ryglewicz, D. Rastenyte, P. Langhorne, M. S. Dennis, C. McKevitt and C. D. Wolfe (2013). "Variations in acute stroke care and the impact of organised care on survival from a European perspective: the European Registers of Stroke (EROS) investigators." *Journal of Neurology, Neurosurgery and Psychiatry* **84**: 604–612.

Balabanova, D., M. McKee, N. Koroleva, I. Chikovani, K. Goguadze, T. Kobaladze, O. Adeyi and S. Robles (2009). "Navigating the health system: diabetes care in Georgia." *Health Policy Planning* **24**(1): 46–54.

Barnett, K., S. W. Mercer, M. Norbury, G. Watt, S. Wyke and B. Guthrie (2012). "Epidemiology of multimorbidity and implications for health care, research, and medical education: a cross-sectional study." *The Lancet* **380**(9836): 37–43.

Beran, D., A. Abdraimova, B. Akkazieva, M. McKee, D. Balabanova and J. S. Yudkin (2012). "Diabetes in Kyrgyzstan: changes between 2002 and 2009." *International Journal of Health Planning and Management* **28**(2): e121–e137.

Berta, P., C. Seghieri and G. Vittadini (2013). "Comparing health outcomes among hospitals: the experience of the Lombardy Region." *Health Care Management Science* **16**(3): 245–257.

Birkmeyer, J. D., A. E. Siewers, E. V. Finlayson, T. A. Stukel, F. L. Lucas, I. Batista, H. G. Welch and D. E. Wennberg (2002). "Hospital volume and surgical mortality in the United States." *New England Journal of Medicine* **346**(15): 1128–1137.

Black, N. (2013). "Patient reported outcome measures could help transform healthcare." *British Medical Journal* **346**: f167.

Black, N. and S. Tan (2013). "Use of national clinical databases for informing and for evaluating health care policies." *Health Policy* **109**(2): 131–136.

Brook, R. H. (2009). "Assessing the appropriateness of care – its time has come." *Journal of the American Medical Association* **302**(9): 997–998.

Busse, R., E. van Ginneken and C. Normand (2012). "Re-examining the cost pressures on health systems." In *Health Systems: Health, wealth and societal well-being.* M. McKee and J. Figueras, Eds. Maidenhead, Open University Press: 37–60.

Carter, P. and B. Jarman (2013). "Who knew what, and when, at Mid Staffs?" *British Medical Journal* **346**: f726.

Colombo, C. and J. Littlewood (2011). "The implementation of standards of care in Europe: state of the art." *Journal of Cystic Fibrosis* **10**(Suppl. 2): S7–S15.

Doyle, Y., M. McKee, B. Rechel and E. Grundy (2009). "Meeting the challenge of population ageing." *British Medical Journal* **339**: b3926.

Girling, A. J., T. P. Hofer, J. Wu, P. J. Chilton, J. P. Nicholl, M. A. Mohammed and R. J. Lilford (2012). "Case-mix adjusted hospital mortality is a poor proxy for preventable mortality: a modelling study." *BMJ Quality and Safety* **21**(12): 1052–1056.

Goldacre, B. (2013). *Bad Pharma: How drug companies mislead doctors and harm patients.* London, Signal.

Hawkes, N. (2012). "Cancer and heart disease networks face cuts, say charities." *British Medical Journal* **345**: e6800.

Healy, J. and M. McKee (2004). *Accessing Healthcare: Responding to diversity.* Oxford, Oxford University Press.

Heller, G., R. Schnell, D. K. Richardson, B. Misselwitz and S. Schmidt (2003). "[Assessing the impact of delivery unit size on neonatal survival: estimation of potentially avoidable deaths in Hessen, Germany, 1990–2000]." *Deutsche Medizinische Wochenschrift* **128**(13): 657–662.

Hunter, D. J., C. M. McKee, N. A. Black and C. F. Sanderson (1995). "Health care sought and received by men with urinary symptoms, and their views on prostatectomy." *British Journal of General Practice* **45**(390): 27–30.

Hunter, D. J., C. M. McKee, C. F. Sanderson and N. A. Black (1994). "Appropriate indications for prostatectomy in the UK – results of a consensus panel." *Journal of Epidemiology and Community Health* **48**(1): 58–64.

Jarman, B. (2012). "When managers rule." *British Medical Journal* **345**: e8239.

Lecky, F., M. Woodford and D. W. Yates (2000). "Trends in trauma care in England and Wales 1989–97. UK Trauma Audit and Research Network." *The Lancet* **355**(9217): 1771–1775.

Legido-Quigley, H., D. Panteli, S. Brusamento, C. Knai, V. Saliba, E. Turk, M. Sole, U. Augustin, J. Car, M. McKee and R. Busse (2012). "Clinical guidelines in the European Union: mapping the regulatory basis, development, quality control, implementation and evaluation across member states." *Health Policy* **107**(2/3): 146–156.

Maringe, C., S. Walters, J. Butler, M. P. Coleman, N. Hacker, L. Hanna, B. J. Mosgaard, A. Nordin, B. Rosen, G. Engholm, M. L. Gjerstorff, J. Hatcher, T. B. Johannesen, C. E. McGahan, D. Meechan, R. Middleton, E. Tracey, D. Turner, M. A. Richards and B. Rachet (2012). "Stage at diagnosis and ovarian cancer survival: evidence from the International Cancer Benchmarking Partnership." *Gynecologic Oncology* **127**(1): 75–82.

McCartney, M. (2012). *The Patient Paradox.* London, Pinter & Martin.

McHugh, C., A. Robinson and J. Chesters (2010). "Health promoting health services: a review of the evidence." *Health Promotion International* **25**(2): 230–237.

McKee, M. (2002). "What can health services contribute to the reduction of inequalities in health?" *Scandinavian Journal of Public Health* Suppl. **59**: 54–58.

McKee, M. (2010). "Citizens' juries: more questions than answers?" *Journal of Epidemiology and Community Health* **64**(9): 750–751.

McKee, M., D. M. J. Delnoij and H. Brand (2004). "Prevention and public health in social insurance systems." In *Social Health Insurance Systems in Western Europe*. R. Saltman, R. Busse and J. Figueras, Eds. Buckingham, Open University Press: 267–280.

McKee, M., A. Gilmore and T. E. Novotny (2003). "Smoke free hospitals." *British Medical Journal* **326**(7396): 941–942.

Mindell, J., E. Klodawski, J. Fitzpatrick, N. Malhotra, M. McKee and C. Sanderson (2008). "The impact of private-sector provision on equitable utilisation of coronary revascularisation in London." *Heart* **94**(8): 1008–1011.

Mohammed, M. A., J. J. Deeks, A. Girling, G. Rudge, M. Carmalt, A. J. Stevens and R. J. Lilford (2009). "Evidence of methodological bias in hospital standardised mortality ratios: retrospective database study of English hospitals." *British Medical Journal* **338**: b780.

Mooney, G. and S. Houston (2004). "An alternative approach to resource allocation: weighted capacity to benefit plus MESH infrastructure." *Applied Health Economics and Health Policy* **3**(1): 29–33.

Nolte, E., C. Bain and M. McKee (2006). "Diabetes as a tracer condition in international benchmarking of health systems." *Diabetes Care* **29**(5): 1007–1011.

Nolte, E. and C. M. McKee (2012). "In amenable mortality – deaths avoidable through health care – progress in the US lags that of three European countries." *Health Affairs (Millwood)* **31**(9): 2114–2122.

Nolte, E. and M. McKee (2004). *Does Health Care Save Lives? Avoidable mortality revisited*. London, Nuffield Trust.

Nolte, E. and M. McKee (2011). "Variations in amenable mortality – trends in 16 high-income nations." *Health Policy* **103**(1): 47–52.

Oliver, M. I., N. Pearson, N. Coe and D. Gunnell (2005). "Help-seeking behaviour in men and women with common mental health problems: cross-sectional study." *British Journal of Psychiatry* **186**: 297–301.

Pearson, G., F. Shann, P. Barry, J. Vyas, D. Thomas, C. Powell and D. Field (1997). "Should paediatric intensive care be centralised? Trent versus Victoria." *The Lancet* **349**(9060): 1213–1217.

Petherick, E. S., N. A. Cullum and K. E. Pickett (2013). "Investigation of the effect of deprivation on the burden and management of venous leg ulcers: a cohort study using the THIN database." *PLoS One* **8**(3): e58948.

Priebe, S., A. Matanov, H. Barros, R. Canavan, E. Gabor, T. Greacen, P. Holcnerova, U. Kluge, P. Nicaise, J. Moskalewicz, J. M. Diaz-Olalla, C. Strassmayr, A. H. Schene, J. J. Soares, S. Tulloch and A. Gaddini (2013). "Mental health-care provision for marginalized groups across Europe: findings from the PROMO study." *European Journal of Public Health* **23**(1): 97–103.

Rare Diseases Task Force (2011). *Patient Registries in the Field of Rare Diseases: Overview of the issues surrounding the establishment, management, governance and financing of academic registries*. Brussels, Orphanet.

Rawlins, M. (2012). "Reflections: NICE, health economics, and outcomes research." *Value in Health* **15**(3): 568–569.

Rechel, B., J. Erskine, B. Dowdeswell, S. Wright and M. McKee (2009). *Capital Investment for Health: Case studies from Europe*. Copenhagen, European Observatory on Health Systems and Policies.

Rechel, B., S. Wright, N. Edwards, B. Dowdeswell and M. McKee (2009). *Investing in Hospitals of the Future*. Copenhagen, European Observatory on Health Systems and Policies.

Rice, N. and P. Smith (2002). "Strategic resource allocation and funding decisions." In *Funding Health Care: Options for Europe*. E. Mossialos, A. Dixon, J. Figueras and J. Kutzin, Eds. Buckingham, Open University Press: 250–271.

Sanderson, C. F., D. J. Hunter, C. M. McKee and N. A. Black (1997). "Limitations of epidemiologically based needs assessment: the case of prostatectomy." *Medical Care* **35**(7): 669–685.

Sant, M., C. Allemani, M. Santaquilani, A. Knijn, F. Marchesi and R. Capocaccia (2009). "EUROCARE-4: Survival of cancer patients diagnosed in 1995–1999. Results and commentary." *European Journal of Cancer* **45**(6): 931–991.

Spanou, C., S. A. Simpson, K. Hood, A. Edwards, D. Cohen, S. Rollnick, B. Carter, J. McCambridge, L. Moore, E. Randell, T. Pickles, C. Smith, C. Lane, F. Wood, H. Thornton and C. C. Butler (2010). "Preventing disease through opportunistic, rapid engagement by primary care teams using behaviour change counselling (PRE-EMPT): protocol for a general practice-based cluster randomised trial." *BMC Family Practice* **11**: 69.

Stead, L. F. and T. Lancaster (2012). "Combined pharmacotherapy and behavioural interventions for smoking cessation." *Cochrane Database of Systematic Reviews* **10**: CD008286.

Stevens, A. and J. Gabbay (1991). "Needs assessment needs assessment." *Health Trends* **23**(1): 20–23.

Sundmacher, L. and R. Busse (2011). "The impact of physician supply on avoidable cancer deaths in Germany: a spatial analysis." *Health Policy* **103**(1): 53–62.

Tempfer, C. B. and P. Nowak (2011). "Consumer participation and organizational development in health care: a systematic review." *Wiener Klinische Wochenschrift* **123**(13/14): 408–414.

Teutsch, S. and B. Rechel (2012). "Ethics of resource allocation and rationing medical care in a time of fiscal restraint – US and Europe." *Public Health Reviews* **34**(1): 1–10.

Tugwell, P., K. Bennett, D. Feeny, G. Guyatt and R. B. Haynes (1984). "A framework for the evaluation of technology: the technology assessment iterative loop." In *Health Care Technology: Effectiveness, efficiency and public policy*. D. Feeny, G. Guyatt and P. Tugwell, Eds. Ottawa, Canadian Medical Association and The Institute for Research on Public Policy: 41–56.

van de Ven, W. P., K. Beck, C. Van de Voorde, J. Wasem and I. Zmora (2007). "Risk adjustment and risk selection in Europe: 6 years later." *Health Policy* **83**(2/3): 162–179.

Velasco Garrido, M., F. B. Kristensen, C. P. Nielsen and R. Busse (2008). *Health Technology Assessment and Health Policy-making in Europe*. Copenhagen, European Observatory on Health Systems and Policies.

Whitehead, D. (2004). "The European Health Promoting Hospitals (HPH) project: how far on?" *Health Promotion International* **19**(2): 259–267.

chapter nine

Screening

Martin McKee, Bernd Rechel

Introduction

Screening as a means to detect disease early is an established public health function throughout Europe. However, it is not without controversy. In theory, the early detection of disease, or a marker of future disease, makes perfect sense. Detection will make it possible to intervene at an early stage and prevent the development or progression of the disease. However, in reality, the situation is much more complicated and there are many screening programmes that either fail to meet their potential or, worse, are completely ineffective or even harmful. There is a crucial distinction between organized screening (based on a defined target population, central organization and planning, systematic monitoring of uptake by different groups within the population, evidence-based screening intervals, and quality assurance systems) and opportunistic screening (offered spontaneously by healthcare providers when patients use health services or at the request of patients) (Holland and Stewart 2005; Hakama, Coleman et al. 2008). Organized screening is almost always more efficient, makes better use of available resources, and is less likely to result in harm.

In this chapter, we focus mainly on screening programmes for cancer but, before looking at them in detail, it should be noted that there are several other categories of screening programmes. The first category includes those undertaken to detect severe foetal abnormalities, such as neural tube defects or chromosomal anomalies such as Down's syndrome. Detection of such a severe anomaly will allow the mother to be counselled and offered termination of pregnancy. Other screening tests are offered to mothers at high risk of specific disorders because of their family history. The most recent European survey of antenatal screening practices, undertaken in 18 countries in 2004, reported that 10 had policies or recommendations in place to screen for Down's syndrome (Table 9.1) and 14 for structural abnormalities (Boyd, Devigan et al. 2008). However, policies vary, both with regard to the methods used and the criteria for identifying those at highest risk. Thus, the incidence of Down's syndrome

Table 9.1 Policies on screening for Down's syndrome in 18 European countries in 2004

Country	National screening programme or recommendation to offer screening to all women	Age (years) at which amniocentesis or CVS is offered
Austria	No	$\geq$35
Belgium	Yes	$\geq$36 (charged if <36)
Croatia	No	$\geq$35
Denmark	Yes	Not offered primarily on basis of maternal age
England and Wales	Yes	Not offered primarily on basis of maternal age
Finland	Yes	$\geq$39
France	Yes	$\geq$38
Germany	Yes	$\geq$35
Ireland	No	—
Italy	Yes	$\geq$35
Malta	No	—
Netherlands	No	$\geq$36
Norway	No	$\geq$38
Poland	Yes	$\geq$35
Portugal	Yes	$\geq$35
Spain	No	$\geq$35
Sweden	No	$\geq$35
Switzerland	Yes	Not offered primarily on basis of maternal age

Source: Boyd, Devigan et al. (2008)

increases with maternal age but there is considerable variation in the age at which amniocentesis or chorionic villous sampling (CVS) is offered. A key consideration is the variation in access to termination of pregnancy within Europe. At the time of writing, there is a virtual ban on termination in Ireland and Malta, requiring those women seeking termination to travel abroad, while it is heavily restricted in Poland.

A second category of screening programmes is administered to newborn babies. These are largely uncontroversial and can be done cheaply and easily using a spot of blood taken at birth. Although the conditions that they are seeking to detect are rare, they have severe consequences if detected late and consequently go untreated. In each case, there is a treatment available that can significantly modify the course of the disease. The range of disorders that can be screened for has increased rapidly with the introduction of new technologies, with some countries offering tests for up to 20 abnormalities. The situation in Europe in 2007 has been reviewed in a recent survey (Bodamer, Hoffmann et al. 2007) but is changing rapidly. Examples of the more common abnormalities sought include phenylketonuria, which will lead to serious and irreversible mental disorders unless the affected child is given a special diet, congenital hypothyroidism, which again leads to severe learning difficulties unless treated with thyroid hormone, a simple oral preparation, and medium-chain acyl-CoA dehydrogenase deficiency (MCADD), again treated with a special diet. In some European countries, the newborn screening regime also includes tests for disorders that, while there is no single effective treatment, it is possible to address with a range of measures that will slow progression of the disease or reduce its consequences – these are cystic fibrosis and sickle cell disease. The latter is an example of a condition for which it is necessary to consider the background prevalence. It occurs almost entirely in persons of Afro-Caribbean origin and thus screening will be most important in countries where this ethnic group is present in significant numbers.

A third category of screening programmes is for infectious disease, particularly tuberculosis (TB), although antenatal screening for syphilis is also widespread. While some countries limit screening for TB to contacts of sputum smear-positive pulmonary TB, others screen people who are HIV-positive, prisoners, and hospital contacts of inpatients (Bothamley, Ditiu et al. 2008). There are also some high-prevalence countries in the eastern part of the WHO European Region, such as Belarus and Ukraine, that still rely on diagnosis through mass screening of the population by X-ray (Atun and Olynik 2008; Richardson, Boerma et al. 2008). Of 50 European countries covered in a survey in 2006, 28 countries screened immigrants for TB (Bothamley, Ditiu et al. 2008). However, the individual and public health benefit of this practice, as well as the ethical issues involved, are highly contested (Wörmann and Krämer 2011).

A fourth category of screening programmes is related to risk factors for non-communicable diseases and their risk factors, such as hypertension, overweight and obesity, lack of physical activity, tobacco and alcohol consumption, high cholesterol and blood glucose levels, and salt in urine. European initiatives, aimed at improving the prevention of cardiovascular disease, include guidelines for clinical practice (Perk, De Backer et al. 2012). These actions are in line with the 2008–2013 Action Plan for the Global Strategy for the Prevention and Control of Non-communicable Diseases, which recommends programmes for the early detection of and screening for hypertension, diabetes, and cardiovascular risk (WHO 2008).

This chapter explores a final category of screening programmes, those aiming to detect cancer in its early stages. We begin by reviewing the established criteria for implementing a screening programme. We then review the evidence for screening for selected conditions, including some of the current controversies. This is followed by a brief overview of screening practices across Europe. Finally, we examine the public health role in the organization and management of screening programmes.

When is a screening programme justified?

Basic criteria for evaluating screening programmes were set out in a 1968 report prepared for the World Health Organization (WHO) (Box 9.1).

Box 9.1   Basic criteria for evaluating screening programmes

1. The condition should be an important health problem.
2. There should be a treatment for the condition.
3. Facilities for diagnosis and treatment should be available.
4. There should be a latent stage of the disease.
5. There should be a test or examination for the condition.
6. The test should be acceptable to the population.
7. The natural history of the disease should be adequately understood.
8. There should be an agreed policy on whom to treat.
9. The total cost of finding a case should be economically balanced in relation to medical expenditure as a whole.
10. Case-finding should be a continuous process, not just a "once and for all" project.

Source: Wilson and Jungner (1968)

It is apparent from studying these criteria that it may be justifiable to set up a screening programme for a given condition in some settings but not in others. It makes little sense to screen for a condition that is extremely rare because this will involve subjecting perhaps tens of thousands of people to an examination just to detect one case. However, the incidence of conditions for which one might wish to screen may vary between populations. Thus, it may be appropriate to screen for a particular form of cancer where it is common but not where it is rare. This may also change over time. The increasingly common practice of immunizing adolescent girls against human papilloma virus will in time make cervical cancer extremely uncommon, so that existing screening programmes for this condition might become superfluous. However, the importance of a condition is not judged simply by its frequency. A further consideration is its impact on the individual concerned. To be important, it should be life threatening or at least pose a risk of significant impairment. As a consequence, screening programmes have focused largely on cancers and inherited errors of metabolism and foetal anomalies. There are increasing calls to screen for cardiovascular disease and associated risk factors, but some argue that the necessary resources would be better spent on population-level initiatives to reduce exposure to these risk factors in the first place (McCartney 2012).

The second and third criteria are equally self-evident but have often been ignored in practice. During the 1980s, a number of then communist countries in central and eastern Europe implemented radiological screening for lung cancer, using equipment that was otherwise under-utilized for the diagnosis of TB. Unfortunately, there was little that could be offered in treatment to those identified as having cancer. The fourth criterion requires that there be a stage in the disease process when treatment can make a difference. As in the example of lung cancer screening, by the time the tumour is detectable, it is likely to no longer be operable. The fifth and sixth criteria relate to the existence of a test for the condition that is feasible and acceptable. It would not make sense to screen people by means of invasive surgery or exposure to excessive amounts of radiation. In practice, however, these criteria are not always adhered to, leading to suboptimal or even adverse outcomes.

The evidence for cancer screening programmes

The Council of the European Union, after reviewing the evidence base on population-based screening programmes for cancer, concluded that there is justification to screen for cancer of the cervix, breast, and colon, provided there are appropriate quality assurance systems (Council of the European Union 2003). These recommendations were endorsed by the WHO Regional Committee for Europe for the 53 member states of the WHO European Region (WHO 2011). These three types of cancer (cervix, breast, and colon) are among the most common and deadly cancers, accounting for almost 20% of cancer deaths in the WHO European Region.

The earliest cancer screening programmes aimed to prevent the development of cervical cancer. It has long been recognized that changes in the cells of the cervix can be identified long before the development of invasive cancer, with a typical interval of 10–12 years (Gustafsson and Adami 1989; van Oortmarssen and Habbema 1991). Initially based on the detection of cancer cells, screening was extended in some countries to detect human papilloma virus, the cause of cervical cancer. Data from observational studies indicate that well-organized cervical screening programmes can reduce mortality from cervical cancer by 80% or more (International Agency for Research on Cancer 2005).

The evidence for the effectiveness of breast cancer screening is more controversial. Although, unlike screening for cervical cancer, breast cancer screening has been subject to a number of randomized controlled trials with long-term follow-up, these have been of low or moderate quality. Data from these trials suggest that biannual mammography (X-ray of the breast) screening programmes in women aged between 50 and 69 years can decrease mortality by approximately 25%. Observational data of routine practice suggest that this may be an overestimate of what can be achieved and some studies even dispute the benefits of screening. A study comparing breast cancer mortality in six European countries found that screening was unlikely to have played a role in mortality reductions (Autier, Boniol et al. 2011). Similar findings in the United States led the Preventive Services Task Force (an independent panel of experts in primary care and prevention) in 2009 to recommend the discontinuation of routine breast cancer screening in women younger than 50 and the reduction of screening intervals from one to two years for those aged 50–74. However, this met with resistance from groups with vested interests in mammography, leading to the so-called "mammography war" (Bleyer 2011). However, a major weakness of these more critical studies is that they have not used longitudinal individual data that would make it possible to distinguish those women who were screened from those who were not. Studies using such longitudinal individual data for Europe have found reductions in mortality of 25–31% for women invited for screening and 38–42% for women screened (Broeders, Moss et al. 2012).

It is now recognized that mammography will identify a significant number of lesions that are either not malignant or will progress very slowly if at all. Concerns have therefore been voiced about the effectiveness of mammography and the consequences of over-diagnosis (Gotzsche, Jorgensen et al. 2012). A study of breast cancer incidence in the United States between 1976 and 2008 found that the mammography programme there was associated with a large increase in the detection of early-stage breast cancer, but only a marginal reduction of late-stage breast cancer, suggesting substantial over-diagnosis and only a small effect of screening on breast cancer mortality (Bleyer and Welch 2012). A recent review undertaken in the United Kingdom concluded that the existing mammography programme should be continued, as it will reduce mortality, although at the cost of a number of women being treated unnecessarily (Independent UK Panel on Breast Cancer Screening 2012).

The third cancer that is the subject of screening programmes in a number of European countries is colorectal cancer, but programmes have only been implemented relatively recently (von Karsa, Anttila et al. 2008). Randomized controlled trials have shown that biannual screening using the faecal occult blood test among those aged 50–74 can reduce mortality by about 16% (Hewitson, Glasziou et al. 2007). This is somewhat smaller than the reduction seen with screening for cervical and breast cancer and there is considerable debate about whether screening programmes for colorectal cancer are cost-effective.

Advances in technology may make it possible to screen for cancers or other diseases for which there is currently no effective means for early diagnosis or treatment. One cancer that is currently attracting attention in this regard is that of the ovary. Another, much more controversial example that has been advocated to be included in future screening programmes is prostate cancer, identified through prostate-specific antigens (PSAs). The European Randomized Study of Screening for Prostate Cancer, involving 162,388 patients in eight European countries, found a reduction in prostate cancer mortality of 20% after 9 years. However, it is necessary to treat almost 50 men with an elevated PSA level to save one life, while many of those treated will be left with potentially severe side-effects. For this reason, there are significant concerns that screening will lead to over-diagnosis and over-treatment (Schröder 2012).

Cancer screening practices in Europe

As mentioned above, the EU and the WHO Regional Office for Europe recommend organized, population-based screening programmes for cervical, breast, and colorectal cancer (Council of the European Union 2003; WHO 2011). Yet, there is still considerable variation across countries in how far they have followed these recommendations. By 2007, 22 of the 27 EU countries were running population-based screening programmes for breast cancer, 15 for cervical cancer and only 12 for colorectal cancer (von Karsa, Anttila et al. 2008).

Few countries in Europe have a single national body to review screening practice and policy, and population registers for call and recall and follow-up of patients are also comparatively rare (Holland, Stewart et al. 2006). Although there are exceptions, such as Slovenia, progress has been in general slowest in countries in central and eastern Europe, in particular the countries of the former Soviet Union, where early detection and prevention of non-communicable disease was virtually lacking in the Soviet era and is still under-developed (Maier and Martin-Moreno 2011). Most countries in south-eastern Europe have also very little systematic screening for cancers (WHO 2009), but are slowly catching up. Croatia, for example, introduced organized, population-based screening programmes for breast cancer in 2006, colorectal cancer in 2008, and cervical cancer in 2012.

In addition to differences between countries, screening practices also vary within countries, in particular where health service provision and thus screening is devolved to regional or local governments (Holland, Stewart et al. 2006), such as in Spain (García-Armesto, Abadía-Taira et al. 2010). In Belgium, the availability of screening programmes for certain types of cancer differs among the country's three communities (Gerkens and Merkur 2010). In Denmark, too, access to screening programmes varies and organized breast cancer screening only takes place in some parts of the country (Strandberg-Larsen, Nielsen et al. 2007). Italy is another country with very pronounced regional differences, leading to cross-regional patient flows. National screening programmes for breast, cervical, and colorectal cancer were only established in 2004 and coverage differs considerably across regions (Lo Scalzo, Donatini et al. 2009).

Cervical cancer screening programmes

Although there is widespread consensus about the technical aspects of undertaking screening for cervical cancer, including the optimal ways of obtaining a high-quality sample and examining it, countries differ widely in the organization of cervical cancer screening programmes. Major differences relate to whether screening programmes have been set up or not, whether they are systematic or opportunistic, and what percentage of the target population they reach (Table 9.2).

Organized, population-based screening takes place in the Czech Republic, Denmark, Estonia, Finland, Hungary, Iceland, Ireland, Italy, Latvia, Lithuania, the Netherlands, Norway, Poland, Slovenia, Sweden, and the United Kingdom (Table 9.2). In most cases, it includes the maintenance of registers of women at risk, covering all women living in a given area within a specified age range who are not otherwise ineligible by, for example, having had a hysterectomy, as well as integrated systems to issue regular invitations and to ensure that any abnormalities are followed up. The interval between successive examinations is typically 3–5 years, depending on the woman's age. The entire system is subject to regular quality assurance. Organized, population-based screening can have a significant impact on disease-specific mortality levels. In Finland, where organized cervical cancer screening was established in the 1960s, age-standardized mortality rates have declined by approximately 80% (Anttila and Nieminen 2007).

In contrast, in some other countries in Europe, such as Armenia, Austria, Belgium, Bosnia and Herzegovina, and Germany, screening is opportunistic. Women are offered examinations, typically when they attend their physician or

Table 9.2 Cervical cancer screening practices in selected European countries, 2012

	Type of screening	Geographical scope of programme	Age range (years)	Screening interval (years)	Coverage of target population
Albania	No data	No data	No data	No data	No data
Armenia	Opportunistic	National	30–60	3	No data
Austria	Opportunistic	National	18–not specified	1	No data
Azerbaijan	No programme	—	—	—	—
Belarus	Opportunistic	National	18–no limit	1	No data
Belgium	Opportunistic	National	25–64	3	70%
Bosnia and Herzegovina	Opportunistic	National	20–no limit	1 (extended to 3 years after 3 consecutive negative smears)	No data
Bulgaria	Opportunistic	National	30–59	3	No data
Croatia	Opportunistic	National	25–64	3	35–42%
Cyprus	No programme	—	—	—	—
Czech Republic	Organized	National	25–60		48%
Denmark	Organized	National	23–65	3 in age 23–50 (5 for 50+)	69%
Estonia	Organized	National	30–59	3	13%
Finland	Organized	National	(25) 30–60 (65)	5	73%
France	Opportunistic, organized in 5 regions	National	20 (25)–not specified	3	71%
Former Yugoslav Republic of Macedonia	Opportunistic	National	30–55	3	15–25%
Georgia	Opportunistic, organized in 1 region	National	25–60	3	20%
Germany	Opportunistic	National	20–not specified	1	No data
Greece	Opportunistic	National	20–not specified	1	No data
Hungary	Organized	National	25–65	3	28–31%
Iceland	Organized	National	20–69	2 up to age 39, 4 years afterwards	80%
Ireland	Organized	Regional, national planned	25–65	3 in age 25–44, 5 years afterwards	62–66%
Italy	Organized	National	25–64	3	>59%

Latvia	Organized	National	25–70	3	42%
Lithuania	Organized	National	25–60	3	9–17% (39%)
Luxembourg	Opportunistic	National	15–not specified	1	No data
Malta	No programme	—	—	—	—
Moldova	Opportunistic	National	20–no limit	2	No data
Montenegro	Opportunistic	National	25–64	3	No data
Netherlands	Organized	National	30–60	5	77%
Norway	Organized	National	25–69	3	75%
Poland	Organized	National	25–59	3	23–27%
Portugal	Organized in 3 regions	National	25–64	3	58%
Romania	Opportunistic, organized in one pilot region	National	25–64	3	18% (10% in pilot region)
Russian Federation	Opportunistic	National	18–no limit	1	15–20%
Serbia	Opportunistic (organized in process of implementation)	National	25–65 (69)	3	20%
Slovakia	Opportunistic	National	23–64	3	17–20%
Slovenia	Organized	National	20–64	3	70–74%
Spain	Opportunistic, organized in regions	Regional	30–65	3	No data
Sweden	Organized	National	23–60	3	73%
Switzerland	Opportunistic	National	20–no limit	3	80% (age 22–44), 65% (age 45–64)
Turkey	Opportunistic	National	18–no limit	1	No data
Ukraine	Opportunistic	National	18–65	1	No data
United Kingdom	Organized	National	(20) 25–60 (64)	3	74%

Source: Adapted from Kesic, Poljak et al. (2012)

gynaecologist for other purposes. As a consequence, they may undergo many more examinations in their lifetime than in those countries with organized screening programmes. In some cases, they may undergo examinations as frequently as every 6 months. In Germany, a woman could have up to 50 smears in her lifetime, while in Finland she is unlikely to have more than seven. However, the age-standardized death rate from cervical cancer in the former is almost twice that in the latter (WHO 2012). Furthermore, because this approach to screening is opportunistic, it will often miss those at greatest risk. Cervical cancer is much more common in women of lower social class, but they are least likely to attend their physicians for other purposes.

While opportunistic screening for cervical cancer has reached coverage rates of 70–71% and resulted in a reduction of cervical cancer mortality in countries where the benefits of screening are now well known, such as Belgium or France (Kesic, Poljak et al. 2012), it is less successful than organized, population-based screening, which is therefore recommended by the European Guidelines for Quality Assurance in Cervical Cancer Screening (Arbyn, Anttila et al. 2008). Despite these guidelines, which are directed at all countries of the WHO European Region (and not only EU member states), by 2012 only 16 European countries had organized population-based screening programmes for cervical cancer (Kesic, Poljak et al. 2012). Furthermore, in western European countries, screening programmes (whether systematic or opportunistic) tend to be more developed than in countries in central and eastern Europe (Hakama, Coleman et al. 2008; Arbyn, Antoine et al. 2010), and reach 80% of women aged 20–69 in Iceland and 80% of women aged 22–44 in Switzerland (Table 9.2). In many new EU member states, as well as the countries of the former Yugoslavia, organized screening programmes have begun, although not all are yet fully functioning. Some of the greatest gaps are in the former Soviet countries, which rely on opportunistic screening, but with a very low coverage in middle-aged and older women and little impact on morbidity and mortality (Kesic, Poljak et al. 2012). Although it is difficult to assess the impact of cervical cancer screening on mortality in the general population, the high mortality rates in many countries of central and eastern Europe and the former Soviet Union seem to be at least in part due to the absence of organized screening programmes (Kesic, Poljak et al. 2012; Anttila and Martin-Moreno 2013).

In addition to the already mentioned differences in cervical cancer screening programmes in Europe, it is noteworthy that the age ranges and screening intervals differ markedly between countries. According to the European Guidelines for Quality Assurance in Cervical Cancer Screening, resources should be concentrated on the age range from 30 or 35 to 60 years and screening intervals should be 3 years for women aged 25–49 and 5 years for those aged 50–64 (Arbyn, Anttila et al. 2008). It is apparent that many countries still need to adapt their national practices to adhere to these recommendations.

Breast cancer screening programmes

Countries in Europe also differ in the extent to which they have implemented organized, population-based screening programmes for breast cancer, based on registers of women at risk, integrated information systems, and quality assurance mechanisms. In 2007, such programmes were in place in Belgium, the Czech Republic, Estonia, Hungary, Finland, France, the Netherlands, Spain, Sweden, and the United Kingdom. A number of countries, including Germany, Italy, Ireland, Poland, and Portugal, were in the process of rolling out nationwide population-based programmes. Others, including Greece, Latvia, Lithuania, and Slovenia, still relied on opportunistic screening (Figure 9.1).

As mentioned above, there are also pronounced regional differences in some countries. In Italy in 2008, breast cancer screening programmes covered 75% of the female population in the northern and central regions, but only 10% in the south (Lo Scalzo, Donatini et al. 2009). In Switzerland, there has been only slow progress in implementing a nationwide breast cancer screening programme, with approaches varying substantially across cantons. Routine mammography

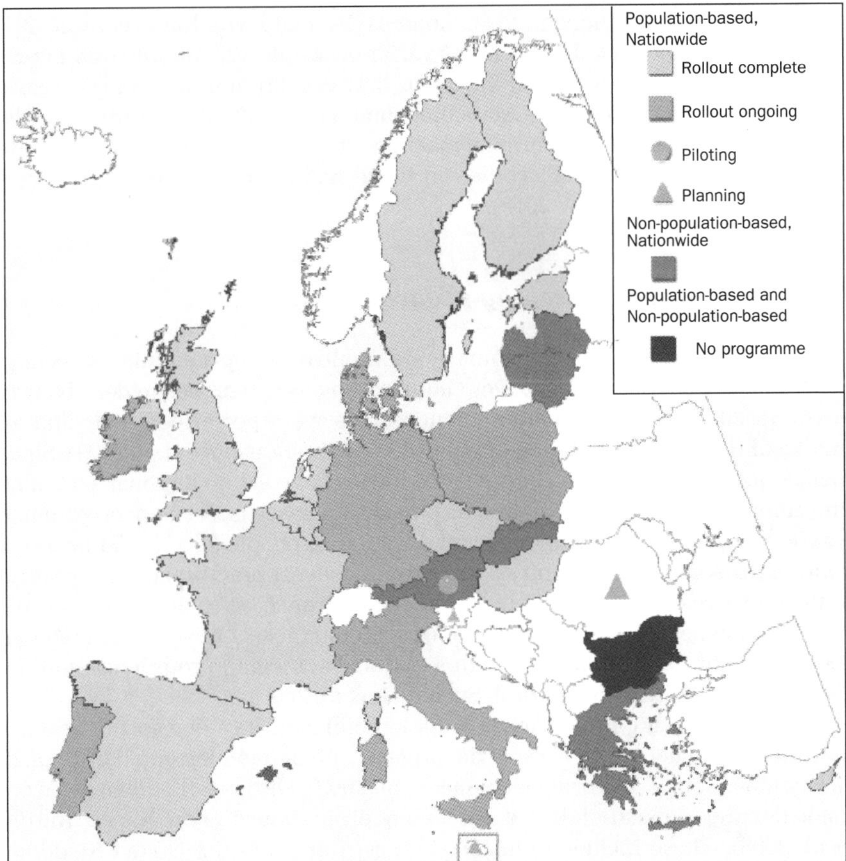

Figure 9.1 Distribution of breast cancer screening programmes based on mammography in the EU in 2007

Source: von Karsa, Anttila et al. (2008)

for target population groups is only paid for by the insurer in the six cantons that run their own prevention programmes (OECD/WHO 2011).

A survey of 10 national and 16 regional breast cancer screening programmes in 18 European countries, comprising a target population of 26.9 million women aged 50–69, found that participation rates of those personally invited ranged among programmes from 19.4% in Poland to 88.9% in the Navarra region of Spain in 2005–2007. Thirteen of the 26 programmes achieved at least 70%, which is the EU benchmark of acceptable participation, and 9 achieved the desirable level of at least 75%. Coverage ranged from 28.4% in Italy to 92.1% in the Navarra region of Spain (Giordano, von Karsa et al. 2012).

There were also differences in the target population. While some of the 26 programmes targeted the female population aged 50–69, in line with the recommendations of the European Council, others, such as Sweden, targeted women from 40 years of age. Furthermore, some had higher upper age limits, such as the Netherlands, which targeted women up to 75 years of age. All of the 26 screening programmes used the recommended interval of 24 months, except the United Kingdom, which used 36 months (Giordano, von Karsa et al. 2012).

The survey also found substantial variation in the volume of tests across screening units, with a 27-fold variation between programmes in the yearly number of examinations per screening unit and a 20-fold variation in the number of tests per mammography machine. It might be challenging to ensure the quality of the tests undertaken in those units with low testing volumes (Giordano, von Karsa et al. 2012).

Colorectal cancer screening programmes

In 1976, Germany was the first country in Europe to set up a national screening programme for colorectal cancer, initially covering persons older than 44 years. In 2003–2005, 1.5 million colonoscopies were performed, reaching an uptake of the target population of about 12% (West, Boustière et al. 2009). Since then, a growing number of European countries have set up national screening programmes. In France, a national, population-based screening programme was set up in 2003, based upon biennial testing of people aged 50–74 years. In contrast to some other countries in Europe, general practitioners are central to the logistics of the screening programme in France, as they are responsible for the implementation and follow-up of screening tests (West, Boustière et al. 2009). Finland followed in 2004 with a national screening programme and the United Kingdom in 2006 (Zavoral, Suchanek et al. 2009).

By 2007, screening programmes for colorectal cancer of one sort or another had been implemented or were in the process of being implemented in 19 of 27 EU member states (Zavoral, Suchanek et al. 2009). Of those, 12 countries were implementing population-based screening programmes (von Karsa, Anttila et al. 2008). These included Finland, France, Italy, and the United Kingdom. Cyprus, Hungary, Portugal, Romania, Slovenia, and Croatia were piloting or planning screening programmes at the time and Sweden and Spain were piloting population-based screening programmes on a regional basis. Opportunistic screening took place in Austria, Bulgaria, the Czech Republic, Germany, Greece,

Latvia, and Slovakia. No programmes existed in Belgium, Bulgaria, Denmark, Estonia, Ireland, Lithuania, the Netherlands or Poland (Figure 9.2).

As with breast cancer screening, there are regional variations in colorectal cancer screening. In Italy, a nationwide campaign was initiated in 2005, but its implementation was left in the hands of 21 regional centres. By 2009, 11 of 21 regions, mostly in the north of the country, had set up screening programmes (Zavoral, Suchanek et al. 2009). Spain has also devolved screening activities to the country's regions, with only limited pilot studies having taken place by 2009 (Zavoral, Suchanek et al. 2009).

Age groups eligible for screening differ across countries. Many countries only include those older than 50 years, while Bulgaria includes those older than 31 years and some countries, such as Finland and Sweden, only start at 60 years of age. Some countries, including Austria, Belgium, Bulgaria, Cyprus, the Czech Republic, Denmark, Germany, Greece, Hungary, Latvia, Slovakia,

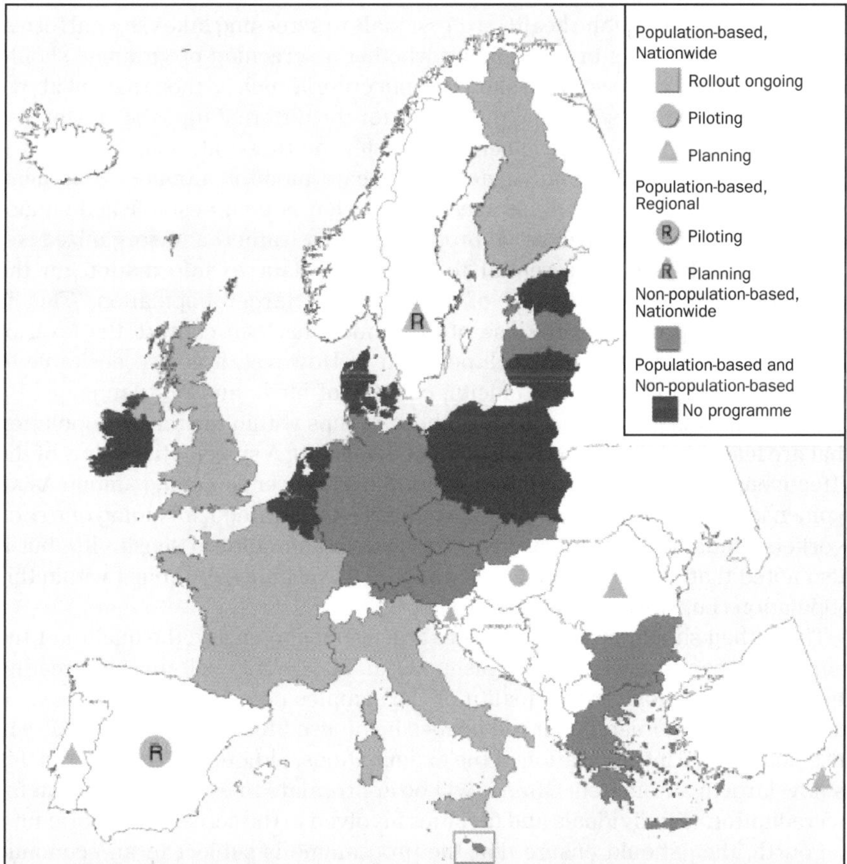

Figure 9.2 Distribution of colorectal cancer screening programmes based on the faecal occult blood test in the EU in 2007

Source: von Karsa, Anttila et al. (2008)

and Slovenia do not have upper age limits, Poland has an upper age limit of 65 years, Slovenia, Spain, and Sweden have a limit of 69 years, Hungary and Portugal of 70 years, and France and Romania of 74 years (Zavoral, Suchanek et al. 2009).

Countries also differ in the testing methods they use. The most common method of testing is the faecal occult blood test, testing stool for occult bleeding, which was the only test recommended by the European Council in 2003 (Council of the European Union 2003). However, several countries have also introduced screening colonoscopy, either as the only method or as the method of choice, such as in Germany and the Czech Republic (Zavoral, Suchanek et al. 2009). European guidelines for quality assurance in colorectal cancer screening and diagnosis were published in 2010 (von Karsa, Segnan et al. 2010).

The role of public health in screening programmes

The contribution of public health professionals to screening takes several forms. First, they have a role in determining whether a screening programme should be offered at all. To do so, they should apply criteria such as those set out above and follow European screening guidelines for the different types of cancer.

Second, they should implement a register of those at risk, linked to a comprehensive information system that can monitor uptake, treatment, and outcomes. Failure to do so means that what is being established cannot legitimately be described as a programme but rather a disorganized set of activities. It will be essential to link these data to information on the socio-economic characteristics of those in the target population. This is most commonly done by the use of postcodes that can capture the level of deprivation in the areas in which people live. However, it is also desirable to record information such as ethnicity, country of birth, and first language. By these means it is possible to identify those groups within the target population that are least likely to avail themselves of screening. A systematic review of the effectiveness of measures to increase uptake of cancer screening among Asian women identified the importance of a multifaceted strategy, including outreach workers, initiatives to increase ease of access, and cultural sensitivity, but it also noted that measures need to be tailored to specific sub-groups within this population (Lu, Moritz et al. 2012).

Third, they should ensure that there are systems to ensure the quality of the screening programme (Sauven, Bishop et al. 2003). This will involve creating mechanisms to monitor the quality of the samples obtained, as in the case of cervical cancer screening, or the images being used for mammography. It will also address the interpretation of the examinations, although in some cases this is now largely automated. Often it will be appropriate to establish a system for accreditation of individuals and facilities involved in the screening programme.

Fourth, they should ensure that the programme is subject to an economic evaluation. It will rarely be appropriate simply to take such an evaluation from another setting, as the baseline prevalence of disease may vary, as will the package of interventions necessary to deliver the screening programme and the cost of each element within the package.

Fifth, they should ensure that there are systems in place for monitoring the outcomes of the screening programme. For cancer screening, as a minimum, there should be a well-organized cancer registry. Unfortunately, even now the coverage of many countries by cancer registration is still inadequate (De Angelis, Francisci et al. 2009). There are, however, a number of challenges in monitoring outcomes. The most important is what is termed "lead time bias". This arises because the early detection of a cancer or a premalignant lesion will automatically increase the apparent incidence, even if there is no beneficial impact on mortality. This is simply because the patient will know that they have the cancer for longer but will die at the same time anyway. Similarly, rates of cancer detection may be misleading because some of those cancers may never progress to kill the patient. Thus, it is necessary to use a variety of variables to form a judgement about the effectiveness of a programme, unless it has been subject to a randomized controlled trial with a high degree of external validity.

Finally, public health professionals have a role to play in informing the public about the rationale for screening programmes, the underlying scientific evidence, clinical, epidemiological, and economic considerations, and clinical outcomes, including, where necessary, advising that they are inappropriate.

Conclusion

This chapter has shown how there have been major improvements in recent years, but, as far as available data make it possible to judge, that there is also much scope for further progress. Many European countries, including some of the wealthiest, have so far failed to set up screening programmes for cervical, breast, and colorectal cancer. Among those that have set up programmes, a major difference across countries is whether screening programmes are opportunistic or systematic. While some opportunistic screening programmes have achieved high coverage rates and resulted in health improvements, there is increasing recognition of the advantages associated with systematic, population-based screening activities.

There are many challenges in setting up screening programmes and moving to an integrated population-based model based on a comprehensive cancer plan to make sure that those diagnosed with cancer can be enrolled in treatment. To do so will require coordinated action by intergovernmental organizations, national and regional governments, health financing bodies, professional associations, health workers, and consumers. Effective communication will be crucial to inform the public about the opportunities and limitations associated with organized screening, helping patients to make informed choices. It will also be important to make the most of existing European networks against cancer. One of these is the European Partnership for Action Against Cancer (EPAAC), launched in 2009 by the European Commission, with the aim of bringing together a range of stakeholders from across Europe to exchange examples of good practice [http://www.epaac.eu/].

While ideally all people in Europe should have access to comprehensive screening programmes for the cancers discussed in this chapter, it is also necessary to acknowledge that financial and professional resources differ vastly across the WHO European Region. One way of dealing with this diversity is to adapt the frequency, diagnostic methods, and target populations of screening programmes to fit available country resources, following a cascade concept (Zavoral, Suchanek et al. 2009). This will make it possible to set up initially less ambitious programmes in resource-poor settings, which will start to provide health benefits to the population and which can then be gradually extended.

References

Anttila, A. and J. M. Martin-Moreno (2013). "Cancer screening." In *Successes and Failures of Health Policy in Europe: Four decades of divergent trends and converging challenges*. J. Mackenbach and M. McKee, Eds. Maidenhead, Open University Press: 179–192.

Anttila, A. and P. Nieminen (2007). "Cervical cancer screening program in Finland with an example on implementing alternative screening methods." *Collegium Antropologicum* **31**(Suppl. 2): 17–22.

Arbyn, M., J. Antoine, Z. Valerianova, M. Mägi, A. Stengrevics, G. Smailyte, O. Suteu and A. Micheli (2010). "Trends in cervical cancer incidence and mortality in Bulgaria, Estonia, Latvia, Lithuania and Romania." *Tumori* **96**(4): 517–523.

Arbyn, M., A. Anttila, J. Jordan, G. Ronco, U. Schenck, N. Segnan, H. G. Wiener, A. Herbert, J. Daniel and L. von Karsa, Eds. (2008). *European Guidelines for Quality Assurance in Cervical Cancer Screening*, 2nd edition. Luxembourg, Office for Official Publications of the European Communities.

Atun, R. and I. Olynik (2008). "Resistance to implementing policy change: the case of Ukraine." *Bulletin of the World Health Organization* **86**(2): 147–154.

Autier, P., M. Boniol and A. Gavin (2011). "Breast cancer mortality in neighbouring European countries with different levels of screening but similar access to treatment: trend analysis of WHO mortality database." *British Medical Journal* **343**: d4411.

Bleyer, A. (2011). "US breast cancer mortality is consistent with European data." *British Medical Journal* **343**: d5630.

Bleyer, A. and H. G. Welch (2012). "Effect of three decades of screening mammography on breast-cancer incidence." *New England Journal of Medicine* **367**: 1998–2005.

Bodamer, O. A., G. F. Hoffmann and M. Lindner (2007). "Expanded newborn screening in Europe 2007." *Journal of Inherited Metabolic Disease* **30**(4): 439–444.

Bothamley, G. H., L. Ditiu, G. B. Migliori, C. Lange and TBNET contributors (2008). "Active case finding of tuberculosis in Europe: a Tuberculosis Network European Trials Group (TBNET) survey." *European Respiratory Journal* **32**: 1023–1030.

Boyd, P. A., C. Devigan, B. Khoshnood, M. Loane, E. Garne and H. Dolk (2008). "Survey of prenatal screening policies in Europe for structural malformations and chromosome anomalies, and their impact on detection and termination rates for neural tube defects and Down's syndrome." *BJOG: An International Journal of Obstetrics and Gynaecology* **115**(6): 689–696.

Broeders, M., S. Moss, L. Nyström, S. Njor, H. Jonsson, E. Paap, N. Massat, S. Duffy, E. Lynge, E. Paci and EUROSCREEN Working Group (2012). "The impact of mammographic screening on breast cancer mortality in Europe: a review of observational studies." *Journal of Medical Screening* **19**(Suppl. 1): 14–25.

Council of the European Union (2003). Council Recommendation of 2 December 2003 on cancer screening. *Official Journal of the European Union* L 327/34–L 327/37.

De Angelis, R., S. Francisci, P. Baili, F. Marchesi, P. Roazzi, A. Belot, E. Crocetti, P. Pury, A. Knijn, M. Coleman and R. Capocaccia (2009). "The EUROCARE-4 database on cancer survival in Europe: data standardisation, quality control and methods of statistical analysis." *European Journal of Cancer* **45**(6): 909–930.

García-Armesto, S., M. Abadía-Taira, A. Durán, C. Hernández-Quevedo and E. Bernal-Delgado (2010). "Spain: health system review." *Health Systems in Transition* **12**(4): 1–295.

Gerkens, S. and S. Merkur (2010). "Belgium: health system review." *Health Systems in Transition* **12**(5): 1–266.

Giordano, L., L. von Karsa, M. Tomatis, O. Majek, C. deWolf, L. Lancucki, S. Hofvind, L. Nystrom, N. Segnan, A. Ponti and The Eunice Working Group (2012). "Mammographic screening programmes in Europe: organization, coverage and participation." *Journal of Medical Screening* **19**(Suppl. 1): 72–82.

Gotzsche, P. C., K. J. Jorgensen, P. H. Zahl and J. Maehlen (2012). "Why mammography screening has not lived up to expectations from the randomised trials." *Cancer Causes and Control* **23**(1): 15–21.

Gustafsson, L. and H. O. Adami (1989). "Natural history of cervical neoplasia: consistent results obtained by an identification technique." *British Journal of Cancer* **60**(1): 132–141.

Hakama, M., M. P. Coleman, D.-M. Alexe and A. Auvinen (2008). "Cancer screening." In *Responding to the Challenge of Cancer in Europe*. M. P. Coleman, D.-M. Alexe, T. Albreht and M. McKee, Eds. Ljubljana, Institute of Public Health of the Republic of Slovenia: 69–92.

Hewitson, P., P. Glasziou, L. Irwig, B. Towler and E. Watson (2007). "Screening for colorectal cancer using the faecal occult blood test, Hemoccult." *Cochrane Database Systematic Reviews* **1**: art. CD001216.

Holland, W. and S. Stewart (2005). *Screening in Disease Prevention: What works?* London, Nuffield Trust.

Holland, W., S. Stewart and C. Masseria (2006). *Screening in Europe*. Policy Brief. Copenhagen, WHO, on behalf of the European Observatory on Health Systems and Policies.

Independent UK Panel on Breast Cancer Screening (2012). "The benefits and harms of breast cancer screening: an independent review." *The Lancet* **380**(9855): 1778–1786.

International Agency for Research on Cancer (IARC) (2005). *Cervix Cancer Screening*. Lyon, IARC.

Kesic, V., M. Poljak and S. Rogovskaya (2012). "Cervical cancer burden and prevention activities in Europe." *Cancer Epidemiology, Biomarkers and Prevention* **21**: 1423–1433.

Lo Scalzo, A., A. Donatini, L. Orzella, S. Profili, A. Cicchetti, l. S. Profi and A. Maresso (2009). "Italy: health system review." *Health Systems in Transition* **11**(6): 1–216.

Lu, M., S. Moritz, D. Lorenzetti, L. Sykes, S. Straus and H. Quan (2012). "A systematic review of interventions to increase breast and cervical cancer screening uptake among Asian women." *BMC Public Health* **12**: 413.

Maier, C. B. and J. M. Martin-Moreno (2011). "Quo vadis SANEPID? A cross-country analysis of public health reforms in 10 post-Soviet states." *Health Policy* **102**(1): 18–25.

McCartney, M. (2012). *The Patient Paradox: Why sexed up medicine is bad for your health*. London, Pinter & Martin.

OECD/WHO (2011). *OECD Reviews of Health Systems: Switzerland*. Paris, OECD Publishing.

Perk, J., G. De Backer, H. Gohlke, I. Graham, Z. Reiner, W. Verschuren, C. Albus, P. Benlian, G. Boysen, R. Cifkova and C. Deaton (2012). "European guidelines on cardiovascular disease prevention in clinical practice (version 2012)." *European Heart Journal* **33**: 1635–1701.

Richardson, E., W. Boerma, I. Malakhova, V. Rusovich and A. Fomenko (2008). "Belarus: health system review." *Health Systems in Transition* **10**(6): 1–118.

Sauven, P., H. Bishop, J. Patnick, J. Walton, E. Wheeler and G. Lawrence (2003). "The National Health Service Breast Screening Programme and British Association of Surgical Oncology audit of quality assurance in breast screening 1996–2001." *British Journal of Surgery* **90**(1): 82–87.

Schröder, F. (2012). "Landmarks in prostate cancer screening." *BJU International* **110**(Suppl. 1): 3–7.

Strandberg-Larsen, M., M. Nielsen, S. Vallgårda, A. Krasnik, K. Vrangbæk and E. Mossialos (2007). "Denmark: health system review." *Health Systems in Transition* **9**(6): 1–164.

van Oortmarssen, G. J. and J. D. Habbema (1991). "Epidemiological evidence for age-dependent regression of pre-invasive cervical cancer." *British Journal of Cancer* **64**(3): 559–565.

von Karsa, L., A. Anttila, G. Ronco, A. Ponti, N. Malila, M. Arbyn, N. Segnan, M. Castillo-Beltran, M. Boniol, J. Ferlay, C. Hery, C. Sauvaget, L. Voti and P. Autier (2008). *Cancer Screening in the European Union: Report on the implementation of the Council Recommendation on cancer screening – First Report.* Brussels, European Commission.

von Karsa, L., N. Segnan and J. Patnick, Eds. (2010). *European Guidelines for Quality Assurance in Colorectal Cancer Screening and Diagnosis.* Luxembourg, Publications Office of the European Union.

West, N. J., C. Boustière, W. Fischbach, F. Parente and R. J. Leicester (2009). "Colorectal cancer screening in Europe: differences in approach; similar barriers to overcome." *International Journal of Colorectal Disease* **24**: 731–740.

Wilson, J. M. G. and G. Jungner (1968). *Principles and Practice of Screening for Disease.* Geneva, WHO.

World Health Organization (WHO) (2008). *2008–2013 Action Plan for the Global Strategy for the Prevention and Control of Noncommunicable Diseases.* Geneva, WHO.

World Health Organization (WHO) (2009). *Evaluation of Public Health Services in South-eastern Europe.* Copenhagen, WHO Regional Office for Europe.

World Health Organization (WHO) (2011). Regional Committee for Europe: Resolution EUR/RC61/12 – Action Plan for implementation of the European Strategy for the Prevention and Control of Noncommunicable Diseases 2012–2016. Baku, Azerbaijan, 15 September 2011. Copenhagen, WHO.

World Health Organization (WHO) (2012). *European Health for All Database*, August 2012 edition. Copenhagen, WHO Regional Office for Europe.

Wörmann, T. and A. Krämer (2011). "Communicable diseases." In *Migration and Health in the European Union.* B. Rechel, P. Mladovsky, W. Devillé, B. Rijks, R. Petrova-Benedict and M. McKee Maidenhead, Open University Press: 121–138.

Zavoral, M., S. Suchanek, F. Zavada, L. Dusek, J. Muzik, B. Seifert and P. Fric (2009). "Colorectal cancer screening in Europe." *World Journal of Gastroenterology* **15**(47): 5907–5915.

chapter ten

Health promotion

Bernd Rechel, Martin McKee

Introduction

This chapter provides an overview of health promotion practice and training in the European region of the World Health Organization (WHO). Many policies from across and beyond government can promote health (Mackenbach and Bakker 2003), but this chapter is limited to what might be termed formal health promotion activities, undertaken in organizations explicitly identified as undertaking health promotion.

The basis of modern health promotion can be traced to the 1974 report of the then Minister of Health in Canada, Marc Lalonde, on "New Perspectives on the Health of Canadians" (the Lalonde Report), which argued that, in order to promote the health of populations, it is necessary to go beyond a biomedical model and address factors such as the environment, as well as individual behaviours and lifestyles (Lalonde 1974). However, it was not until the 1980s that the term entered into widespread use (Minkler 1989), receiving a major boost from the 1986 Ottawa Charter for Health Promotion, which recognized the limits of traditional approaches to public health in the face of the rise of chronic and non-communicable diseases (Dempsey, Barry et al. 2011). Health promotion also embraced and developed the notion of "positive health", inspired by Aaron Antonovsky's work on "salutogenesis", which emphasizes factors that support human health and well-being, rather than those that cause disease (Antonovsky 1979). The Alma Ata Conference in 1978, with its emphasis on intersectoral action, was also instrumental in developing a new understanding of health and health promotion (Lloyd 2012).

The Ottawa Charter set out one of the best known and most widely used definitions of health promotion as "the process of enabling people to increase control over, and to improve, their health" (WHO, Health and Welfare Canada et al. 1986). In line with the Lalonde Report, it moved beyond the narrow focus on individual behaviours towards a positive conceptualization of health and a much broader concern with a wide range of social and environmental interventions. Furthermore, in line with the Alma Ata Declaration, the Ottawa Charter emphasized that health improvements depend on the existence of basic conditions and resources, including "peace, shelter, education, food, income, a stable eco-system, sustainable resources, social justice and equity" (WHO, Health and Welfare Canada et al. 1986). The charter identified the following key areas for action (WHO, Health and Welfare Canada et al. 1986):

- building healthy public policies in all sectors;
- creating supportive environments;
- strengthening community action;
- developing personal skills;
- reorienting health services towards health promotion.

A subsequent series of global health promotion conferences has advanced the thinking behind health promotion further (Baum, Ollila et al. 2013). There has also been an increasing recognition of the concerns of low- and middle-income countries. The Bangkok Charter for Health Promotion in a Globalized World, adopted at the Sixth Global Conference on Health Promotion in Bangkok in 2005, defined health promotion as "the process of enabling people to increase control over their health and its determinants, and thereby improve their health" (WHO 2005), placing a stronger emphasis on health determinants than the definition of health promotion contained in the Ottawa Charter. The Bangkok Charter further emphasized the importance of healthy public policies, government action across all sectors, and placing health promotion at the centre of the global development agenda.

The most recent Global Conference on Health Promotion, in Finland in 2013, further emphasized the concept of Health in All Policies, promoted previously by a Finnish government during its presidency of the European Union. This concept is defined as "an approach to public policies across sectors that systematically takes into account the health implications of decisions, seeks synergies, and avoids harmful health impacts in order to improve population health and health equity" (WHO 2013). The concept of Health in All Policies (HiAP) goes beyond the traditional intersectoral action, with more emphasis on multi-level policy-making and the need for understanding of the level of governance at which decisions are taken and the actors involved (Baum, Ollila et al. 2013).

The new European health policy framework and strategy, Health 2020, builds on these developments. It calls for action across government and society to achieve health and well-being, with the strategic objectives of improving health for all and reducing health inequities, and improving leadership and participatory governance for health (WHO 2012).

It is evident from these seminal documents that health promotion goes far beyond educating individuals about potentially harmful consequences of risky behaviours. Instead, it embraces many of the principles of modern public health, including a wider understanding of the determinants of health (the "causes of the causes") and new approaches to solving public health problems, such as through intersectoral action, healthy public policies, and HiAP (Dempsey, Barry et al. 2011). These aspects of modern public health are dealt with in greater depth in other chapters of this book (see Chapter 11, "Tackling the social determinants of health"; Chapter 12, "Intersectoral working"; Chapter

13, "Health impact assessment"). This chapter provides an overview of the organizational structures in place in Europe for health promotion activities, the integration of health promotion in health service provision, and the training of health promotion professionals.

Organizational structures

Almost every Ministry of Health in Europe has a unit responsible for health promotion and disease prevention. However, in some countries, in particular in central and eastern Europe, health promotion is still underdeveloped, with a narrow and often fragmented focus on topics such as HIV/AIDS or tobacco control, with little or no attention to non-communicable diseases and mental health (WHO 2009b). Furthermore, despite the international declarations on health promotion mentioned above and their emphasis on upstream approaches that address the determinants of health, most health promotion practice is concerned with individual lifestyles, risks, and behaviours (Lloyd 2012). In particular, in countries with conservative or neoliberal governments or political cultures, there has been a tendency, although with some notable exceptions, to take an individualistic approach, constraining health promotion to health education and the provision of other forms of information to allow healthier choices, while opposing what are often more effective approaches, such as regulation and fiscal measures.

Mapping capacity for health promotion at a national level is difficult because there is often considerable local variation (Mittelmark, Wise et al. 2006). Thus, the descriptions included in this chapter are, of necessity, generalizations. That said, it is clear from a study reviewing public health capacity in European Union (EU) member states that capacity for addressing health promotion and social determinants of health is generally viewed as comparatively weak (Aluttis, Chiotan et al. 2012). Furthermore, responsibilities for broader public health issues, such as action on behavioural and social determinants of health and health inequalities, were often less clearly defined than those for "traditional" areas of public health, such as communicable disease control, hygiene, and immunization (Aluttis, Baer et al. 2012). Not surprisingly, a review of health promotion research literature in the European Economic Area (EEA) in the period 1995–2005 found major differences in output across countries (Clarke, Gatineau et al. 2007). Nordic countries had the highest research output per head of population, while the United Kingdom had the highest overall output in health promotion literature. There was a weak inverse relationship of the number of publications with health need (measured as disability-adjusted life years per million population) ($r^2 = 0.07$) and a slightly stronger relationship with gross domestic product ($r^2 = 0.45$). This suggests that the quantity of health promotion research literature is not related to health needs, but instead is greater in richer countries where the need may be less, but the capacity to undertake public health research is greater. Major differences among European countries were also found with regard to mental health promotion policies. A study reviewing regions in 10 EU member states found that only three had started to develop mental health promotion policies (Ozamiz 2011).

Additional insights have been provided by a study on the political economy of health promotion. This found that statements supporting health-promoting activities were strongest in the "liberal" (e.g. United Kingdom and other English-speaking countries) and "social democrat" (e.g. Nordic countries) welfare states and weakest in the "Latin" (e.g. Spain, Italy, Greece) and "conservative" (e.g. France, Germany, Belgium) welfare states (Raphael 2013a). However, these statements were much more likely to be translated into policies in the social democrat states than in the others (Raphael 2013b). These findings are consistent with the analyses of performance on public health policy presented in Chapter 2, "The changing context of public health in Europe" (see also Mackenbach and McKee 2013).

In western Europe, some countries where health care is funded from social health insurance are expanding health promotion activities, which had previously been relatively weak (see Chapter 14, "Organization and financing of public health"). Countries such as Austria and Switzerland have established new foundations for health promotion (Schang, Czabanowska et al. 2011; Saltman, Allin et al. 2012). In Austria, there is now a national competence centre for health promotion, the Fund for a Healthy Austria. While these initiatives seek to strengthen health promotion, their overall impact has yet to be evaluated. Concerns include the placing of health promotion outside the public arena for policy-making, an emphasis on individual behaviours rather than structural measures to address health determinants, and the potential for conflicts of interest where funds are raised from activities such as gambling or sales of health-damaging products.

These developments reflect long-standing practice in Austria and Switzerland whereby health promotion activities have been outsourced to external institutions such as non-governmental organizations (NGOs) (Hofmarcher and Rack 2006; Ladurner, Gerger et al. 2011; OECD 2012). A similar situation exists in some other European countries where NGOs play a prominent role in areas such as tobacco control, prevention of drug use and hazardous alcohol consumption, suicide prevention, and promotion of mental health, with financing from national budgets, sometimes supplemented with EU funding. One of the challenges is how to evaluate the effectiveness and quality of these activities. Other challenges include how activities should be planned to reflect the needs of the population and ensure equitable access, and how to achieve sustainability and cooperation between NGOs and professional organizations. A number of European networks have emerged to exchange experience and advocate for action, including EuroHealthNet (originally the European Network for Health Promotion Agencies) and the European Public Health Alliance (EPHA).

As noted above, some of the most successful and most widely known health promotion activities have been implemented in the Nordic countries (Glenngård, Hjalte et al. 2005), although less so in Denmark (Strandberg-Larsen, Nielsen et al. 2007). In Finland, health promotion and disease prevention have been a main focus of health policy for decades, such as in the oft-cited North Karelia Project (Vuorenkoski, Mladovsky et al. 2008).

In central and eastern Europe and the countries of the former Soviet Union, health promotion was underdeveloped in the Soviet period (Saltman, Allin et al. 2012). Although the SANEPID services initially made huge progress in the fight against communicable diseases, they largely neglected health promotion and intersectoral action (WHO 2009b; Maier and Martin-Moreno 2011). However, paradoxically, preventive medicine was considered a key strength of the Semashko system. This largely relied on secondary prevention, aiming to detect diseases through a large number of often ineffective screening initiatives, rather than on primary prevention of non-communicable diseases (Richardson, Boerma et al. 2008; Gotsadze, Chikovani et al. 2010). In a number of countries of the region, such as Belarus (Richardson, Boerma et al. 2008), this approach has been retained and health promotion tends to be one of the most underdeveloped and underfinanced domains of public health (Maier, Palm et al. 2009). Public health services in many countries of the region continue to be more concerned with hygiene, sanitation, and traditional methods of communicable disease control, and less with health promotion and intersectoral action for health (Rechel and McKee 2006; Armenian, Crape et al. 2009; WHO 2009b).

There are, however, attempts to overcome this legacy. One example is Kazakhstan, which has established a wide-ranging programme of activity to encourage healthy lifestyles, although unhealthy lifestyles remain rampant (Katsaga, Kulzhanov et al. 2012). Most post-Soviet states have either enlarged the remits of existing public health systems to include health promotion or established new health promotion structures (Maier and Martin-Moreno 2011; Ministry of Health of the Republic of Uzbekistan 2011). In Kyrgyzstan, a Republican Centre for Health Promotion has been established, as well as a range of health promotion initiatives organized by village health communities with the participation of large numbers of volunteers (Maier, Palm et al. 2009; Ibraimova, Akkazieva et al. 2011; Maier and Martin-Moreno 2011). In countries such as Kyrgyzstan and Tajikistan, community health workers are key frontline providers of public health services, including health promotion (see Chapter 15, "Developing the public health workforce"). In Uzbekistan, health promotion, mainly consisting of the dissemination of information on public health issues, is entrusted to the Institute of Health and Medical Statistics (Ministry of Health of the Republic of Uzbekistan 2011). In Armenia, limited financial and human resources together with poorly defined roles and responsibilities mean that there are few state-sponsored health promotion activities and health promotion is most commonly conducted by international agencies, often on a sporadic and short-term basis (Armenian, Crape et al. 2009). In Estonia, systematic health promotion activities were launched in 1993, when the Ministry of Social Affairs decided to create a system for financing national and community-based health promotion projects (Koppel, Leventhal et al. 2009). The demand-driven system was financed from an earmarked share of the budget of the Estonian Health Insurance Fund and managed by a committee of experts making funding decisions and coordinating evaluation (see Chapter 14, "Organization and financing of public health").

In south-east Europe, most countries have some sort of health promotion activity in the area of communicable disease, in particular HIV/AIDS, as well as programmes on alcohol and tobacco use, but health promotion on non-communicable diseases is far less common and even non-existent in some countries (WHO 2009b). Despite many individual activities, health promotion is so far underdeveloped in this part of Europe, in particular with regard to non-communicable diseases and conventional risk factors (WHO 2007a, 2009b). In Croatia, the institutes of public health, at county level, are responsible for the majority of health-promoting activities. Croatia and Slovenia have been involved in the European Network of Health Promoting Schools since the early 1990s (WHO 2009b). For the adult population, health promotion activities in Croatia are more project-oriented, supported by local authorities and provided either by healthcare providers or NGOs (WHO 2007b). In Slovenia, health promotion was undertaken by public health institutes throughout the 1990s, but this was only formalized in 2003 (WHO 2009a). In the former Yugoslav Republic of Macedonia, a National Committee for Health Promotion was established in 2000 as an expert body with a multidisciplinary approach, but by 2007 was still not functioning (WHO 2007e). In Romania, there is a National Programme for Health Promotion (WHO 2007d). A particular challenge identified in several countries in south-east Europe is the lack of long-term and sustainable financing for health promotion activities, which is not linked to the financing of the rest of the health system (WHO 2009b).

Health promotion in health service provision

Historically, health services have focused on curative aspects and the treating of diseases. Only recently has there been increasing recognition that health services (both at primary care level and in hospitals) should pursue the wider objective of improving overall health. As the first point of contact with the health system, primary healthcare workers can play a crucial role in health promotion activities. In several countries, such as Bosnia and Herzegovina (WHO 2007c), they have been identified as the main implementers of health promotion activities. However, in many countries primary healthcare workers are insufficiently involved in health promotion activities, including in some countries of south-east Europe (WHO 2007a, 2009b), Uzbekistan (Ministry of Health of the Republic of Uzbekistan 2011), and Armenia (Armenian, Crape et al. 2009). Major barriers include a lack of incentives, as well as a high workload but limited resources (Armenian, Crape et al. 2009).

A survey of general practitioners in 11 European countries (Croatia, Estonia, Georgia, Greece, Ireland, Malta, Poland, Slovakia, Slovenia, Spain, and Sweden) found that more than half faced barriers in carrying out health promotion activities, such as lack of time and lack of additional reimbursement. There was substantial variation by countries (Brotons, Björkelund et al. 2005). Similar findings emerged in a survey of patients attending primary healthcare practices in 22 European countries in 2008–2009. The survey found that a high proportion of patients engaging in unhealthy lifestyles (especially those with high levels of alcohol consumption) did not perceive the need to change their lifestyle, and about half the patients reported not having had any discussion on healthy lifestyles with their GPs (Brotons, Bulc et al. 2012).

The importance of health promotion has also been recognized at other levels of care, including health-promoting hospitals and health services (HPH). The primary focus is on patients, but health workers and the local community are also targeted. This recognizes that hospitals and other healthcare settings are not only places where healing takes place, but can also cause harm to patients and health workers alike, such as through hospital-acquired infections or occupational health injuries (Rechel, Wright et al. 2009). The WHO has established an International Network on Health Promoting Hospitals and Health Services, consisting of coordinating institutions, participating hospitals and health services, and WHO Collaborating Centres. The network aims to facilitate information exchange, using tools such as newsletters, conferences, websites, an online library and activity database, as well as working groups and taskforces (WHO 2007f). Most hospitals and health service providers that are members of the network, however, are located in western Europe, where the initiative began. Coverage in the eastern part of the WHO European Region, where arguably the need is greatest, is still very thin.

Going beyond health services, many other health promotion innovations have emanated from Europe, including such initiatives as Healthy Cities and Health Promoting Schools, which have become global movements that support the implementation of innovative health promotion activities at the local level (Ziglio, Hagard et al. 2000). Another example is the European Network for Workplace Health Promotion (ENWHP), established in 1996 as an informal network of national occupational health and safety institutes, public health, health promotion, and statutory social insurance institutions. The network promotes good practice in workplace health promotion and advocates the adoption of such practice in all European workplaces (see Chapter 5, "Occupational health and safety"). These initiatives are consistent with the Ottawa Charter, which states that "health is created and lived by people within the settings of their everyday life; where they learn, work, play and love" (WHO, Health and Welfare Canada et al. 1986), also known as the settings-based approach. Healthy public policy was another principal objective of the Ottawa Charter, but intersectoral action is still limited in many countries (see Chapter 11, "Tackling the social determinants of health"; Chapter 12, "Intersectoral working"; Chapter 13, "Health impact assessment").

Training

A number of chapters in this volume show how diverse the training of public health workers is across Europe (see Chapter 6, "Environmental health"; Chapter 15, "Developing the public health workforce"). This also applies to the area of health promotion, where the workforce comes from a wide range of disciplines, often without any agreed training structure or career pathway (Dempsey, Barry et al. 2011). To date, there is no overall body to ensure quality standards for the training and professional practice of those involved in health promotion activities in Europe. At the same time, greater professionalization of health promotion practice has occurred in many countries, with the creation of posts at national, regional, and local level, with titles such as "local health planner", "public health coordinator", and "public health strategist". One area of skills development is "social marketing", the application of marketing techniques to change behaviour for social purposes, such as addressing smoking, alcohol consumption, and illicit drug use (French, Blair-Stevens et al. 2010).

Several attempts have been made to achieve more comparable qualifications and improved professional standards of health promotion workers in Europe. One of the most recent initiatives, funded by the European Commission and implemented between 2009 and 2012, was the project on "Developing competencies and professional standards for health promotion capacity building in Europe (CompHP)". The project aimed to develop competency-based standards and an accreditation system for health promotion practice, education, and training in the EU member and candidate countries. The project resulted in a framework of core competencies, consisting of 11 core domains and 68 core competency statements. The core competencies formed the basis for the development of professional standards and an accreditation framework (Barry, Battel-Kirk et al. 2012a, 2012b; Battel-Kirk, Van der Zanden et al. 2012). The PROMISE Project has developed guidelines for training of social and health professionals in mental health promotion (Greacen, Jouet et al. 2012). However, the multisectoral nature of health promotion suggests that the focus should be on achieving an appropriate mix of competencies in teams or organizations rather than requiring that each individual working in health promotion have all the relevant competencies.

Attempts by the International Union for Health Promotion and Education to establish a pan-European accreditation system aim to build on the experience in those European countries, such as Estonia, the Netherlands, and the United Kingdom, that have developed competencies, standards, and accreditation systems for health promotion, although these systems differ considerably from one country to the next. A European accreditation system could be a boost for the quality of health promotion training and practice across Europe (Santa-María Morales, Battel-Kirk et al. 2009).

Conclusion

Health promotion is an essential part of public health. However, as this chapter has shown, countries in Europe differ widely in how far they promote the health of their populations. This applies to health promotion activities, the integration of health promotion in health service provision, and the ways that countries have moved towards healthy public policies in other sectors. The training of professionals involved in health promotion activities also differs widely across countries. The scope for improvement seems to be largest in countries in central and eastern Europe and the former Soviet Union, but there is also much room for improvements in western Europe. In particular, it will be necessary to ensure the quality of health promotion programmes, with more equitable coverage and better use of emerging technologies.

To achieve progress in promoting the health of populations, it will also be essential to mobilize public support and engage all sectors of society in a coordinated manner. One of the most pressing challenges is to move beyond a narrow focus on individual lifestyles, risks, and behaviours towards upstream approaches that address the underlying determinants of health, whichever sector they emanate from. This is as much a political as a practical challenge.

References

Aluttis, C. A., C. Chiotan, M. Michelsen, C. Costongs, H. Brand, on behalf of the Public Health Capacity Consortium (2012). *Reviewing Public Health Capacity in the EU.* Maastricht, Maastricht University.

Antonovsky, A. (1979). *Health, Stress and Coping.* San Francisco, CA, Jossey-Bass.

Armenian, H. K., B. Crape, R. Grigoryan, H. Martirosyan, V. Petrosyan and N. Truzyan (2009). *Analysis of Public Health Services in Armenia.* Yerevan, American University of Armenia.

Barry, M. M., B. Battel-Kirk, H. Davison, C. Dempsey, R. Parish and M. Schipperen (2012a). *The CompHP Project Handbooks.* Paris, IUHPE.

Barry, M. M., B. Battel-Kirk and C. Dempsey (2012b). "The CompHP core competencies framework for health promotion in Europe." *Health Education and Behavior* **39**(6): 648–662.

Battel-Kirk, B., G. Van der Zanden, M. Schipperen, P. Contu, C. Gallardo, A. Martinez, S. Garcia de Sola, A. Sotgiu, M. Zaagsma and M. M. Barry (2012). "Developing a competency-based Pan-European accreditation framework for health promotion." *Health Education and Behavior* **39**(6): 672–680.

Baum, F., E. Ollila and S. Pena (2013). "History of HiAP." In *Health in All Policies: Seizing opportunities, implementing policies.* K. Leppo, E. Olilla, S. Pena, M. Wismar and S. Cook, Eds. Helsinki, Ministry of Social Affairs and Health, Finland: 25–42.

Brotons, C., C. Björkelund, M. Bulc, R. Ciurana, M. Godycki-Cwirko, E. Jurgova, P. Kloppe, C. Lionis, A. Mierzecki, R. Pineiro, L. Pullerits, M. R. Sammut, M. Sheehan, R. Tataradze, E. A. Thireos and J. Vuchak (2005). "Prevention and health promotion in clinical practice: the views of general practitioners in Europe." *Preventive Medicine* **40**: 595–601.

Brotons, C., M. Bulc, M. R. Sammut, M. Sheehan, C. Manuel da Silva Martins, C. Björkelund, A. J. Drenthen, D. Duhot, S. Görpelioglui, E. Jurgova, S. Keinanen-Kiukkanniemi, P. Kotányi, V. Markou, I. Moral, A. Mortsiefer, L. Pas, I. Pichler, D. Sghedoni, R. Tatardze, E. Thireos, L. Valius, J. Vuchak, C. Collins, E. Cornelis, R. Ciurana, P. Kloppe, A. Mierzecki, K. Nadaraia, M. Godycki-Cwirko (2012). "Attitudes toward preventive services and lifestyle: the views of primary care patients in Europe. The EUROPREVIEW patient study." *Family Practice* **29**: i168–i176.

Clarke, A., M. Gatineau, M. Thorogood and N. Wyn-Roberts (2007). "Health promotion research literature in Europe 1995–2005." *European Journal of Public Health* **17**(Suppl. 1): 24–28.

Dempsey, C., M. M. Barry, B. Battel-Kirk and CompHP Project Partners (2011). *Literature Review: Developing competencies for health promotion.* Paris, IUHPE.

French, J., C. Blair-Stevens, D. McVey and R. Merritt, Eds. (2010). *Social Marketing and Public Health: Theory and practice.* Oxford, Oxford University Press.

Glenngård, A., F. Hjalte, M. Svensson, A. Anell and V. Bankauskaite (2005). *Health Systems in Transition: Sweden.* Copenhagen, WHO Regional Office for Europe on behalf of the European Observatory on Health Systems and Policies.

Gotsadze, G., I. Chikovani, K. Goguadze, D. Balabanova and M. McKee (2010). "Reforming sanitary-epidemiological service in Central and Eastern Europe and the former Soviet Union: an exploratory study." *BMC Public Health* **10**: 440.

Greacen, T., E. Jouet, P. Ryan, Z. Cserhati, V. Grebenc, C. Griffiths, B. Hansen, E. Leahy, K. M. da Silva, A. Sabic, A. De Marco and P. Flores (2012). "Developing European guidelines for training care professionals in mental health promotion." *BMC Public Health* **12**: 1114.

Hofmarcher, M. and H.-M. Rack (2006). "Austria: health system review." *Health Systems in Transition* **8**(3): 1–247.

Ibraimova, A., B. Akkazieva, A. Ibraimov, E. Manzhieva and B. Rechel (2011). "Kyrgyzstan: health system review." *Health Systems in Transition* **13**(3): 1–152.

Katsaga, A., M. Kulzhanov, M. Karanikolos and B. Rechel (2012). "Kazakhstan: health system review." *Health Systems in Transition* **14**(4): 1–154.

Koppel, A., A. Leventhal and M. Sedgley, Eds. (2009). *Public Health in Estonia 2008: An analysis of public health operations, services and activities.* Copenhagen, WHO Regional Office for Europe.

Ladurner, J., M. Gerger, W. Holland, E. Mossialos, S. Merkur, S. Stewart, R. Irwin and J. Soffried, Eds. (2011). *Public Health in Austria: An analysis of the status of public health.* Copenhagen, WHO Regional Office for Europe on behalf of the European Observatory on Health Systems and Policies.

Lalonde, M. (1974). *A New Perspective on the Health of Canadians: A working document.* Toronto, Minister of Supply and Services Canada.

Lloyd, L. (2012). *Health and Care in Ageing Societies: A new international approach.* Bristol, Policy Press.

Mackenbach, J. P. and M. J. Bakker (2003). "Tackling socioeconomic inequalities in health: analysis of European experiences." *The Lancet* **362**(9393): 1409–1414.

Mackenbach, J. and M. McKee, Eds (2013). *Successes and Failures of Health Policy in Europe.* Buckingham, Open University Press.

Maier, C. B. and J. M. Martin-Moreno (2011). "Quo vadis SANEPID? A cross-country analysis of public health reforms in 10 post-Soviet states." *Health Policy* **102**(1): 18–25.

Maier, C., W. Palm, J. M. Martin-Moreno, D. Mircheva and M. Haralanova (2009). *The Reform of Public Health and the Role of the Sanitary-epidemiolgical Services (Sanepid) in the Newly Independent States.* Meeting report, Bishkek, Kyrgyzstan, 10–12 November 2008. Copenhagen, WHO Regional Office for Europe.

Ministry of Health of the Republic of Uzbekistan (2011). *Self-Assessment of Public Health Services in the Republic of Uzbekistan.* Technical report. Copenhagen, WHO Regional Office for Europe.

Minkler, M. (1989). "Health education, health promotion and the open society: an historical perspective." *Health Education Quarterly* **16**(1): 17–30.

Mittelmark, M. B., M. Wise, E. W. Nam, C. Santos-Burgoa, E. Fosse, H. Saan, S. Hagard and K. C. Tang (2006). "Mapping national capacity to engage in health promotion: overview of issues and approaches." *Health Promotion International* **21**(Suppl. 1): 91–98.

OECD (2012). *Health Data 2012* [stats.oecd.org, accessed 8 December 2012]. Paris, OECD.

Ozamiz, J. (2011). "Mental health promotion policies in Europe." *Journal of Mental Health* **20**(2): 174–184.

Raphael, D. (2013a). "The political economy of health promotion: Part 1, national commitments to provision of the prerequisites of health." *Health Promotion International* **28**(1): 95–111.

Raphael, D. (2013b). "The political economy of health promotion: Part 2, national provision of the prerequisites of health." *Health Promotion International* **28**(1): 112–132.

Rechel, B. and M. McKee (2006). "Health systems and policies in South-Eastern Europe." In *Health and Economic Development in South-Eastern Europe.* WHO, Ed. Paris, WHO: 43–69.

Rechel, B., S. Wright, N. Edwards, B. Dowdeswell and M. McKee, Eds. (2009). *Investing in Hospitals of the Future.* Copenhagen, WHO on behalf of the European Observatory on Health Systems and Policies.

Richardson, E., W. Boerma, I. Malakhova, V. Rusovich and A. Fomenko (2008). "Belarus: health system review." *Health Systems in Transition* **10**(6): 1–118.

Saltman, R., S. Allin, E. Mossialos, M. Wismar and E. van Ginneken (2012). "Assessing health reform trends in Europe." In *Health Systems, Health, Wealth and Societal Wellbeing*. J. Figueras and M. McKee, Eds. Maidenhead, Open University Press: 209–246.

Santa-María Morales, A., B. Battel-Kirk, M. Barry, L. Bosker, A. Kasmel and J. Griffiths (2009). "Perspectives on health promotion competencies and accreditation in Europe." *Global Health Promotion* **16**(2): 21–31.

Schang, L., K. Czabanowska and V. Lin (2012). "Securing funds for health promotion: lessons from health promotion foundations based on experiences from Austria, Australia, Germany, Hungary and Switzerland." *Health Promotion International* **27**(2): 295–305.

Strandberg-Larsen, M., M. Nielsen, S. Vallgårda, A. Krasnik, K. Vrangbæk and E. Mossialos (2007). "Denmark: health system review." *Health Systems in Transition* **9**(6): 1–164.

Vuorenkoski, L., P. Mladovsky and E. Mossialos (2008). "Finland: health system review." *Health Systems in Transition* **10**(4): 1–168.

World Health Organization (WHO) (2005). *The Bangkok Charter for Health Promotion in a Globalized World*. Geneva, WHO.

World Health Organization (WHO) (2007a). *Evaluation of Public Health Services in Bulgaria*. Draft National Report. Copenhagen, WHO Regional Office for Europe.

World Health Organization (WHO) (2007b). *Evaluation of Public Health Services in South-eastern Europe: Croatia*. Draft National Report. Copenhagen, WHO Regional Office for Europe.

World Health Organization (WHO) (2007c). *Evaluation of Public Health Services in South-eastern Europe: Federation of Bosnia and Herzegovina*. Draft National Report. Copenhagen, WHO Regional Office for Europe.

World Health Organization (WHO) (2007d). *Evaluation of Public Health Services in South-eastern Europe: Romania*. Draft National Report. Copenhagen, WHO Regional Office for Europe.

World Health Organization (WHO) (2007e). *Evaluation of Public Health Services in South-eastern Europe: The former Yugoslav Republic of Macedonia*. Draft National Report. Copenhagen, WHO Regional Office for Europe.

World Health Organization (WHO) (2007f). *The International Network of Health Promoting Hospitals and Health Services: Integrating health promotion into hospitals and health services. Concept, framework and organization*. Copenhagen, WHO Regional Office for Europe.

World Health Organization (WHO) (2009a). *Evaluation of Public Health Services in Slovenia*. Copenhagen, WHO Regional Office for Europe.

World Health Organization (WHO) (2009b). *Evaluation of Public Health Services in South-eastern Europe*. Copenhagen, WHO Regional Office for Europe.

World Health Organization (WHO) (2012). *Health 2020 Policy Framework and Strategy*. Copenhagen, WHO Regional Office for Europe.

World Health Organization (WHO) (2013). *Helsinki Statement on Health in All Policies*, adopted at the 8th Global Conference on Health Promotion, Helsinki, Finland, 10–14 June 2013. Geneva, WHO.

World Health Organization (WHO), Health and Welfare Canada and Canadian Public Health Association (1986). *Ottawa Charter for Health Promotion: An International Conference on Health Promotion. The Move Towards a New Public Health*, 17–21 November, Ottawa, Ontario, Canada [http://www.phac-aspc.gc.ca/ph-sp/docs/charter-chartre/pdf/charter.pdf, accessed 11 March 2013].

Ziglio, E., S. Hagard and J. Griffiths (2000). "Health promotion development in Europe: achievements and challenges." *Health Promotion International* **15**(2): 143–154.

chapter eleven

Tackling the social determinants of health

EuroHealthNet

Introduction

The social determinants of health belong to the so-called "wicked problems" (Rittel and Webber 1973) for public policy-makers and practitioners. Despite overwhelming evidence of the impact of social determinants on health, the need for complex, multisectoral solutions has presented a major challenge to action in every country in Europe. This chapter sets out how the necessary practical steps are nevertheless achievable, providing examples from the local, national, and international level.

The social determinants of health can be broadly defined as those factors that impact on health, or, as the WHO Commission on Social Determinants of Health put it:

> the conditions in which people are born, grow, live and age, including the health system. These circumstances are shaped by the distribution of money, power and resources at global, national and local levels. (Commission on Social Determinants of Health 2008)

The main causes of death, morbidity, and health inequalities are conditioned by social, environmental, and economic factors. Health systems play an important role, and access to healthcare, disease prevention, and health promotion services is a vital component of interventions, but the importance of coordinated and comprehensive policies and programmes to address the social determinants of health is increasingly being recognized.

It is clear that social, economic, and environmental factors play a significant part in determining individual and population health and its distribution. Having a sense of control over one's life and being free to choose, for example, has a positive impact on health and well-being (WHO 2013c). In 1978, the Alma Ata Declaration recognized the importance of economic and social development on health (WHO/UNICEF 1978). Healthy public policy was a key component of the 1986 Ottawa Charter for Health Promotion (WHO 1986), and was understood to include policies that have a health impact, such as those related to transport, education, and the economy (see Chapter 12, "Intersectoral working"; Chapter 13, "Health impact assessment"). More recent examples of the recognition of the importance of addressing the social determinants of health include the 2009 World Health Assembly resolution on "Reducing health inequities through action on the social determinants of health" (WHA 2009), the European Commission's 2009 communication on "Solidarity in health: Reducing health inequalities in the EU" (Commission of the European Communities 2009), and the WHO European Region's report on the social determinants of health in Europe (Marmot, Allen et al. 2012).

When addressing the social determinants of health, it is useful to distinguish between health inequalities and health inequities. Health inequalities are differences in health status or in the distribution of health determinants between different population groups. Examples include differences in morbidity between older and younger people, or differences in mortality between people from different social classes. Some health inequalities are due to biological variations, while others are related to individual choice or external conditions largely outside the control of individuals. Crucially, there are some health inequalities that are avoidable and result from unfair social and economic policies. These disparities in health can be defined as health inequities. Health equity, therefore, incorporates a notion of fairness and implies the aspiration that no one should be prevented from achieving his or her full health potential.

Since 1990, the WHO Regional Office for Europe has commissioned a series of technical documents and studies, clarifying concepts and principles on social determinants and equity in health, including work illustrating the major determinants of health and their interrelationships. Based on this concept, Dahlgren and Whitehead also set out a framework for action to reduce health inequities, including four broad areas (indicated by numbers 1–4 in Figure 11.1): strengthening individuals, strengthening communities, improving access to essential services, and encouraging macroeconomic and cultural change. Although implementation of the measures recommended was fragmented, a growing body of evidence and a series of recommendations for action were drawn up in the 2000s. In 2003, the WHO publication "The social determinants of health: Solid facts" (Wilkinson and Marmot 2003) presented decision-makers with clear evidence and policy options.

The impact of social determinants on health

The social, economic, and political conditions within a society determine the extent of its social stratification and, consequently, influence the extent of its health inequalities. Policies for sustainable economic growth and more equal income distribution, for example, have been shown to have a positive impact on health.

Material circumstances (e.g. housing, environment), psychosocial factors (e.g. negative life events, job insecurity), and the interactions between behavioural factors (e.g. diet, smoking, alcohol consumption) and biological

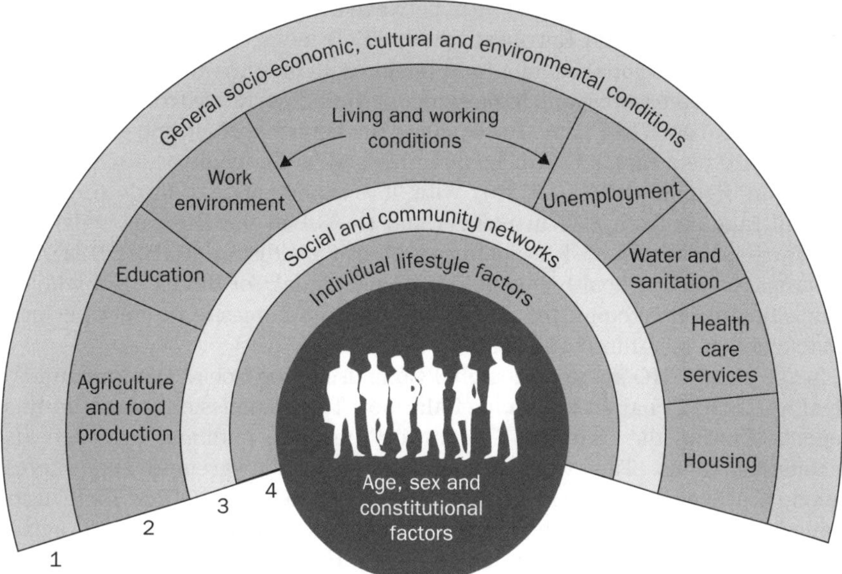

Figure 11.1 The main determinants of health

Source: Dahlgren and Whitehead (1993)

factors influence the distribution of health and well-being. The health system is a social determinant that can mitigate or worsen the effects that different material, psycho-social, and behavioural conditions can have on health.

People in lower social classes are exposed to greater risks to their health, including poorer living conditions (Eurofound 2007; Royal Commission on Environmental Pollution 2010), greater exposure to traffic and noise (European Environment State and Outlook UBA 2009), and feelings of stress and lack of control (Friedli 2009). Furthermore, the lower an individual's socio-economic status, the greater the likelihood of them engaging in risky behaviours, such as smoking (ASPECT Consortium 2004; Mackenbach, Meerding et al. 2007), poor diet, and low levels of physical activity. The poorest people in western Europe are also most likely to be obese (Robertson, Lobstein et al. 2007); more affluent people are more likely to have healthier diets (Nelson, Erens et al. 2007).

The unequal distribution of wealth and power leads to major variations within countries in terms of health and well-being. The relationship between socio-economic status and health has been described as the "social gradient": "a stepwise or linear decrease in health that comes with decreasing social position" (Marmot 2004). This social gradient has been identified in all countries as a common pattern for health and illness: the lower one's socio-economic position, the worse is one's health (Commission on Social Determinants of Health 2008).

Differences in life expectancy at birth between the lowest and the highest socio-economic groups within European Union (EU) member states (e.g. between manual and professional occupations, people with primary and post-secondary education, and the lowest and highest income quintiles) range from 4 to 10 years for men and from 2 to 7 years for women (Mackenbach, Meerding et al. 2007).

There are also major health inequalities across the countries of the WHO European Region (WHO 2013b), with life expectancy at birth for males in 2010 ranging from 80.4 in Switzerland to 63.1 in the Russian Federation and for females from 85.4 in Spain to 73.5 in Kazakhstan (WHO 2013a). The economic impact of health inequalities is substantial; for the EU as a whole it was estimated to account for a 9.5% loss in gross domestic product per year (Mackenbach, Meerding et al. 2007).

In 2005, the WHO set up the Global Commission on Social Determinants of Health (CSDH), chaired by Michael Marmot. The commission issued its final report, "Closing the Gap in a Generation", in 2008, outlining evidence and recommendations. This work stimulated renewed awareness and interest among European countries. In 2009, the WHO Regional Office for Europe commissioned a study on the impact of social determinants of health across Europe as part of its European health policy, Health 2020 (WHO 2011). When the final report is published (a summary is already available in *The Lancet*: Marmot, Allen et al. 2012), it will set out the current state of knowledge for work on social determinants of health in Europe. Its second interim report, published in 2011, included the following findings and recommendations (WHO Regional Office for Europe 2011):

- There are major health inequalities within and between all countries in Europe.
- These inequalities are mostly avoidable.
- Action is needed in view of the significant human and economic costs associated with poor health and premature mortality.
- Unless urgent action is taken, gaps between and within countries will widen.
- Action must be both systematic and sustained and is critical in responding to the global economic downturn, allocating resources for health and developing a new health policy for Europe.
- Action to reduce health inequalities is needed across all government sectors. Health ministries have a vital role to play, both in ensuring the contribution of the health system and in advocating for health equity in development plans, policies, and actions in other sectors. However, the health system alone cannot reduce health inequalities.
- Realizing the potential of health for all in Europe requires scaling up and systematizing action on social determinants of health and reducing health inequalities.

At a global level, the CSDH is also being followed up. A declaration on the required future steps has been agreed by WHO member states, together with a further resolution of the World Health Assembly, the 2012 Rio Political Declaration on Social Determinants of Health (WHA 2012), as well as online resources and case studies, incorporating approaches within and beyond health systems (WHO 2013a).

From evidence into action

The stark and persisting inequalities in health create an imperative to act; differences in social, economic, and environmental conditions are strongly influenced by the actions of governments, the private sector, and local communities. The CSDH report stated that: "We know enough to act" (Commission on Social Determinants of Health 2008). But what should this action entail?

Descriptions of health inequalities can focus on the poor health of socio-economically disadvantaged groups, health gaps between different groups of the population, and social gradients across whole populations (Graham 2004). This is not simply a technical matter, as the choice of approach can influence perceptions of success or failure (Judge, Platt et al. 2006). It is important for decision-makers to be clear about the rationale for focusing on particular aspects of inequality, taking account of their specific cultural, political, and social environment. Ideally, a holistic approach built around measures to tackle the "3 Gs" of inequities – groups, gaps, and gradient – is desirable. Taking a life-course perspective directs attention to how social determinants of health operate at every stage of development, from early childhood to adolescence and adulthood, to both immediately influence health (offering politically important short-term opportunities to evaluate the success of policies) and provide the basis for health or illness at later stages of the life-course (Davey Smith 2003).

The gradient concept argues that approaches should be based on "proportionate universalism": actions should be directed at all, but proportionate to the degree of disadvantage (*The Lancet* 2010). The universalism element is also important in view of the politically charged debate about social determinants of health. In some European countries, there is a powerful neoliberal agenda that portrays socially disadvantaged groups as the "undeserving" poor (McKee and Stuckler 2011).

The CSDH report provided some further guidance for approaches to address health inequities. It included the following priority recommendations (Commission on Social Determinants of Health 2008):

- Measure and understand the problem and assess the impact of action.
- Improve daily living and working conditions.
- Tackle the inequitable distribution of power, wealth, and resources.

The "causes of the causes" of ill health, and possible policy solutions, often require coordinated multisectoral action (see Chapter 12, "Intersectoral working"). For example, the current high levels of youth unemployment in many European countries have been called "a public health emergency" (Marmot 2012) because of their expected adverse impact on health inequities, already manifest as rising suicide rates in those facing job losses (Barr, Taylor-Robinson et al. 2012). The complex mechanisms and causal pathways that link these underlying causes with disease and premature death need to be understood to ensure the implementation of effective policies for reducing health inequities. Public health advocates need to play a leadership role within health systems, but also a facilitating, coordinating or "stewardship" role in wider public governance (see Chapter 16, "Developing public health leadership") and act as advocates for the poor and dispossessed.

International initiatives and support

The WHO Regional Office for Europe has played an important role in advising member states on approaches to reducing health inequities. In addition to its work on social determinants of health (see above), the establishment of the WHO European Office for Investment in Health, opened in Venice in 2003 (WHO Regional Office for Europe 2013), has given member states of the WHO Regional Office for Europe a focal point for guidance and support. Its publications "Concepts and principles for tackling social inequities in health: Levelling up Part 1" and "European strategies for tackling social inequities in health: Levelling up Part 2" (Dahlgren and Whitehead 2006; Whitehead and Dahlgren 2006) remain important reference documents.

For the EU, achieving a high level of health protection has been a stated objective since the 1992 Maastricht Treaty, even while leaving responsibility for the organization and delivery of health care with member states. However, the EU has the power, under the Treaties, to facilitate cooperation for the exchange of knowledge and one example has been a collaboration between willing states in 2011–2013, called the Joint Equity Action. It brings together participating states, regions, stakeholders, and experts to identify and take forward activities and initiatives in four specific areas:

- building evidence and monitoring systems;
- developing tools, such as equity impact assessments;
- strengthening sub-national and regional cooperation and contributions;
- partnering multisectoral stakeholders from civil society, the private sector, and other potential bodies.

At the level of both the EU and the wider WHO European Region, evidence, tools, and policy advice for addressing the social determinants of health are now more easily available than ever before. A web portal with searchable case studies and links (www.health-inequalities.eu) was developed by EuroHealthNet, a network of agencies involved in health promotion in Europe. It provides a resource of relevant EU research outcomes, as well as links to databases and other sources of information and evidence. Another web portal provides a policy evaluation tool developed by EU-funded research on "Tackling the gradient" (www.health-gradient.eu), specifically addressing inequities for young people and families. Policy-makers can also make use of health in all approaches (Olilla 2010) or methodologies from the project on "Crossing bridges", co-funded by www.eurohealthnet.eu from the EU Public Health Action Programme.

Other international stakeholders have also emerged. A People's Movement for Health has been set up in Europe, the European Public Health Alliance has launched a Charter for Health Equity (EPHA 2010), and regional networks and stakeholder initiatives are collaborating using such tools as the web portal of EuroHealthNet and the EU Joint Equity Action. Such partnerships are also being explored in EU joint actions and projects.

National policies and practices

By endorsing the World Health Assembly Resolution on Social Determinants of Health in 2009, countries worldwide have expressed a commitment to addressing health inequities "within and across countries through political commitment" (WHA 2009) and "to coordinate and manage intersectoral action for health in order to mainstream health equity in all policies, where appropriate, by using health and health equity assessment tools" (World Health Assembly 2009), even if the reality is somewhat different, especially in the wake of the global financial crisis (McKee, Karanikolos et al. 2012), as some governments seek to dismantle their welfare states.

This is alarming, given evidence that policy and practice can make a difference to health inequalities. A report published by the Scottish Government in 2010, "Long-term monitoring of health inequalities" (Scottish Government 2011) (Box 11.1), shows how health inequalities can decrease, remain stable, or

Box 11.1 National policies and practices: Scotland

Reducing inequalities has become a major government priority (EuroHealthNet 2013). In 2008 and 2009, the Scottish Government issued three related policy documents – "Equally Well", "The Early Years Framework", and "Achieving Our Potential"; each deals with the causes of health and social inequalities. A cross-ministerial working group for reducing inequalities is responsible for the preparation, implementation, and evaluation of strategic policy frameworks, led by the Ministry of Public Health and Sport. An initial report highlights the need for setting priorities at the local level. Community Planning Partnerships work to transform local services and address the causes that give rise to inequality.

Actions aimed at reducing inequalities in early childhood include a new framework for maternity care in Scotland and an accompanying policy for improving antenatal health. These policies aim to:

- reduce inequalities in maternal and infant health outcomes at birth and across the life course;
- measure improved access, care, and experience for all women, and prioritizing improvements for those at risk of poor health outcomes;
- develop tailored, proportionate, universal provision that identifies and facilitates access to specialist provision where needed.

"Improving Maternal and Infant Nutrition: A Framework for Action 2011–16" aims to improve the nutrition of mothers and infants in the broader context of improving the health and well-being of all. This framework is aimed at a variety of organizations with a role in improving maternal and infant nutrition, primarily the National Health Service (NHS), local authorities, employers, the community, and the voluntary sector, who have the most opportunity to influence culture and behaviour change.

increase over time. So who should be taking the responsibility to initiate policies addressing the social determinants of health? The baton rests, at least initially, with public health authorities and ministries of health, to draw public attention to the scale of the problem and advocate for action.

There are examples of proportionate universalism in action, such as enforcement of car seatbelt legislation or traffic calming measures in dense neighbourhoods. They offer benefits for the majority, while tackling in particular inequities along the social gradient. These policies also offer co-benefits for other sectors, such as housing or transport, and to health systems.

Approaches have varied greatly from one country to another, due to varying national contexts and political ideologies. They include measures in areas such as income redistribution, improvement of childhood conditions, work and working environments, health-related behaviours, health services, social inclusion, and territorial approaches (Mackenbach and Bakker 2003). One of the most notable national reviews on social determinants of health is the "Fair Society, Healthy Lives" report on England (Marmot, Allen et al. 2010). It encouraged a network of local authorities to take forward its recommendations, with the establishment of an Institute for Health Equity at University College London.

In some countries, provisions related to health inequalities and the social determinants of health are included in national health strategies, such as the National Population Health Plan in Estonia and the National Health Programme 2007–2015 in Poland. The Finnish Government resolution on the public health programme "Health 2015" contains explicit lines of action on health inequalities. Slovenia adopted a national strategy on health and development in 1996 and several of its regions have since adopted regional strategies on reducing health inequalities (Box 11.2). However, in several countries health policies that were once seen as a way forward have since been abandoned, due to a change of government.

Health strategies or policies alone, however, are insufficient. Most European countries claim to be doing something about inequalities, but this is often confined to identifying vulnerable groups or improving access to services. In contrast, Norway offers examples of approaches embedded across public policies. The education and employment sectors in Ireland, Norway (Box 11.3), Finland, and Spain are examples of European countries that have developed strategies promoting equal opportunities and inclusion for all. Strategies developed in the economic sector, the environment, urban and regional planning, neighbourhood renewal and housing in the United Kingdom, Netherlands, and Estonia are other examples of how it is possible to address the social determinants of health (EuroHealthNet 2008).

Many interventions and implementation mechanisms developed and implemented in European countries focus on the most disadvantaged, without considering the differences across the entire social gradient. As noted above, it can be crucial to sustainability, ownership, engagement of all partners, and political commitment that gradients are acknowledged; this benefits everybody.

Box 11.2   National policies and practices: Slovenia

Slovenia has a coordinated approach for reducing inter-regional health inequalities resulting from poor socio-economic status. Each region in Slovenia has prepared a regional strategy for tackling health inequalities, built on similar aims and objectives, but including also specific objectives, based on a methodology developed within the programme on "Investment in health and development in Pomurje – MURA".

The public health section of the Ministry of Health took the lead on advocacy and the raising of awareness, identifying concrete ways to integrate health into broader development agendas, and creating partnership with other sectors. The programme includes three approaches to reducing health inequities: the population approach (which works across the entire social gradient with the aim of improving the health status for all), action for reducing the gap between the most economically disadvantaged and the most privileged groups, and targeted interventions for vulnerable groups.

Intersectoral collaboration was supported by coordination mechanisms at the national and regional levels and joint policy planning of priorities, i.e. improving healthy lifestyles, increasing healthy food production and distribution, developing healthy tourism, preserving the natural and cultural heritage, and reducing the ecological burden. A new strategic action plan was prepared for each financial period (2000–2006 and 2007–2013), as well as integrated key working areas for the regional development programme (Buzeti, Djomba et al. 2011; EuroHealthNet 2013).

It will also be important to improve the availability of data. Few countries in Europe engage in the systematic monitoring and analysis of social inequities in health and, in some, such as France and Germany, there are severe obstacles to collecting any data on ethnic minorities, among whom social disadvantage is often concentrated. Beyond these extreme examples, comparable data and indicators that could be used to measure and describe health inequities are not routinely collected across Europe (Aluttis, Chiotan et al. 2013). Those data that do exist are under-utilized, and in many countries there is little capacity to perform complex analyses and identify health inequalities.

It is also important to realize that the power of central governments is far from absolute. In many countries, power to act on health determinants have been devolved to regional, city or local administrations, where the impact of social determinants is most keenly felt. The CSDH recommendation to improve living and working conditions across the social gradient is being addressed actively by numerous bodies in many European countries. This includes localized reviews (as in southern Sweden) or scaling up well-evaluated regional initiatives (such as the national strategic approach in Slovenia, following pilot

Box 11.3   National policies and practices: Norway

The Norwegian national strategy for reducing social inequalities in health is a good example of a comprehensive intersectoral policy (EuroHealthNet 2013). The Norwegian Directorate for Health and Social Affairs has developed an intervention map that identifies strategic entry points taking into account universal and selective approaches:

	Social reform Upstream	Risk reduction Midstream	Effect reduction Downstream
Universal measures	Public system for education, taxes, labour market policies, etc.	Working and living environment, broad lifestyle measures, etc.	Health system
Selective measures	Means-tested social benefits, etc.	Targeted lifestyle measures, etc.	Targeted health services

Source: Torgersen, Giæver et al. (2007)

The priorities of the Norwegian strategy are to:

- reduce social inequalities that contribute to inequalities in health, including in the areas of income, education, employment and working conditions;
- reduce social inequalities in health-related behaviour and use of health services;
- provide targeted initiatives to promote social inclusion;
- develop knowledge and cross-sectoral tools.

In the National Health and Care Plan (2011–2015), the Norwegian government outlined further specific policy measures and goals for an increase in quality-adjusted life years and a reduction of social inequalities in health.

work in Mursk-Sobota and other regions). The WHO "Healthy Cities" and "Regions for Health" networks champion and support such approaches as part of the European health policy Health 2020.

Public health professionals play a vital role for initiating interventions, providing the evidence base, leadership and advocacy, supporting planning and monitoring, and sustaining efforts over time. However, it can be more effective to set up cross-departmental or cross-sectoral initiatives with mutual goals, supported by public health professionals, but led at senior levels by non-health professionals. This can bring new perspectives to difficult challenges, widen accountability and ownership, and remove barriers of terminology and culture that actions led primarily by public health professionals often encounter.

Conclusions

Tangible steps are being taken at international, national, and sub-national level towards measuring and understanding the problem of social determinants of health. However, so far, progress has been slow, variable and insufficient, and ambitious national or international targets have not been achieved. Reasons include the lack of sustained political commitment and the failure to secure the involvement of relevant stakeholders. Localized or community-based approaches have shown promising outcomes, but scaling them up to whole countries is complex and requires additional structures and legislation; strategies alone are insufficient. Yet, methodologies on the implementation of systematic approaches to health equity impact assessments (see Chapter 13), intersectoral collaboration (see Chapter 12), private–public partnerships, and health in all policies are increasingly available.

The current economic crisis is likely to have a strong impact on health inequalities, with a human cost that is as yet difficult to gauge (Figueras and McKee 2012). Its magnitude and effects vary between and within countries, as does the capacity of welfare systems to provide adequate protection. The crisis has aggravated poverty and social exclusion, affecting mental and physical health, and pressure is increasing on public and voluntary services. The economic crisis threatens to deepen health inequalities, especially in countries and regions where protective measures and policies are not in place (European Commission 2010).

The CSDH argued that processes of globalization and marketization, driven largely by powerful corporate vested interests, are another social determinant of poor health, although some critics have argued that this fails to recognize the benefits the private sector could bring. While acknowledging the many risks associated with private–public partnerships, and the need to build partnerships on top of a strong regulatory framework, there remains scope for involving some private and third-sector actors without infringing public health values. If, for example, local entrepreneurs and public health bodies can be brought as partners into the planning of community initiatives that improve employment and the local environment, this is likely to benefit health equity without having negative impacts. Crucially, the CSDH recommendation to reduce the inequitable distribution of power, wealth, and resources underlines the importance of addressing those factors behind the social gradient. Until that is achieved, inequities will persist.

However, the lack of adequate information and evaluation systems means that much of the impact still remains poorly understood. In view of the broader lack of data on social inequities, European countries should aim to introduce disaggregated indicators for equity, as well as equity impact assessments for planning and audit processes (see Chapter 13).

While better data systems are being established, existing knowledge can be used to inform short-term interventions that meet goals within the time-frames of political cycles. These interventions usually focus on equitable approaches to lifestyle factors such as smoking, obesity or alcohol, or on early child development. However, community-based interventions involving multisectoral planning and implementation offer promising pathways, particularly when closely integrated with clear societal and economic needs, such as tackling poverty, youth unemployment, migration, ageing, education, crime, transport or housing. Involvement of public health, by engaging within and beyond health systems (for example, in human resources planning for health and care systems or integrated neighbourhood policies), is a crucial way of demonstrating mutual benefits for policy and investment. Whether public health advocates, who can only direct very small proportions of public expenditure, have the capacity and political support to initiate the required measures is however in many countries doubtful.

References

Aluttis, C., C. Chiotan, K. Michelsen, C. Costongs and H. Brand (2013). *Review of Public Health Capacity in the EU*. Luxembourg, European Commission Directorate General for Health and Consumers.

ASPECT Consortium (2004). *Tobacco or Health in the European Union: Past, present and future*. Brussels, European Commission [http://ec.europa.eu/health/ph_determinants/life_style/Tobacco/Documents/tobacco_fr_en.pdf, accessed 9 May 2013].

Barr, B., D. Taylor-Robinson, A. Scott-Samuel, M. McKee and D. Stuckler (2012). "Suicides associated with the 2008–2010 recession in the UK: a time-trend analysis." *British Medical Journal* **345**: e5142.

Buzeti, T., J. Djomba, M. Blenkus and M. Ivanusa (2011). *Health Inequalities in Slovenia*. Copenhagen, WHO Regional Office for Europe.

Commission of the European Communities (2009). Communication from the Commission to the European Parliament, the Council, the European Economic and Social Committee and the Committee of the Regions on solidarity in health: reducing health inequalities in the EU. Brussels, Commission of the European Communities [http://ec.europa.eu/health/ph_determinants/socio_economics/documents/com2009_en.pdf, accessed 9 May 2013].

Commission on Social Determinants of Health (2008). *Closing the Gap in a Generation: Health equity through action on the social determinants of health*. Final Report of the Commission on Social Determinants of Health. Geneva, WHO.

Dahlgren, G. and M. Whitehead (1993). *Tackling Inequalities in Health: What can we learn from what has been tried?* Working paper prepared for the King's Fund International Seminar on Tackling Inequalities in Health, September 1993, Ditchley Park, Oxfordshire. London, King's Fund.

Dahlgren, G. and M. Whitehead (2006). *Levelling Up (Part 2): A discussion paper on European strategies for tackling social inequities in health*. Brussels, WHO Collaborating Centre for Policy Research on Social Determinants of Health, University of Liverpool [http://www.who.int/social_determinants/resources/leveling_up_part2.pdf, accessed 9 May 2013].

Davey Smith, G. (2003). *Health Inequalities: Lifecourse Approaches*. Bristol, Policy Press.

Eurofound (2007). *European Foundation for Living and Working Conditions Second Survey* [http://www.eurofound.europa.eu/surveys/eqls/2007/index.htm, accessed 9 May 2013].

EuroHealthNet (2008). *DETERMINE Consortium: Policies and actions addressing the socio-economic determinants of health inequalities – examples of activity in Europe* [http://www.publichealth.ie/sites/default/files/documents/files/Working%20 document%201%20%5BExamples%20of%20activity%20in%20Europe%5D.pdf].

EuroHealthNet (2013). *European Portal for Action on Health Inequalities* [http://www. health-inequalities.eu/HEALTHEQUITY/EN/policies/policy_database/, accessed 11 July 2013].

European Commission (2010). *Draft Joint Report on Social Protection and Social Inclusion* [http://ec.europa.eu/social/keyDocuments.jsp?pager.offset=10&langId=e n&mode=advancedSubmit&advSearchKey=Joint Report on Social protection and social inclusion, accessed 9 May 2013].

European Environment State and Outlook UBA (2009). *The German Environmental Survey (GerES) for Children 2003/2006: Noise.* Environment 7 Health 01/200.

European Public Health Alliance (EPHA) (2010). *Launch of the European Charter for Health Equity: Together for more equity in health* [http://www.epha.org/spip. php?article4333, accessed 9 May 2013].

Figueras, J. and M. McKee (2012). *Health Systems, Health, Wealth and Societal Well-being: Assessing the case for investing in health systems.* Maidenhead, Open University Press [http://www.euro.who.int/__data/assets/pdf_file/0007/164383/ e96159.pdf, accessed 9 May 2013].

Friedli, L. (2009). *Mental Health, Resilience and Inequalities.* Copenhagen, WHO Regional Office for Europe.

Graham, H. (2004). "Tackling health inequalities in England." *Journal of Social Policy* **33**(1): 115–131.

Judge, K., S. Platt, C. Costongs and K. Jurczak (2006). *Health Inequalities: A challenge for Europe.* Independent expert report commissioned by the UK Presidency of the EU. London, COI for the Department of Health.

Mackenbach, J., W. J. Meerding and A. Kunst (2007). *Economic Implications of Socio-economic Inequalities in Health in the European Union* [http://ec.europa.eu/ health/ph_determinants/socio_economics/documents/socioeco_inequalities_en.pdf, accessed 9 May 2013]. Brussels, European Commission.

Mackenbach, J. P. and M. J. Bakker (2003). "Tackling socioeconomic inequalities in health: analysis of European experiences." *The Lancet* **362**(9393): 1409.

Marmot, M. (2004). *Status Syndrome.* London, Bloomsbury.

Marmot, M. (2012). Presentation to the 8th Annual World Health Care Congress Europe, Amsterdam, 23–24 May.

Marmot, M., J. Allen, R. Bell, E. Bloomer and P. Goldblatt (2012). "WHO European review of social determinants of health and the health divide." *The Lancet* **380**(9846): 1011–1029.

Marmot, M., J. Allen, P. Goldblatt, T. Boyce, D. McNeish, M. Grady and I. Geddes (2010). *Fair Society, Healthy Lives: Strategic review of health inequalities in England post-2010* [http://www.instituteofhealthequity.org/Content/FileManager/pdf/ fairsocietyhealthylives.pdf, accessed 9 May 2013].

McKee, M., M. Karanikolos, P. Belcher and D. Stuckler (2012). "Austerity: a failed experiment on the people of Europe." *Clinical Medicine* **12**: 346–350.

McKee, M. and D. Stuckler (2011). "The assault on universalism: how to destroy the welfare state." *British Medical Journal* **343**: d7973.

Nelson, M., B. Erens, B. Bates, S. Church and T. Boshier (2007). *Low Income Diet and Nutrition Survey 2007.* London, Foods Standards Agency.

Olilla, E. (2010). "Health in all policies from rhetoric to action." *Scandinavian Journal of Public Health* **39**(6): 11–18.

Rittel, H. W. J. and M. M. Webber (1973). "Dilemmas in a general theory of planning." *Policy Sciences* 4(2): 155–169.

Robertson, A., T. Lobstein and C. Knai (2007). *Obesity and Socio-economic Groups in Europe: Evidence review and implications for action*. Brussels, European Commission [http://ec.europa.eu/health/ph_determinants/life_style/nutrition/documents/ev20081028_rep_en.pdf, accessed 9 May 2013].

Royal Commission on Environmental Pollution (2010). *The European Environment, State and Outlook, Synthesis 2010: The urban environment*, 26th Report. London, Royal Commission on Environmental Pollution.

Scottish Government (2011). *Long-Term Monitoring of Health Inequalities* [http://www.scotland.gov.uk/publications/2011/10/21133633/0, accessed 9 May 2013]. Edinburgh, The Scottish Government.

The Lancet (2010). "Health equity – an election manifesto?" *The Lancet* **375**(9714): 525.

Torgersen, T. P., Ø. Giæver and O. T. Stigen (2007). *Developing an Intersectoral National Strategy to Reduce Social Inequalities in Health – The Norwegian case*. Copenhagen, WHO Regional Office for Europe.

Whitehead, M. and G. Dahlgren (2006). *Levelling Up (Part 1): A discussion paper on concepts and principles for tackling social inequities in health*. Liverpool, WHO Collaborating Centre for Policy Research on Social Determinants of Health [http://www.who.int/social_determinants/resources/leveling_up_part1.pdf, accessed 9 May 2013].

Wilkinson, R. and M. Marmot (2003). *Social Determinants of Health: The solid facts*. Copenhagen, WHO Regional Office for Europe [http://www.euro.who.int/__data/assets/pdf_file/0005/98438/e81384.pdf, accessed 9 May 2013].

World Health Assembly (WHA) (2009). *Reducing Health Inequities through Action on the Social Determinants of Health* [http://apps.who.int/gb/ebwha/pdf_files/A62/A62_R14-en.pdf, accessed 9 May 2013]. Geneva, WHA.

World Health Assembly (WHA) (2012). W*orld Health Assembly Endorses the Rio Political Declaration on Social Determinants of Health* [http://www.who.int/sdhconference/background/en/index.html, accessed 9 May 2013]. Geneva, WHA.

World Health Organization (WHO) (1986). *The Ottawa Charter for Health Promotion* [http://www.who.int/healthpromotion/conferences/previous/ottawa/en/index4.html]. Geneva, WHO.

World Health Organization (WHO) (2011). *Health 2020* [http://www.euro.who.int/en/what-we-do/event/first-meeting-of-the-european-health-policy-forum/health-2020]. Copenhagen, WHO Regional Office for Europe.

World Health Organization (WHO) (2013a). *European Health for All Database*, January 2013 edition. Copenhagen, WHO Regional Office for Europe.

World Health Organization (WHO) (2013b). *The European Health Report 2012: Charting the way to well-being*. Copenhagen, WHO Regional Office for Europe.

World Health Organization (WHO) (2013c). *Social Determinants of Health – Action: SDH* [http://www.who.int/social_determinants/actionsdh/en/, accessed 9 May 2013]. Geneva, WHO.

World Health Organization (WHO)/UNICEF (1978). Report of the International Conference on Primary Health Care Geneva, World Health organization, UNICEF (http://www.unicef.org/about/history/files/Alma_Ata_conference_1978_report.pdf accessed 09 May 2013).

World Health Organization (WHO) Regional Office for Europe (2011). *Interim Second Report on Social Determinants of Health and the Health Divide in the WHO European Region*. Copenhagen, WHO Regional office for Europe [http://www.euro.who.int/__data/assets/pdf_file/0010/148375/id5E_2ndRepSocialDet-jh.pdf, accessed 9 May 2013].

World Health Organization (WHO) Regional Office for Europe (2013). *WHO European Office for Investment for Health and Development, Venice, Italy* [http://www.euro.who.int/en/who-we-are/who-european-office-for-investment-for-health-and-development,-venice,-italy, accessed 9 May 2013]. Copenhagen, WHO Regional Office for Europe.

chapter twelve

Intersectoral working and Health in All Policies

Matthias Wismar,
Jose M. Martin-Moreno

Introduction

Intersectoral working is common in public health practice in Europe, as several chapters in this volume demonstrate. Environmental health, occupational health, health promotion, tackling the social determinants, food security, and health impact assessment all imply some degree of intersectoral action. The need for intersectoral working has been politically acknowledged by many international documents and resolutions, such as the Declaration of Alma-Ata (WHO 1978). More recently, conceptual debate and political action on intersectoral work has focused on Health in All Policies (HiAP) (Box 12.1).

Many of the determinants of health are shaped by other ministries (see Chapter 11, "Tackling the social determinants of health"), which often

Box 12.1   Definition of HiAP

Health in All Policies (HiAP) is an approach to public policies across sectors that systematically takes account of the health and health systems implications of decisions, seeks synergies, and avoids harmful health impacts, in order to improve population health and health equity. A HiAP approach is founded on health-related rights and obligations. It emphasizes the consequences of public policies on health determinants, and aims to improve the accountability of policy-makers for health impacts at all levels of policy-making.

Source: Ollila, Baum et al. (2013), adapted from WHO Working Definition prepared for the 8th Global Conference on Health Promotion, Helsinki, 10–14 June 2013

have objectives that are unrelated to or at odds with those of ministries of health. Alcohol control policy illustrates this point (Kemm 2007). The causal links influencing alcohol consumption, health, and behaviour provide multiple entry points for alcohol control policies. However, most of these entry points fall within the remit of the ministries responsible for taxes, retail trade, transport, education, economic development, criminal justice, agriculture, and social welfare. These ministries pursue different objectives – they may want to stimulate economic activity, enhance mobility or provide security. Some of these objectives may be conducive to health, whereas others are unrelated or even detrimental to health. An added complication for national ministries of health may be that certain competencies, such as for education and trade, are outside the scope of national governments and are the responsibility of regional governments or supranational organizations, such as the European Union or the World Trade Organization.

Development of intersectoral health policies

Intersectoral health policies have a long history, dating back to the vision of Health for All (HFA) set forth in the Alma Ata Declaration (WHO 1978), the European HFA policy (WHO Regional Office for Europe 1985), and its later revisions (WHO Regional Office for Europe 1999). The new European health policy Health 2020, adopted in 2012, also emphasizes the need to tackle the social determinants of health (WHO Regional Office for Europe 2013). This continuing interest in tackling the social determinants of health has necessitated a better understanding of intersectoral work, in particular intersectoral governance. Health in All Policies (HiAP), the whole-of-government approach (Box 12.2), and the whole-of-society approach (Box 12.3) are part of this debate.

Box 12.2   WHO definition of the whole-of-government approach

Whole-of-government activities are multi-level (from local to global) government actions, which are also increasingly involving groups outside government. This approach requires building trust, common ethics, a cohesive culture, and new skills. It stresses the need for better coordination and integration, centred on the overall societal goals for which the government stands. In countries with federal systems or in which the regional and local levels are politically autonomous, extensive consultations across levels of government can strengthen whole-of-government approaches. Accountability is required at all levels and in all systems.

Source: WHO Regional Office for Europe (2013)

Box 12.3 WHO definition of the whole-of-society approach

A whole-of-society approach goes beyond institutions: it influences and mobilizes local and global culture and media, rural and urban communities, and all relevant policy sectors, such as the education system, the transport sector, the environment and even urban design, as demonstrated in the case of obesity and the global food system. Whole-of-society approaches are a form of collaborative governance that can complement public policy. They emphasize coordination through normative values and the building of trust among a wide variety of actors. By engaging the private sector, civil society, communities, and individuals, the whole-of-society approach can strengthen the resilience of communities to withstand threats to their health, security, and well-being.

Source: WHO Regional Office for Europe (2013)

Several exercises to map intersectoral policies in European countries have been conducted, with varying geographical foci and analytical dimensions (van de Water and van Herten 1998; Busse and Wismar 2002; Wismar and Busse 2002). For the update of the European HFA policy in 2005, WHO commissioned an exercise to map uptake of HFA policies (WHO Regional Office for Europe 2005). To be included in the mapping exercise, policies had to cover several sectors, be value-based, use health targets, and be stipulated in a document. This study found that many countries had drawn up and adopted HFA policies, while some were in the course of developing such policies at the time of the research. The mapping exercise also collected health policy developments from the regional and local level, finding that many countries that have HFA policies at the national level also have sub-national HFA policies.

The new European health policy, Health 2020, identified four interlinked priority areas for specific action, based on priorities of member states, as well as their capacities to address them:

- investing in health throughout the life-course;
- tackling non-communicable and communicable diseases;
- strengthening people-centred health systems, public health capacity and emergency preparedness, surveillance and response; and
- creating resilient communities and supportive environments.

By creating and strengthening partnerships, including those with important supranational actors such as the EU, the WHO Regional Office for Europe hopes to foster a political and social environment in which health occupies a more prominent place in policy-making across the spectrum of government.

Health 2020 places the responsibility for health on society as a whole, but recognizes the particular role governments need to play. Ambitious in its scope, but cognizant of the inherent difficulties in making leaders from different sectors – as well as industry, communities, and individuals – responsible for population health, Health 2020 offers a touchstone for intersectoral policies

Box 12.4   The Millennium Development Goals

- MDG 1: Eradicate extreme poverty and hunger
- MDG 2: Achieve universal primary education
- MDG 3: Promote gender equality and empower women
- MDG 4: Reduce child mortality rates
- MDG 5: Improve maternal health
- MDG 6: Combat HIV/AIDS, malaria, and other diseases
- MDG 7: Ensure environmental sustainability
- MDG 8: Develop a global partnership for development

across the European region. Operationally, however, it has to overcome a number of difficulties, including the vast differences between European countries in public health capacities, before its strategic objectives can be translated into national policies.

The United Nations (UN) has also influenced intersectoral work in the countries of the WHO European Region, in particular in some of the poorer countries in the former Soviet Union. At the heart of the UN's approach to development lie the Millennium Developments Goals (MDGs). In 2000, the 193 UN member states, along with 23 international organizations, agreed to work towards the eight MDGs (see Box 12.4) and 21 associated targets by 2015.

MDGs 4–6 are health goals, recognizing the role of health as a precondition for development. The remaining MDGs, in particular those related to poverty and hunger, but also primary education and gender equality, are health-related and address key social determinants of health.

For EU member states, the EU's mandate for intersectoral work is stipulated in Article 168 of the Treaty on the Functioning of the European Union, according to which a "high level of human health protection shall be ensured in the definition and implementation of all Union policies and activities" (European Union 2010). The article was introduced by the Maastricht Treaty on European Union, which was adopted in 1992 and entered into force in 1993. The article was revised several times, but the "Health in All Policies" element was kept intact, constituting a mandate for intersectoral working (Merkel 2010).

Furthermore, the Finnish presidency of the European Council in 2006 promoted the development and implementation of Health in All Policies, by which governments would consider the health and health policy implications of policies outside the health system (Ståhl, Wismar et al. 2006). This initiative resulted in council conclusions (Council of the European Union 2006) and was followed by the Rome Declaration (Ministerial Conference 2007), in which member states pledged to actively promote Health in All Policies. Perhaps inevitably, these words have not always been matched by actions (Koivusalo 2010).

With the aim of further specifying and implementing its public health mandate, the EU has formulated the health strategy "Together for Health: A strategic

Box 12.5 Together for Health

Principles

- Strategy based on shared values
- Health is the greatest wealth
- Health in All Policies
- Strengthening the EU's voice in global health

Objectives

- Fostering good health in an ageing Europe
- Protecting citizens from health threats
- Supporting dynamic health systems and new technologies

approach for the EU 2008–2013" (Commission of the European Communities 2007). The strategy is based on four principles and contains three objectives (Box 12.5).

Several EU-funded programmes, either led by the European Commission directorate responsible for health, the Directorate General for Health and Consumers (DG SANCO), or by other directorates, have been aligned with this health strategy. These include the Second Programme of Community Action in the Field of Health, with a budget of €300 million for the policy's period, and the Seventh Framework Programme 2007–2013 (FP7), which lists research on health as a priority.[1] This, however, is a small amount since the budget of the EU equals roughly 1% of the member states' GDP and the lion's share of the EU budgets goes into the Common Agricultural Policy and the Structural Funds. The EU's health strategy also plays a role in its regional policy, its information and communication programmes, employment and social affairs, health security preparedness, and the 6th Environment Action Programme of the European Community 2002–2012.[2]

The EU's health strategy builds on 25 years of experience with public health programmes and strategies, even predating the formal introduction of its public health mandate. "Europe against Cancer" was the EU's first public health programme, running from 1987 to 2000; it was later complemented by seven other vertical programmes, concerned with health promotion, health monitoring, communicable diseases, rare diseases, injury prevention, pollution-related diseases, and drug prevention. In 2003, the vertical programmes were replaced by a more horizontal approach, introduced with the Programme of Community Action in the field of Public Health 2003–2008. This programme rested on three horizontal planks: improving health information and knowledge, responding rapidly to health threats, and addressing health determinants (European Parliament and Council of the European Union 2002).

Overall, while some things have been achieved, especially with regard to including health in the EU's Structural Funds, intersectoral policy development has been difficult and at times prone to failure (Merkel 2010). For example, Europe 2020, the EU's 10-year growth strategy following the Lisbon Agenda, does not touch upon health in its five targets or its seven flagship initiatives. This means that the role of health in the EU's future is left undefined.

Intersectoral working across ministries, sectors, and civil society

Intersectoral policy formulation and implementation requires ministries of health to engage with other ministries, sectors, and civil society. In this section, we discuss intersectoral governance structures, actions, and strategies that can be used in this process.[3]

Intersectoral governance structures

At the Adelaide International Meeting on Health in All Polices in 2010, co-organized by WHO and the Government of South Australia, participants summarized some of the existing tools that can facilitate intersectoral working (Box 12.6).

Some of these tools can be regarded as intersectoral structures. We use the term "intersectoral structure" to refer to a tangible medium (going beyond personal relationships) that can facilitate intersectoral action. Although the term may appear abstract, it is of practical relevance (Mulgan 2010). It may be based on explicit terms of reference or specified in an organization's organigram. Intersectoral governance structures can be found everywhere, including cabinets, parliaments, and public administration. They can be established for specific purposes, such as funding, or for reaching out beyond government and public administration.

Box 12.6   Tools for intersectoral working

- inter-ministerial and inter-departmental committees
- community consultations and citizens' juries
- cross-sectoral action teams
- partnership platforms
- integrated budgets and accounting
- health lens analysis
- cross-cutting information and evaluation systems
- impact assessments
- joined-up workforce development
- legislative frameworks

Source: Adelaide Statement on Health in All Policies (WHO 2010)

Ministerial linkages bring together policy fields at the highest decision-making level that would otherwise be separated, if not isolated. There are different approaches to establishing policy coherence at cabinet level. In South Australia, cabinet ministers developed a joint policy in which each of them "owned" a number of aligned targets (Wismar and Ernst 2010). Another way of handling ministerial linkages can be illustrated by the United Kingdom during Tony Blair's time as Prime Minister. Blair commissioned the Treasury to develop policy frameworks, which in turn were further developed by each of the ministries (Smith 2008). Other examples for issue-driven ministerial linkages include the French cancer plans under presidents Jacques Chirac (Paris and Polton 2008) and Nicolas Sarkozy.

Cabinet sub-committees, either standing or ad hoc, are another intersectoral structure that facilitates dialogue and collaboration at government level. While it is difficult to trace the work of these cabinet sub-committees due to confidentiality issues, emerging evidence underscores the importance of setting the context for policy change by developing a common understanding of issues and solutions (Metcalfe and Lavin 2012). Thus, in England a cabinet sub-committee for public health was abandoned in 2012 as ministers failed to turn up for meetings.

Public health ministers are another way of establishing ministerial linkages, though not necessarily at the cabinet table. The mandate of such ministers can vary. Tessa Jowell, the first minister given the designation "public health" in the United Kingdom (although in reality simply the renaming of an existing minister of state, or sub-cabinet level post), played a role in forging tobacco control policy. In Sweden, the post of public health minister was created in the context of the new national health policy, which focused entirely on the social determinants of health (Hogstedt, Lundgren et al. 2004). The minister of public health was responsible for implementation of the policy, with access to a high-level national steering committee composed of directors general from key state agencies and representatives of regional and local authorities (Pettersson 2010). However, the positions have since been abolished in both countries.

Parliamentary committees can also facilitate intersectoral action. Their role can be illustrated by the inquiry into health inequalities of the House of Commons Health Select Committee in the United Kingdom (2009). It showed that Parliament can be an important advocate for intersectoral governance in line with a HiAP approach. Overcoming partisan divisions, grounds for cross-party consensus and policy were developed in Parliament (Earwicker 2012).

Intersectoral committees are one of the most frequently used intersectoral governance structures. There is ample literature on how these committees should be run, including appropriate terms of reference, an adequate level of seniority. and a suitable frequency of meetings. While these technical issues must be considered when managing intersectoral committees, they are only part of the story. Such committees are often unpopular among members, and can be ineffective or even used as a mechanism for delay or sabotage. Intersectoral committees only work effectively under very specific circumstances; while useful to overcome bureaucratic issues, they cannot resolve political ones. They work best for important issues on which a wide consensus already exists, and worst when consensus is lacking or when the issue is not considered a priority (Greer 2012b).

Mega-ministries and ministerial mergers may be created with the hope that they might enhance the efficiency and coherence of political and administrative work. One example is the Hungarian Ministry for National Resources, which comprises six ministries that may exist as individual ministries in other countries. It remains unclear how far the stated goals have been met (Greer 2012a).

Joint budgets are an intersectoral structure that can facilitate the funding of health-related activities. The pooling takes place within government and funds come from different sources for joint projects. England has utilized this tool, and Sweden is also piloting several projects. A particularly difficult hurdle is assigning accountability, which creates an insurmountable barrier for ministries of health in a number of countries (McDaid, Drummond et al. 2008; McDaid 2012).

Delegated finance is an intersectoral governance structure that pools resources outside of government, allowing for additional funds to be raised. Examples include the health promotion foundations in Switzerland, Austria, Australia, and Thailand. Germany also planned to set up a health promotion foundation, with an annual budget of 250 million; however, it failed twice, in 2005 and 2007, to secure support in Parliament. Health promotion foundations may be co-financed from tax revenues, "sin taxes" or health insurance contributions. Often branded as institutional duplications that undermine established health promotion agencies, foundations can help to increase health promotion expenditure of other sectors (Schang, Czabanowska et al. 2011; Schang and Lin 2012).

Public consultation aims to reach out and engage with the wider public (Gauvin 2012). Different structures have been used. Austria, for instance, used a public consultation process to communicate and discuss its new intersectoral public health policy. With inputs from almost 4500 people, non-governmental agencies (NGOs), and other stakeholders,[4] it was considered a relatively successful consultation. Another example is the European Commission, which, as part of its general decision-making process, submits all legislative and policy proposals to a public consultation process.

Health conferences organized by national or regional governments are a governance structure that helps to reach out to a range of stakeholders. Examples can be found in Austria, Germany, and France. The best analysed system is in the German state of North Rhine-Westphalia, where the state health conference is mirrored by health conferences in the state's municipalities. Evaluations have been positive, suggesting that the system has some relevance for agenda-setting, coordination, and joint implementation (Brand and Michelsen 2012).

Private–public partnerships (PPPs) can facilitate industry engagement in health matters. The EU Platform on Diet, Physical Activity, and Health is an example of such a PPP, facilitating joint action between the European Commission, industry, and a large number of NGOs. Some European countries have mirrored these activities with similar national PPPs (Kosinska and Palumbo 2012). However, such mechanisms have also attracted substantial criticism for giving corporate vested interests undue influence on policy-making (see Chapter 7, "Food security and healthier food choices").

Intersectoral governance actions

Different intersectoral actions need to be employed to tackle the social determinants of health through intersectoral action, depending on the country, the subject, and the state of policy development (Box 12.7). Ensuring that there is a common understanding and interpretation of facts is a prerequisite, helping to generate support throughout government and beyond. The WHO Tallinn Charter (WHO Regional Office for Europe 2008), for example, stressed that health and health care should be considered not only as expenditure but also as investment. Similarly, the Wanless Report commissioned by the Treasury of the United Kingdom set out the benefits of engaging people in living healthier lives (Wanless 2012).

Setting goals and targets is another intersectoral activity that requires a solid understanding of win–win situations, the commonalities between different ministries and sectors, and the differences in their missions. Examples include HFA policies, Health 2020, the MDGs, as well as national and sub-national goals and targets. Other actions facilitated by intersectoral structures include advocacy, monitoring and evaluation, financial support, provision of a legal mandate, implementation and management.

Box 12.7 Examples for intersectoral action and HiAP

In 2013, the German Government launched a framework for global health policy at cabinet level, to ensure that Germany is actively and consistently contributing to global health. The framework focuses on tackling effectively cross-border health threats, strengthening health systems worldwide, expanding intersectoral cooperation, strengthening health research and health economy, and strengthening the global health architecture.[5]

France implemented two subsequent intersectoral programmes to combat cancer. The first ran from 2004 to 2007 and included measures on prevention and screening, patient care and support, modernization of cancer services, access to innovative treatments, research and training (Paris and Polton 2008). The new cancer plan, running from 2009 to 2013, focused on health inequalities, coordination and integration of care, and medical and community health initiatives for patient support.[6]

Finland has a track record in intersectoral working, even predating the Alma Ata Declaration of 1978. The famous North-Karelia Project to curb cardiovascular disease in Finnish men and women started in 1972. All major public health and societal problems have been dealt with from an intersectoral perspective, including diet and nutrition, physical activity, road traffic safety, tobacco and alcohol consumption, extending working lives, occupational health and safety, and suicide prevention. Epidemiological evidence has played an important role in supporting negotiations with other sectors. This was only possible because of the public health capacity of the National Institute for Health and Welfare (THL) and its predecessors (Melkas 2013).

Israel introduced a national programme to tackle obesity, a leading cause of ill-health and preventable death. The programme has ambitious, quantified goals. The key strategies to achieve these goals are increasing knowledge, fostering health-promoting environments, and incentivizing organizations and municipalities to engage in health promotion. Attention is given to intersectoral structures for collaborating with ministries and stakeholders. The programme also includes a comprehensive legislative agenda (Kranzler, Davidovich et al. 2013).

Sweden invests about 1.7% of its GDP in child and family-friendly policies. The system is one of universal access featuring: high-quality prenatal care; near-monthly developmental monitoring in the first 18 months of life, so that vision, hearing, speech/language, and dental problems are identified and addressed before the child starts school; and universal, non-compulsory access to publicly funded high-quality early learning and care programmes. These programmes and services are complemented by an income policy that brings virtually all families with young children above the poverty line, as well as up to 18 months of paid parental leave with incentives for the participation of fathers (Mercer, Hertzmann et al. 2013).

Intersectoral strategies and windows of opportunity for policy change

Political strategies to change policy will differ from case to case. Ministries of health will need to adopt different strategies when confronting the tobacco industry or when collaborating with the transport sector to promote road safety.

Four political strategies can help ministries of health to achieve their objectives; they are related to the extent that health objectives or objectives of other ministries and sectors are pursued (Ollila 2011):

- The *health strategy* is adopted to ensure that other ministries and sectors adopt policies and interventions that contribute to the aims and objectives of the Ministry of Health. The health strategy is therefore based on the agenda of the Ministry of Health.
- The *win–win strategy* pursues policies and actions where substantial mutual benefit is guaranteed. Policies and measures are compatible with the objectives of all ministries and sectors involved.
- The *cooperation strategy* comes to the fore when the health sector provides evidence and intelligence to help other ministries or sectors achieve their aims. Much of the discussion on the return on investing in health is based on this strategy.

- Finally, the *damage limitation* strategy is a more defensive approach. While the aims of different ministries and sectors may not be reconciled, at least negative health effects can be minimized.

Health policy-makers and activists can become frustrated when, despite a pressing problem and the availability of solutions, policy change does not take place. For example, there are effective tobacco and alcohol control policies, but there are wide variations in the uptake between and within countries. Why has Ireland more advanced tobacco control measures than Germany, and why is Bavaria lagging behind other Länder in Germany? This experience has led to a critique of the public health action cycle, which assumes a cyclical policy development, in which assessment is followed by policy development, implementation and evaluation, after which the cycle starts again (Institute of Medicine 1988). While the policy cycle has some analytical value, it may not always provide adequate descriptions of policy change. Public health promoters who rely on classic knowledge transfer techniques and try to convince policy-makers to pass legislation often fail because policy change is often achieved through coalition-building, mobilizing public opinion, lobbying and influencing political values, and not through disseminating research findings alone (De Leeuw and Clavier 2011). Evidence on existing problems and available solutions is important, but it is often not enough to bring about policy change.

One of the alternative approaches to understanding and achieving policy change is the concept of "policy windows" (Kingdon 1984), which has been derived from political science and adapted to the health policy debate (Ollila 2011). This model emphasizes the role of policy entrepreneurs who take advantage of agenda-setting opportunities, described as windows of opportunities or "policy windows". Policy change is seen as emerging from three independent processes or "streams": the problem stream, the policy stream, and the political stream (Figure 12.1).

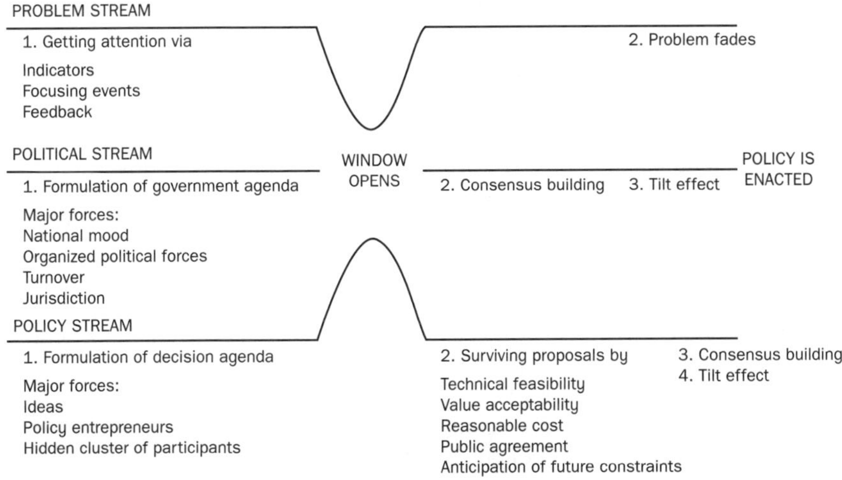

Figure 12.1 Windows of opportunity

Source: Ollila, Baum et al. (2013)

Kingdon's model suggests that the policy process is non-linear and non-sequential. In contrast to what the public health action cycle suggests, problem assessment, policy development, and politics can move in parallel and be relatively unconnected. For example, there may be solutions, but the problem is not yet generally perceived as such.

The question remains how policy windows can be created. In the past, it was often public health crises that led to policy change. For example, the BSE crisis led to the introduction of the EU's health policy mandate,[7] and WHO's International Health Regulations were only reformed after the threat of the SARS epidemic (see Chapter 4, "The health security framework in Europe").

Intersectoral governance structures in practice

Having analysed intersectoral governance structures, actions, and strategies in isolation, it is useful to examine real contexts, where they are sometimes used in combination (Box 12.8). While there is no complete mapping exercise for Europe, a recent report to the Dutch Council for Public Health and Health Care summarizes intersectoral governance structures for England, Finland, New Zealand, Norway, Sweden, and Quebec, showing wide variations in the use and focus of these structures (St.-Pierre, Hamel et al. 2009).

In the EU, key aspects of intersectoral governance were integrated into the legislative process by the European Commission as a response to criticism of its opaque and inconsistent policy-making. The decision-making process was reformed, and all proposals are now included in a road map that informs all other Directorates General and the public. A proposal not on the

Box 12.8 Intersectoral governance structures in action: Finland

In Finland, there are ministerial committees on issues such as foreign policy, macro-economic and financial policy, and social policy, in order to allow ministerial representatives of multi-party governments to participate in the preparatory processes of high-level government policies. At the level of the members of the government, the ministers, the Minister of Health and her core staff for health promotion policy, the inter-ministerial tools to enhance health promotion policies in other ministries are:

- the official decision-making sessions and (particularly) the unofficial preparatory sessions of the whole government;
- the permanent ministerial committee on social policy;
- a temporary ministerial working group, set up until the next election to guide the government policy programme on health promotion.

Source: Lehto (2012)

roadmap cannot be submitted for approval. This allows early input from all major stakeholders into potentially health-relevant proposals, at a time when the plans are still at an early stage of development. Furthermore, an Internet-based public consultation process allows for participation of governments, individuals, and other stakeholders. All legislation and major policy proposals need to be submitted to the Commission's internal integrated impact assessment. This assessment focuses on the economic, environmental, and social (including health) impact of proposals. It makes use of consultations between the different Directorates General. Finally, the Impact Assessment Board needs to formally clear the validity of impact assessments, which are then approved by the College of Commissioners (Commission of the European Communities 2002).

The new decision-making procedure has undoubtedly increased transparency, but it has also attracted some criticism. While the Internet-based consultation process is public, the input beyond governments and other stakeholders has remained limited. Furthermore, the impact assessment procedure has been criticized for not mentioning health appropriately (Salay and Lincoln 2008; Ståhl 2010). While these observations are valid, it is important to go beyond impact assessment reports when assessing the effectiveness of the EU's intersectoral working. The interactions between Commission staff from different directorates and at different levels might be much more important in this regard.

The Commission stressed the need for effective cooperation with member states, health professionals, and civil society in the implementation of its health strategy "Together for Health" (Merkel 2010). To this end, two intersectoral coordination mechanisms were implemented. First, the EU Health Policy Forum brings together NGOs, health professionals, healthcare providers, and businesses. Second, the Working Party on Public Health at Senior Level, a Council body formed of member state representatives, serves as a mechanism to collaborate with member states. According to the mid-term evaluation of "Together for Health", the coordinating mechanisms have not yet realized their full potential. It found the strategy to be coherent with other EU policies, activities, and funding processes, but lacking discernible direct impact on a number of those. Indeed, in most EU member states the influence of the EU health strategy on national health strategies has so far been limited (PHEIAC 2011). However, there are many other forms of intersectoral working at EU level, including various intersectoral platforms, joint policy programmes, and intersectoral actions programmes. A full review of all these activities has not yet been attempted.

Conclusions

How can we create situations and contexts that are conducive to intersectoral working? How can we support the emergence of political will and leadership? What are the implications regarding the intersectoral tasks and skills of public health professionals and how does the training of public health professionals need to be revised to accommodate these new tasks?

Reaching out to other ministries and sectors and engaging them in constructive dialogue that results in intersectoral action requires political will and strong leadership, not only from the health minister but also from the cabinet or the head of government. Examples are the rapid and effective introduction of tobacco control measures in Turkey under Minster of Health Recep Akdağ, supported by the Prime Minister.[8] Yet all too often political will and leadership is weak. The heads of state and cabinet do not deal with health determinants and the minister of health may already be entangled in contentious health reforms, trying to avoid additional controversies with cabinet colleagues. In these situations, windows of opportunities will only open if a so-called "focusing event" is taking place. This can be a health crisis or a public scandal, but there have also been influential reports or coordinated events that have helped to put intersectoral working on the political agenda, such as the Finnish presidency of the European Council in 2006, which resulted in Council conclusions on HiAP and the integration of HiAP in the second health strategy of DG SANCO. Another example for moving intersectoral issues on the political agenda is the report of the WHO Commission on the Social Determinants of Health, which was widely read and contributed to some reorientation.

Intersectoral working and HiAP extend the scope of tasks and skills for public health professionals, in particular with regard to policy analysis, health economics, and communication. They need to analyse and understand policies and politics of other sectors, map stakeholder interests, and communicate effectively with non-health professionals. They will also need to develop some basic understanding of the economics of prevention, which may help to illustrate the mutual benefits of collaboration. In addition, public health professionals need to adopt a strategic attitude. This includes the above-mentioned health, win–win, cooperation, and damage limitation-strategies, in order to push back tobacco, join forces with the education and other sectors, commit industry to more social responsibility, and help to avoid the worst when it comes to seemingly unavoidable issues such as trade liberalization. It would be of great help for HiAP if public health training could better incorporate policy analysis and intersectoral governance in curricula. However, there are other ways to improve professional competence, such as through the posting of health ministry staff in other ministries or training staff of other ministries in health issues.

Notes

1   Health for Growth is the designated but not yet ratified new Public Health Programme for the period 2014–2020. It is explicitly designed to support the broader competitiveness and growth objectives of the Commission. The four objectives of the new proposed programme are to contribute to innovative and sustainable health systems, increase access to better and safer health care for EU citizens, to prevent diseases and promote good health, and to protect citizens from cross-border health threats.

2   For an overview, see: http://ec.europa.eu/health/strategy/implementation/index_ en.htm.

3   This sub-section on intersectoral governance structures and actions draws on a joint study conducted by the European Observatory on Health Systems and Policies and

the International Union for Health Promotion and Education (IUHPE), while the discussion on political strategies and windows of opportunities links to a joint project between the Finnish Ministry of Social Affairs and Health, the Finnish National Institute for Health and Welfare, the UN Research Institute for Social Development and the European Observatory on Health Systems and Policies.

4 http://www.gesundheitsziele-oesterreich.at/ideen-sammlung/ergebnisse-der-ideensuche-mai-bis-august-2011/(accessed 06 June 2012).

5 https://www.bundesgesundheitsministerium.de/fileadmin/dateien/Publikationen/ Gesundheit/Broschueren/Globale_Gesundheitspolitik-Konzept_der_Bundesregierung. pdf (accessed 19 November 2013).

6 http://www.epaac.eu/from_heidi_wiki/France_National_Cancer_Plan_English.pdf.

7 The EU's first public health programme "Europe Against Cancer" started well before the introduction of the public health mandate. Rumour has it that Francois Mitterrand, suffering from prostate cancer, was behind the initiation of the programme.

8 http://www.euro.who.int/en/countries/turkey/news/news/2011/06/turkey-shares-experience-on-tobacco-control-with-neighbouring-and-midincome-countries.

References

Brand, H. and K. Michelsen (2012). "Collaborative governance: the example of health conferences." In *Intersectoral Governance for Health in All Policies*. D. McQueen, V. Lin, M. Wismar, L. St.-Pierre and M. Davies, Eds. Copenhagen, WHO Regional Office for Europe on behalf of the European Observatory on Health Systems and Policies.

Busse, R. and M. Wismar (2002). "Health target programmes and health care services – any link? A conceptual and comparative study (part 1)." *Health Policy* **59**(3): 209–221.

Commission of the European Communities (2002). Communication from the Commission on impact assessment, COM(2002) 276 final [http://ec.europa.eu/governance/impact/ docs/key_docs/com_2002_0276_en.pdf].

Commission of the European Communities (2007). *Together for Health: A strategic approach for the EU 2008–2013*, White Paper COM(2007) 630 final [http://ec.europa. eu/health/ph_overview/strategy/health_strategy_en.htm].

Council of the European Union (2006). *Council Conclusions on Health in All Policies* (HiAP) (EPSCO), 30 November 2006.

De Leeuw, E. and C. Clavier (2011). "Healthy public in all policies." *Health Promotion International* **26**(Suppl. 2): ii237–ii244.

Earwicker, R. (2012). "Parliamentary committees." In *Intersectoral Governance for Health in All Policies*. D. McQueen, V. Lin, M. Wismar, L. St.-Pierre and M. Davies, Eds. Copenhagen, WHO Regional Office for Europe on behalf of the European Observatory on Health Systems and Policies.

European Parliament and Council of the European Union Decision No. 1786/2002/EC of the European Parliament and of the Council of 23 September 2002 adopting a programme of community action in the field of public health (2003–2008).

European Union (2010). "Consolidated Version of the Treaty on the Functioning of the European Union." *Official Journal of the European Union* C 83–C 47.

Gauvin, F.-P. (2012). "Public engagement." In *Intersectoral Governance for Health in All Policies*. D. McQueen, V. Lin, M. Wismar, L. St.-Pierre and M. Davies, Eds. Copenhagen, WHO Regional Office for Europe on behalf of the European Observatory on Health Systems and Policies.

Greer, S. L. (2012a). "Mega-ministries." In *Intersectoral Governance for Health in All Policies*. D. McQueen, V. Lin, M. Wismar, L. St.-Pierre and M. Davies, Eds. Copenhagen,

WHO Regional Office for Europe on behalf of the European Observatory on Health Systems and Policies.

Greer, S. L. (2012b). "Interdepartmental committees and support units." In *Intersectoral Governance for Health in All Policies*. D. McQueen, V. Lin, M. Wismar, L. St.-Pierre and M. Davies, Eds. Copenhagen, WHO Regional Office for Europe on behalf of the European Observatory on Health Systems and Policies.

Hogstedt, C., B. Lundgren, H. Moberg, B. Pettersson and G. Agren (2004). "The Swedish public health policy and the National Institute of Public Health." *Scandinavian Journal of Public Health Supplement* **64**: 6–64.

House of Commons Health Committee (2009). *Health Inequalities*. London, TSO.

Institute of Medicine (1988). *The Future of Public Health*. Washington, D.C.: National Academy Press.

Kemm, J. (2007). "What is HIA and why might it be useful?" In *The Effectiveness of Health Impact Assessment: Scope and limitations of supporting decision-making in Europe*. M. Wismar, J. Blau and K. Ernst, Eds. Copenhagen, WHO: 3–14.

Kingdon, J. W. (1984). *Agendas, Alternatives and Public Policies*. Glenview, IL, Scott, Foresman.

Koivusalo, M. (2010). "The state of Health in All Policies (HiAP) in the European Union: potential and pitfalls." *Journal of Epidemiology and Community Health* **64**(6): 500–503.

Kosinska, M. and L. Palumbo (2012). "Industry engagement." In *Intersectoral Governance for Health in All Policies*. D. McQueen, V. Lin, M. Wismar, L. St.-Pierre and M. Davies, Eds. Copenhagen, WHO Regional Office for Europe on behalf of the European Observatory on Health Systems and Policies.

Kranzler, Y., N. Davidovich, Y. Fleischman, I. Grotto, D. S. Moran and R. Weinstein (2013). "A health in all policies approach to promote active, healthy lifestyle in Israel." *Israel Journal of Health Policy Research* **2**(1): 16.

Lehto, J. (2012). "Joined-up government: the Finnish Government system." In *Intersectoral Governance for Health in All Policies*. D. McQueen, V. Lin, M. Wismar, L. St.-Pierre and M. Davies, Eds. Copenhagen, WHO Regional Office for Europe on behalf of the European Observatory on Health Systems and Policies.

McDaid, D. (2012). "Joined budgets." In *Intersectoral Governance for Health in All Policies*. D. McQueen, V. Lin, M. Wismar, L. St.-Pierre and M. Davies, Eds. Copenhagen, WHO Regional Office for Europe on behalf of the European Observatory on Health Systems and Policies.

McDaid, D., M. Drummond and M. Suhrcke (2008). *How can European Health Systems Support Investment in and the Implementation of Population Health Strategies?* Copenhagen, WHO Regional Office for Europe on behalf of the European Observatory on Health Systems and Policies.

Melkas, T. (2013). "Health in All Policies as a priority in Finnish health policy: a case study on national health policy development." *Scandinavian Journal of Public Health* **41**(11 Suppl.): 3–28.

Mercer, P., C. Hertzmann, H. Molina and Z. Vaghri (2013). "Promoting equity from the start through early child development and Health in All Policies." In *Health in All Policies: Seizing opportunities, implementing policies*. K. Leppo, E. Ollila, S. Peña, M. Wismar and S. Cook, Eds. Helsinki, Ministry of Social Affairs and Health: 105–124.

Merkel, B. (2010). "Health in All Policies: European Union experience and perspectives." *Public Health Bulletin SA* **7**(2): 14–17.

Metcalfe, O. and T. Lavin (2012). "Cabinet committees." In *Intersectoral Governance for Health in All Policies*. D. McQueen, V. Lin, M. Wismar, L. St.-Pierre and M. Davies, Eds. Copenhagen, WHO Regional Office for Europe on behalf of the European Observatory on Health Systems and Policies.

Ministerial Conference (2007). *Declaration on Health in All Policies*, Rome, 18 December.

Mulgan, G. (2010). "Holistic government and what works." *Public Health Bulletin SA* **7**(2): 12–14.

Ollila, E. (2011). "Health in All Policies: From rhetoric to action." *Scandinavian Journal of Public Health* **39**(Suppl. 16): 11–18.

Ollila, E., F. Baum and S. Peña (2013). "Introduction to Health in All Policies and the analytical framework." In *Health in All Policies: Seizing opportunities, implementing policies*. K. Leppo, E. Ollila, S. Peña, M. Wismar and S. Cook, Eds. Helsinki, Ministry of Social Affairs and Health: 3–24.

Paris, V. and D. Polton (2008). "France: targeting investment in health." In *Health Targets in Europe: Learning from experience*. M. Wismar, M. McKee, K. Ernst, D. Srivastava and R. Busse, Eds. Copenhagen, WHO Regional Office for Europe on behalf of the European Observatory on Health Systems and Policies: 101–122.

Pettersson, B. (2010). "Health in All Policies across jurisdictions – a snapshot from Sweden." *Public Health Bulletin SA* **7**(2): 17–20.

Public Health Evaluation and Impact Assessment Consortium (PHEIAC) (2011). *Final Report, 2011* [http://ec.europa.eu/health/programme/docs/mthp_final_report_oct2011_en.pdf, accessed 12 February 2014].

Salay, R. and P. Lincoln (2008). "Health impact assessments in the European Union." *The Lancet* **372**(9641): 860–861.

Schang, L. K., K. M. Czabanowska and V. Lin (2011). "Securing funds for health promotion: lessons from health promotion foundations based on experiences from Austria, Australia, Germany, Hungary and Switzerland." *Health Promotion International* dar023.

Schang, L. and V. Lin (2012). "Delegated financing." In *Intersectoral Governance for Health in All Policies*. D. McQueen, V. Lin, M. Wismar, L. St.-Pierre and M. Davies, Eds. Copenhagen, WHO Regional Office for Europe on behalf of the European Observatory on Health Systems and Policies.

Smith, P. C. (2008). "England: intended and unintended effects." In *Health Targets in Europe: Learning from experience*. M. Wismar, M. McKee, K. Ernst, D. Srivastava and R. Busse, Eds. Copenhagen, WHO Regional Office for Europe on behalf of the European Observatory on Health Systems and Policies.

St.-Pierre, L., G. Hamel, G. Lapointe, D. McQueen and M. Wismar (2009). *Governance Tools and Framework for Health in All Policies*. Quebec, National Collaborating Centre for Healthy Public Policy.

Ståhl, T. (2010). "Is health recognized in the EU's policy process? An analysis of the European Commission's impact assessments." *European Journal of Public Health* **20**(2): 176–181.

Ståhl, T., M. Wismar, E. Ollia, E. Lahtinen and K. Leppo (2006). *Health in All Policies: Prospects and potentials*. Helsinki, Ministry of Social Affairs and Health.

van de Water, H. P. A. and L. M. van Herten (1998). *Health Policies on Target? Review of health target and priority setting in 18 European countries*. Leiden, TNO.

Wanless, D. (2012). *Securing Our Future Health: Taking a long-term view* [http://webarchive.nationalarchives.gov.uk/+/http://www.hm-treasury.gov.uk/consult_wanless_final.htm, accessed 6 June 2012]. London, Department of Health.

Wismar, M. and R. Busse (2002). "Outcome-related health targets – political strategies for better health outcomes: A conceptual and comparative study (part 2)." *Health Policy* **59**(3): 223–241.

Wismar, M. and K. Ernst (2010). "Health in All Policies in Europe." In *Implementing Health in All Policies: Adelaide 2010*. I. Kickbusch and K. Buckett, Eds. Adelaide, SA, Department of Health, Government of South Australia: 53–64.

World Health Organization (WHO) (1978). *Declaration of Alma-Ata* [http://www.who.int/ publications/almaata_declaration_en.pdf].

World Health Organization (WHO) (2010). *Adelaide Statement on Health in All Policies.* Geneva, WHO.

World Health Organization (WHO) Regional Office for Europe (1985). *Targets for Health for All: Targets in support of the European regional strategy for Health for All.* Copenhagen, WHO Regional Office for Europe.

World Health Organization (WHO) Regional Office for Europe (1999). *Health21: The Health for All Policy framework for the WHO European Region.* Copenhagen, WHO Regional Office for Europe.

World Health Organization (WHO) Regional Office for Europe (2005). *The Health for All Policy Framework for the WHO European Region: 2005 update.* European Health for All series No. 7 [http://www.euro.who.int/_data/assets/pdf_file/0008/98387/ E87861.pdf]. Copenhagen, WHO Regional Office for Europe.

World Health Organization (WHO) Regional Office for Europe (2008). *The Tallinn Charter: Health systems for health and wealth* [http://www.euro.who.int/document/ E91438.pdf]. Tallinn, WHO Regional Office for Europe.

World Health Organization (WHO) Regional Office for Europe (2013). *Health 2020: A European policy framework supporting action across government and society for health and well-being.* Copenhagen, WHO Regional Office for Europe.

chapter thirteen

Health impact assessment

Nichola Davies, Paul Lincoln

Introduction

Within Europe, but also elsewhere, health impact assessment (HIA) is used to identify the potential health consequences (intentional or unintentional) of policies, projects, programmes, and plans inside and, increasingly often, outside the health sector. According to the widely used definition provided in the "Gothenburg Consensus", HIA is "any combination of procedures or methods by which a proposed policy or program may be judged as to the effects it may have on the health of a population" (WHO European Centre for Health Policy 2001).

The purpose of HIA is to ensure that considerations relevant to health and well-being are seamlessly factored into the daily decision-making and planning processes, something that is essential if policies are to impact positively on health. HIA can be a means of facilitating collaboration and other forms of intersectoral working between policy-makers and other stakeholders. An advantage of this participatory element of HIA is that it can increase the awareness of health in areas outside the health sector, and help to identify how health inequalities can be reduced.

However, while HIA is gaining traction in some countries as a means to improve public health, HIA in general is coming under powerful attack from those taking advantage of the current financial crisis to pursue a deregulatory ideology based on supply-side economics and from those powerful vested interests, such as multinational corporations and their front organizations, seeking to set the rules in ways that benefit them (Mindell, Reynolds et al. 2012).

This chapter provides a brief overview of the literature on health impact assessments, highlighting emerging trends and developments in the use of HIA both within Europe and internationally. Some examples are given to illustrate the ways in which HIA can be applied to influence policy at all levels.

Why and when to undertake HIA?

Health impact assessment is designed to take into account the best available evidence from a range of sources, including both qualitative and quantitative methods, in order to produce a set of evidence-based recommendations that can be used to inform the decision-making process for a proposed policy. The participative and inclusive nature of HIA facilitates practical suggestions on how to enhance positive aspects of proposals, including positive outcomes for health and well-being, while mitigating or eliminating any potential negative impacts. Unlike other impact assessments, which typically focus only on the negative impacts that may result from a proposed project, programme or policy (such as environmental impact assessments, EIAs), HIA also highlights positive impacts. Health is broadly defined in a HIA, based on a holistic view that includes well-being, recognition of the wider social determinants of health, and the need to reduce health inequalities.

HIAs are most effective when they are applied to proposals prospectively (before) or concurrently (alongside) with any key decisions or commitments being made. The obvious value of using HIAs before or alongside the development of policies or programmes is that they provide an opportunity to modify proposals in ways that will optimize health and well-being. However, HIAs are also conducted retrospectively (after a proposal has been put in place), allowing for the evaluation of policies and programmes. Retrospective HIAs can also be used as a means of influencing future proposals, as they provide an opportunity to look back at the impacts of past actions and consider what could be done differently in the future.

Through these processes, HIA can assist policy-makers in assessing the impact of their decisions on health, while also facilitating coordinated cross-government action, stakeholder involvement, and health in all policies (see Chapter 12, "Intersectoral working"). The literature on HIA identifies at least five key stages (Figure 13.1).

In practice, however, HIAs need not always include all of these stages. Often, after completing the screening stage, it may be determined that a HIA is not required, or that a smaller, less extensive process, such as a rapid HIA, may be more appropriate for that specific proposal. Consequently, HIAs take on a variety of forms, and are used in very different contexts and for a variety of purposes. Emerging trends in the use of HIA discussed in this chapter include:

- Integrated impact assessments (IIAs), which typically combine HIA with other impact assessments, such as an EIA, strategic environmental assessment (SEA) or sustainability assessment (SA)
- Rapid HIAs
- Community-led HIA
- Equity-focused HIAs

Public health and HIA are both multidisciplinary fields, and this might help to explain why there are often diverging views over how to interpret the purpose of HIA, define health, and assess evidence (Harris-Roxas and Harris 2010). Variations in the use of HIA across Europe also reflect political, socio-economic, and institutional differences among countries (Blau, Ernst et al. 2007). Whether

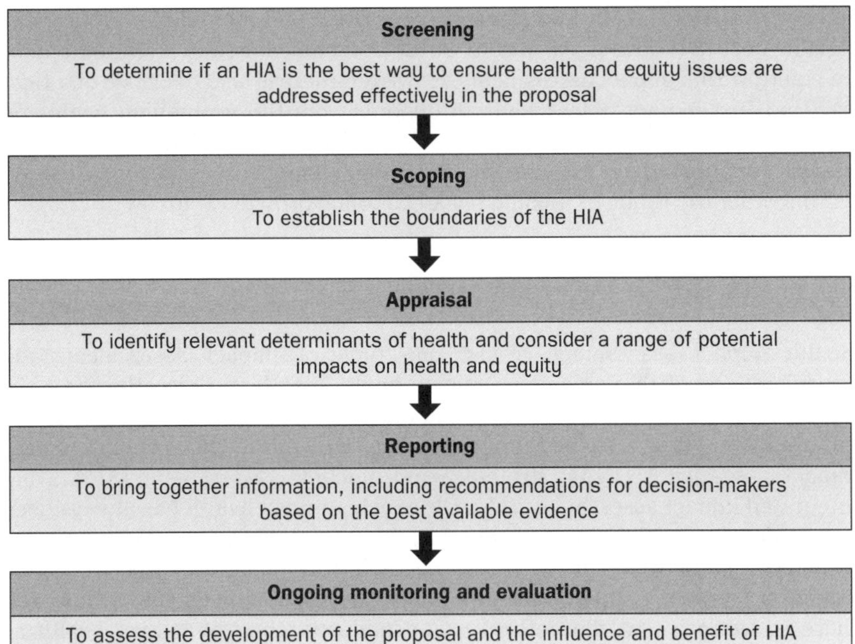

Figure 13.1 Key stages of HIAs

Source: Adapted from Public Health Advisory Committee (2007: 13)

HIAs are undertaken by dedicated HIA agencies or by units within ministries is of lesser importance than that they should always be accessible, transparent, independent, and competent. Furthermore, the appreciation of HIAs should be a core competence of public health professionals.

Several important trends in the use of HIAs in Europe can be distinguished. First, there is increasing use of HIA outside the health sector, where it is being used to assess the potential health implications of a broad range of issues, including urban planning, regeneration and development, transport and housing. Second, IIA is also gaining in popularity, as it is being viewed as an effective way of reducing the burden of impact assessments, combing shared goals into a single process. Third, there is a shift towards HIAs being undertaken outside the formal decision-making processes, often by non-governmental organizations (NGOs) and other civil society organizations, taking the form of community-driven HIAs. In this way, HIA is being used primarily as a means of advocacy, giving voice to perspectives that might otherwise be excluded from the decision-making process. There has been a renewed focus on the use of HIA as a tool for improving equity and reducing health inequalities. Building capacity for health equity impact assessment among policy-makers and planners, and including an equity impact assessment of all government policies, were some of the recommendations made in 2008 by the World Health Organization (WHO) Commission on Social Determinants of Health (CSDH 2008). The Marmot

Review in 2010 (The Marmot Review Team 2010) and the following European Review in 2012 (Marmot, Allen et al. 2012) also contributed to a renewed focus on equity within impact assessments. However, there is also evidence of a fight back against impact assessments in general from those pursuing neoliberal political views. Thus, in November 2012 the British Prime Minister vowed to abolish equality impact assessments, describing impact assessments in general as "bureaucratic rubbish" holding back economic growth (Sparrow 2012).

Use of HIA outside the health sector

Health impact assessment is just one type of impact assessment, and considerations of the impacts on human health also feature in other types of impact assessment. This is most commonly seen in impact assessments in the environmental sector. In the European Union (EU) this includes environmental impact assessment (EIA), strategic environmental assessment (SEA), and integrated impact assessment (IIA). Obviously, human health has always been a consideration within environmental health, and many of the environmental disasters that have resulted in EIA becoming a regulatory process gained attention because of their impact on human health (Caldwell 1988). However, there is concern that the definition and understanding of human health as applied in environmental health, and specifically EIAs, is too narrow and does not include a broader, holistic interpretation of health and well-being, or the wider social determinants of health.

The WHO Regional Office for Europe (2011) suggests that SEAs are a more appropriate tool to assess the potential range of impacts on health within environmental assessments. In Europe, SEAs are supported by two key legal frameworks: the 2004 SEA Directive of the European Commission (2001/42/EC), and the UN Economic Commission for Europe (UNECE) Protocol on SEA. Importantly, SEAs aim for a strategic assessment of high-level decisions on the development and implementation of policies (Wright, Parry et al. 2005), so determining the scope of any subsequent EIAs (Wright, Parry et al. 2005). This means that SEA is undertaken much earlier in the decision-making process than EIA, making it a much more powerful tool to prevent ill health and tackle health inequalities.

At the national level, HIAs are very unevenly distributed. Some countries have shown a much greater willingness to use them than others. Outside of Europe, the Canadian province of British Columbia was one of the first jurisdictions that started to conduct routine impact assessments of public policies, producing the first checklist for HIAs. The Canadian experience showed that HIAs are particularly effective when measurable health targets have been set that can guide the assessment process (Frankish, Green et al. 2001).

Within Europe, the EU has made it a priority to undertake assessments that capture the potential social, economic, and environmental impacts of all new proposals and the impacts on health are considered a key part of this procedure (Wismar, Blau et al. 2007). Nevertheless, only a few European countries have used HIA extensively (Blau, Ernst et al. 2007). This has been attributed in part to a greater awareness and governmental commitment to multisectoral action in the more actively engaged countries (Ståhl, Wismar et al. 2006), as well as to differences in funding and capacity. Some countries have made HIAs mandatory as part of a regulatory process or through legislation (Lee, Robbel et al. 2013). The capacity to undertake or review a HIA influences the extent to which different regulatory and legislative approaches have resulted in HIAs being undertaken. The capacity to respond and take advantage of opportunities within other impact assessments can strategically contribute to further intersectoral working. Public health professionals, for example, are provided with strong levers and opportunities for breaking down some of the silos existing both within and across sectors, when HIA or intersectoral working is made mandatory (St.-Pierre, Hamel et al. 2009; Koivusalo 2010).

Within the EU, some of the post-2004 member states in central and eastern Europe, where public health had been relatively weak, have now started to adopt multisectoral approaches to public health, including the greater use of HIA (Lock and McKee 2005). In this context, HIA is seen as a useful tool for more integrated policy-making across sectors (Lock, Gabrijelcic-Blenkus et al. 2003). In Slovenia, a leader in the field, the need for better intersectoral working between health and agriculture was identified through a HIA of agriculture and food policies in the context of the country's accession to the EU (Lock, Gabrijelcic-Blenkus et al. 2003).

The influence of a country's overall political context on the development of HIA could partly explain why its use is still limited in some European countries, including the young democracies of southern Europe (Bacigalupe, Esnaola et al. 2009) such as Spain, where, until recently, intersectoral approaches to include health within non-health policies had not been common in political decision-making. However, this is slowly changing, as some regional governments in Spain have started to recognize the value of such processes, although whether this will survive the austerity policies being pursued by the Spanish Government in the wake of the current economic crisis remains to be seen. In the Basque country (one of Spain's autonomous communities), the first HIA guidelines were published in Spanish, building on a regional health policy (for the period 2002–2010) designed on the basis of a model of health that actively promoted the inclusion of health in non-health policies (Bacigalupe, Esnaola et al. 2009). An example was a HIA of a local regeneration intervention in the city of Bilbao (Bacigalupe, Esnaola et al. 2009), commissioned by the regional Ministry of Health. Crucially, HIAs require knowledge about what proposals are on the way. They are far easier to conduct in countries with high levels of transparency and access to information.

The uneven development of HIA across Europe and its apparent lack in some countries could also be a reflection of the difficulty of demonstrating its usefulness to other sectors. This might explain why it is often implemented on an ad hoc basis rather than being a systematic part of the policy-making process (Blau, Ernst et al. 2007). In the Netherlands, a more systematic approach was chosen. HIA was originally the responsibility of the Intersectoral Policy Office, set up in 1996 in the Netherlands School of Public Health (Put, Broeder et al. 2001). It was then outsourced to a university department that assessed all proposals for their health implications. However, this approach proved to be unsustainable owing to the high number of proposals and workload associated with impact assessments. Scotland has implemented several HIAs outside the health sector, including the City of Edinburgh Council's Land Transport Strategy and the North Edinburgh Area Renewal Housing Strategy, but barriers to HIA are still experienced (Kemm, Perry et al. 2004). These barriers include heavy workloads and the large number of new initiatives, challenges that are also experienced in other European countries, leading to an increasing drive from some organizations for HIA to be incorporated into other impact assessment processes.

Integrated impact assessment

Integrated impact assessment (IIA) is increasingly being used as a means of bringing together cross-cutting themes and issues. This trend is partly due to the barriers described above, but also due to the increasing use of HIA to assess health impacts from initiatives outside the health sector, such as the urban development of housing, transport, and areas targeted for regeneration. By integrating multiple assessments, IIA has the potential to simplify and reduce the work for policy, programme, and project developers, cutting red tape and reducing the perceived burdens of assessments (Association of Public Health Observatories 2007).

IIA can be described as any process that attempts to cover more than one type of impact assessment in a single process (Association of Public Health Observatories 2007). It "is an approach that assesses the potential impact of proposals (strategies, policies, programmes, projects, plans or other developments) on issues that previously may have been assessed separately, such as economic, environmental, sustainability, equal opportunities, health, wellbeing, and quality of life" (NICE 2005).

Most commonly, IIA combines an EIA (environmental impact assessment) or SIA (social impact assessment) with a HIA, a logical development as the outputs of EIA and SIA can be inputs to HIA (Birley 2003). SEA also has many features of IIA (Association of Public Health Observatories 2007). Incorporating HIA into SEA can offer increased scope for the consideration of the determinants of health in policy-making (Wright, Parry et al. 2005). The UNECE views the inclusion of health in SEAs as an effective strategy to address health impacts without the need for a separate HIA (UN/Regional Environmental Center for Central and Eastern Europe 2006).

IIA considers the social determinants of health, such as housing or transport (NHS Health Development Agency 2003; NICE 2005). Similar to HIA, IIA also aims to take account of inequalities and improve health by comparing how proposals may impact upon the most vulnerable groups in a population (NHS Health Development Agency 2003). Combining impact assessments also ensures the involvement of many sectors, which is considered one of the advantages of IIA. For example, Nottingham City Council in England has described an IIA used in the development of the Nottingham Local Transport Plan 2011–2026 (Nottingham City Council 2011) designed to ensure that the links between environmental, equality, and health impacts are identified. The council believes that this single IIA approach will streamline the processes of SEA, HIA, and equity impact assessment, enabling them to meet the statutory requirements for an SEA and an equity impact assessment, and drawing on good practice for its HIA (Nottingham City Council 2011). In Quebec, Canada, the basis for the systematic practice of HIA in EIA resulted from public health involvement in public hearings about pesticide use, which then led to a memorandum of understanding between the Ministry of Health and Social Services and the Ministry of Environment (Lee, Robbel et al. 2013).

The primary output of IIAs is a set of evidence-based recommendations that should inform the decision-making process associated with the proposal. As with HIA, IIA is most effective when applied to proposals prospectively, but reviewing and mitigating the impacts of proposals that are already underway is also important, and assessments can also be undertaken retrospectively, taking on the form of evaluations. This monitoring and evaluation of proposals allows for inequalities to be mitigated, and practical ways for enhancing health and well-being to be identified and embedded in policy. Although a lack of capacity often means that these evaluative processes are not always completed in practice, they highlight areas where HIA and IIA practices could be strengthened and improved in the future. Perceived disadvantages of IAA include a potential neglect of health. Thus, "Integrated impact assessments cover such a large number of issues that health, considered as part of overall 'social impacts', is often overlooked while other top-line issues, more easily expressed in economic terms, are emphasised" (Salay and Lincoln 2009). Another disadvantage is related to those HIAs that are conducted after other impact assessment processes, as this provides limited scope for the collection of new data upon which to base an assessment (Harris-Roxas et al. 2012).

There is a clear danger of superficial treatment of a wide range of issues, encouraging a "tick box approach" (Association of Public Health Observatories 2007). There is also some debate as to whether IIA itself creates more work, due to the multiplicity of areas covered and the need to involve people representing each of these areas.

Rapid health impact assessment

The costs associated with HIAs can vary considerably (Lee, Robbel et al. 2013) and depend on the context in which the HIA is undertaken. The resourcing of HIAs within IIA, for example, can present challenging practical issues (Birley 2007). Within the EU, research grants play an important role in enabling research and developing techniques and capacity for HIA (Committee on Health Impact Assessment 2011).

One solution to the perceived burden of impact assessments, and the time and resources they require is what is referred to as a rapid HIA. A rapid HIA consists of a brief investigation of the main health impacts of a proposal, building on existing knowledge and research from previous HIAs (NHS Health Development Agency 2002). The primary output of a rapid HIA is a report identifying the potential health impacts of the proposal in question, and providing recommendations for decision-makers. Typically, but not always, a rapid HIA involves a participatory stakeholder workshop. Due to the limited time within which a rapid HIA is completed, it rarely includes wider public consultation or involvement.

Rapid HIAs can be popular with government departments, as their short time-frame can be more easily aligned with the cycle of local government planning. Many organizations also use rapid assessments as an entry point for a full HIA. Essentially, the screening component of a HIA (that aims to determine if a HIA is the best way to ensure that health and equity issues are addressed effectively in the proposal – see Figure 13.1) should also determine whether a full or a rapid HIA is more appropriate for a particular proposal, or whether an alternative impact assessment such as IIA would be a better option. However, in practice, restrictions on time and resources, or a limited opportunity to influence the decision-making process, may dictate that a rapid HIA is the only viable option.

While a rapid HIA can be less resource-intensive than a full HIA, there are several factors that affect the feasibility of conducting this type of HIA within a short period (Furber 2007). They include capacity and resource issues, such as the need to involve someone with experience in conducting a HIA (Furber 2007), but also access to existing literature reviews on health determinants on which the rapid HIA can draw.

The lack of human resources dedicated and available for HIA is often an issue. Slovakia and Lithuania have both seen the health services in charge of reviewing, screening, and scoping documents of an HIA being under-staffed (Lee, Robbel et al. 2013). Tight time-scales and access to a narrow evidence base have also contributed to criticisms around the rigour of evidence used within HIA (Mindell, Biddulph et al. 2010). This consequently presents another challenge for rapid HIAs, which are inevitably always time-restricted. One solution to this may be through practical tools or guides that enable better use of publicly available evidence. In improving the quality of evidence used in HIA, the credibility of HIA itself becomes enhanced (Mindell, Biddulph et al. 2010). Tools that strengthen the involvement of professionals from different sectors in public health approaches are key for reducing cost and establishing buy-in.

One major disadvantage of a rapid HIA is that the less time and resources are available to the process, the less likely it is that a range of stakeholders and communities will be consulted (Milner 2004). Other research suggests that the in-house screening within a rapid appraisal process virtually rules out any chance of involving the public, undermining the fundamental participatory element and principle of HIA (Blau and Mahoney 2005). A review of ten examples of health-related impact assessments in Germany found that participation of specific stakeholders or the general public was often underdeveloped or entirely absent, but that it produced valuable input when present (Rainer and Mekel 2010).

Another disadvantage of a rapid HIA is the reduced scope and depth of the information gathered. A more detailed HIA usually involves collecting new data that can provide deeper insights into the effects that the proposal can have on specific aspects of health within the given context (Furber 2007). More time also allows for greater collaboration between sectors, which can enhance mutual understanding. Finally, wider consultation also provides an opportunity for qualitative evidence and expert opinion to be considered, something which is not always possible or practical in a rapid HIA.

Local approach

Health impact assessment deals not only with predicting the health impact that an activity will have on a population, it also suggests ways to modify the activity to maximize health and mitigate harm (Kemm 2004). However, ensuring that HIA is implemented systematically in routine decision-making has often been difficult, particularly at the local level (Ståhl 2010). Greater involvement, responsibility, and active participation at the local level may help to overcome this problem. Furthermore, in some countries, such as Sweden and some other Nordic countries, it has been easier to engage the local than the national level in conducting HIA.

Within a community or local government context, HIA is often used as a decision-support tool and NGOs or community groups can use it in this way as an advocacy tool to influence decision-making. However, the role of NGOs in influencing healthy planning and policy development within local government can go further. Experience in Australia that is also of relevance to Europe shows how NGOs not only provide input to local governments on health planning issues, but also actively work with communities to influence their local councils, provide local support for councils to include healthy planning in their business, and adopt an advocacy role at the state and local government level (Harris, Wise et al. 2010). NGOs and civil society organizations can often use their recognized credibility and influence, based on strong connections to communities (Harris, Wise et al. 2010). In doing so, they can take leadership roles in working with communities, councils, and other sectors to influence the planning of healthy environments.

Within this local approach to HIA, communities are helping to define issues and contribute to decisions that have a direct impact on them (Harris-Roxas and Harris 2010). While there is a long tradition of local decision-making in some countries, such as those in Scandinavia, others are more centralized. However, this has been changing, with greater localism in some traditionally centralized countries such as France. A common challenge across countries is to maintain HIA teams at local level that have sufficient skills and knowledge.

Community-driven or community-led HIA aims to build the capacity of local residents to become active participants in decisions that impact on the health and well-being of their community. Community-led HIA processes do, however, depend on the community's awareness of the social determinants of health and the development of analytical skills that can be used to identify their own development strategies and priorities to ensure the health and well-being of their community (Cameron, Ghosh et al. 2010). However, this local approach has not been as prevalent in Europe as it has been in countries such as Australia. One of the reasons for this is lack of capacity. Another is the strong participative nature of local HIAs and communities' perception of the limited extent to which they can influence the decision-making process and the improvement of public policies (Bacigalupe, Esnaola et al. 2009). This is particularly the case in countries of southern Europe that share a history of relatively recent dictatorial regimes (Bacigalupe, Esnaola et al. 2009), which have made citizens sceptical of the influence they have to shape government decisions. The same might be true for many post-communist countries in central and eastern Europe and the former Soviet Union.

Equity-focused health impact assessment

A primary goal of all public health is to address health inequalities. The Marmot Review and the publication of "Fair Society, Healthy Lives" (The Marmot Review Team 2010) has brought a renewed interest in and focus on the impact of health inequalities, as has the more recent European review (Marmot, Allen et al. 2012). This has fostered a growing recognition of the need to tackle health inequalities through addressing the social determinants of health at the local, regional, national, and European level.

Equity is a core principle in HIA, with a recent review of policy-oriented HIA arguing that there is now a consensus that HIA is incomplete if it does not consider equity impacts within its process (Gunther 2011). The review also suggested that the equity focus of current HIA guidance needs to be strengthened (Gunther 2011).

Various names for equity-oriented HIAs are used in practice and in the academic literature, but for the purpose of this chapter all HIAs with a focus on equity or health equality will be referred to collectively as equity-focused HIAs. Equity-focused HIA uses HIA methodology to determine the differential impacts of a policy or practice on the health of a population and assesses whether these differential impacts are inequitable (Mahoney, Simpson et al. 2004). This type of HIA is based on the premise that there is currently no standardized or mandated way to identify differential health impacts or to assess whether these differential impacts are inequitable. In general, all equity-focused HIAs seek to provide a means to incorporate evidence about inequalities and their consequences into decision-making processes at all levels. As an extension of a "traditional" HIA they also aim to provide a flexible, yet structured approach to routinely and consistently identifying the possible impacts of policies and practices on different population groups.

However, it could be argued that, in high-quality HIAs, issues of equity and reducing health inequalities are already embedded in the framework and process. At a time when people are looking at streamlining processes, and combining multiple assessments, an additional assessment may not be looked upon that favourably. There may be more value in ensuring that the depth, quality, and scope of HIAs and IIAs allow inequalities to be addressed, and that equity is recognized as a wider social determinant that has a significant and long-lasting impact on health and well-being.

Regulating HIAs? Mandated versus voluntary impact assessments

There is debate as to whether HIA should be mandated, in line with environmental impact assessments in many countries, to fulfil a statutory or regulatory requirement. There are both advantages and disadvantages to this. HIAs that are not mandated, such as community-driven HIAs, allow for more flexibility. The process for undertaking these types of HIAs is often less formalized than for mandated HIAs or other impact assessments (Harris-Roxas and Harris 2010), which tend to place more importance on following tightly prescribed processes. This includes a degree of flexibility around the methods used (for example, not all stages of the HIA are necessarily completed) and there is also a degree of flexibility around what is considered acceptable evidence of impacts (Harris-Roxas and Harris 2010). This higher degree of flexibility can allow for more community involvement and make the HIA more easily adaptable to varying groups and stakeholders. It also discourages the perception of HIA as simply another tick-box exercise. Furthermore, by more easily transcending disciplinary traditions and boundaries, there may be greater opportunity for the assessment of underlying social, economic, and political factors that may be influencing the proposal (Harris-Roxas and Harris 2010).

On the other hand, it can be argued that mandating HIAs ensures that health is always considered as part of the process. Compared with the use of EIA and SEA within Europe, HIAs tend to be under-utilized and their results often overlooked (Salay and Lincoln 2009). This might in part be due to the fact that the European Commission has established formal requirements for EU member states to carry out EIA and SEA, while no similar explicit and detailed requirement exists for HIA (Salay and Lincoln 2009). Also, while the EU has a Treaty obligation to ensure that the health consequences of its policies are considered and the concept of Health in All Policies (HiAP) is adopted (Ståhl, Wismar et al. 2006), in practice these have received scant attention. The question of whether HIA is an EU competence could be clarified through a well-selected legal test case, but to date no one has done this. A related question is how accurately and holistically health is considered in different types of impact assessments. For example, there is much debate around how health is being considered within EIAs. The WHO Regional Office for Europe (2011) claims that although EIA legislation is supposed to deal with health effects, in reality they are assessed poorly or not at all.

Another issue to consider is the risk of capture by vested interests if HIAs become mandatory. As long as they are only voluntary, and do not need to be taken into consideration in important decisions, powerful interests such as the food, tobacco, alcohol, and other industries may feel they can ignore them. The role of the tobacco industry in shaping impact assessments undertaken by the European Commission is a cautionary tale (Smith, Fooks et al. 2010).

Other considerations to take into account when mandating HIA are the implications for practice. With the use of mandated HIA come more rigid and standardized methods of practice. Practitioners may have to be accredited and roles, responsibilities, and accountabilities of proponents, regulators, and practitioners will have to be more clearly articulated (Harris-Roxas and Harris 2010). This has both benefits and considerable risks, in particular if it leads to over-bureaucratization of the process, creating more delays. Capacity issues will arise, as there is currently no clear role for public or corporate institutions in training HIA practitioners. The establishment of permanent structures, such as dedicated units supporting the practice of HIA, would typically require significant investment. However, this could help to ensure a more stable and long-term commitment than ad hoc networks (Government of South Australia 2010).

Conclusions

Health impact assessment is increasingly regarded as a means for identifying the impact of policies on health determinants and as a key strategy for implementing intersectoral action. The approaches to HIA and, more recently, HiAP are seen as strategies for integrating health considerations into other (non-health) policies (Ståhl and Perttilä 2010).

Increased recognition of the wider determinants of health and the importance of building cross-sectoral capacity is vital to ensuring healthy public policy is a goal shared by all sectors. The trend towards integrating impact assessments that share similar methods and goals can serve as a strategy to tackle both health and sustainability challenges.

Each of the impact assessments discussed in this chapter is a legitimate mechanism for influencing decision-making. However, at a time of increasing pressure to reduce the resources and time associated with impact assessments, an integrated approach may have practical value and still, if done properly, ensure that health impacts are adequately considered at all stages of the process.

There is concern that in integrating or combining impact assessments a reductionist approach to health will be adopted. However, all approaches work best when a wide variety of stakeholders are involved, and when there is an opportunity to draw from the best available research, including qualitative data, in order to inform and influence the decision-making process. Incorporating a holistic understanding of health has the advantage of providing an overlap with the priorities of different sectors and illustrating the benefits that exist for all sectors when health is taken into consideration.

Of fundamental importance to this process will be to ensure that the following factors are addressed:

- quality – methods used, experience of practitioners, capacity, available evidence;
- scope – who initiated the assessment, what questions are being asked, whether there is a recognition of unintentional effects;
- depth – concept of health and the wider determinants of health;
- equity – should always be a consideration, with the aim of reducing health inequalities;
- stakeholder and public involvement and participation – opportunity for a range of sectors to be involved, as well as public and expert involvement.

Incorporating HIA within other impact assessments does not necessarily imply a loss of focus on health issues. As long as appropriate criteria related to the above factors are met, integrating health into other impact assessments can in fact reflect a recognition and acceptance of the wider determinants of health. It can also help to establish new ways of working together, involving a range of people across many sectors. Many of the impact assessments discussed in this chapter share a similar range of methods used to gather, synthesize, and communicate information. The determinants of health, for example, are used as a basis for assessing proposals in both HIA and IIA, and there is a growing call for the social determinants of health to be more widely, and consistently, applied in SEAs as well.

Embedding health in the decision-making processes of organizations is crucial to the sustainability and effectiveness of HIA and other approaches that integrate health into assessment processes. However, HIA needs to be viewed as more than the drawing up of a report, with recommendations for action. Including considerations of health within impact assessments and decision-making processes – at all levels, and at all stages – should be regarded as a crucial avenue for building relationships across sectors and a means for collective action on key issues of concern.

References

Association of Public Health Observatories (2007). *Integrated Impact Assessment (IIA)* [http://www.apho.org.uk/resource/view.aspx?RID=48174].

Bacigalupe, A., S. Esnaola, C. Calderon, J. Zuazagoitia and E. Aldasoro (2009). "Health impact assessment of an urban regeneration project: opportunities and challenges in the context of a Southern European city." *Journal of Epidemiology and Community Health* **64**: 950–955.

Birley, M. (2007). "A fault analysis for health impact assessment: procurement, competence, expectations, and jurisdictions." *Impact Assessment and Project Appraisal* **25**(4): 281–289.

Birley, M. H. (2003). "Health impact assessment, integration and critical appraisal." *Impact Assessment and Project Appraisal* **21**(4): 313–321.

Blau, G. and M. Mahoney (2005). *The Positioning of Health Impact Assessment in Local Government in Victoria.* Melbourne, VIC, Deakin University.

Blau, J., K. Ernst, M. Wismar, F. Baro, M. Gabrijelcic Blenkus, K. von Bremen and R. Fehr (2007). "The use of HIA across Europe." In *The Effectiveness of Health Impact Assessment: Scope and limitations of supporting decision-making in Europe.* M. Wismar, J. Blau, K. Ernst and J. Figueras, Eds. Copenhagen, WHO Regional Office for Europe on behalf of the European Observatory on Health Systems and Policies.

Caldwell, L. (1988). "Environmental impact analysis (EIA): origins, evolution and future directions." *Policy Studies Review* **8**: 75–83.

Cameron, C., S. Ghosh and S. Eaton (2010). "Facilitating communities in designing and using their own community health impact assessment tool." *Environmental Impact Assessment Review* **31**(4): 433–437.

Commission on Social Determinants of Health (CSDH) (2008). *Closing the Gap in a Generation: Health equity through action on the social determinants of health.* Final Report of the Commission on Social Determinants of Health. Geneva, WHO.

Committee on Health Impact Assessment (2011). *Appendix A: Experiences with health impact assessment. Improving health in the United States: the role of health impact assessment.* Committee on Health Impact Assessment of the National Academy of Sciences. Washington, D.C., National Academies Press: 130–177.

Frankish, C., L. Green, P. Ratner, T. Chomik and C. Larsen (2001). "Health impact assessment as a tool for health promotion and population health." *WHO Regional Publications, European Series* **92**: 405–437.

Furber, S. E. (2007). "Rapid versus intermediate health impact assessment of foreshore development plans." *NSW Public Health Bulletin* **18**(9/10): 174–176.

Government of South Australia (2010). "Health in All Policies: Adelaide 2010 International Meeting." *Public Health Bulletin SA* **7**(2) [http://www.health.sa.gov.au/pehs/publications/publichealthbulletin-pehs-sahealth-1007.pdf].

Gunther, S. (2011). *A Rapid Review of Enhancing the Equity Focus on Policy Orientated Health Impact Assessment*. Birmingham, Equity Action: EU Joint Action on Health Inequalities.

Harris-Roxas, B. and E. Harris (2010). "Differing forms, differing purposes: a typology of health impact assessment." *Environmental Impact Assessment Review* **31**: 396–403.

Harris, P., M. Wise, S. Dunn and E. Harris (2010). *Influencing Healthy Planning and Policy Development in Local Government: Summary report*. Sydney, NSW, UNSW Research Centre for Primary Health Care and Equity, University of New South Wales.

Kemm, J. (2004). "What is HIA? Introduction and overview." In *Health Impact Assessment: Concepts, theory, techniques and applications*. J. Kemm, J. Parry and S. Palmer, Eds. Oxford, Oxford University Press: 1–13.

Kemm, J., J. Perry and S. Palmer, Eds. (2004). *Health Impact Assessment: Concepts, theory, techniques and applications*. Oxford, Oxford University Press.

Koivusalo, M. (2010). "The state of Health in All policies (HiAP) in the European Union: potential and pitfalls." *Journal of Epidemiology and Community Health* **64**: 500–503.

Lee, J., N. Robbel and C. Dora (2013). *Cross-country Analysis of the Institutionalization of Health Impact Assessment*. Social Determinants of Health Discussion Paper Series 8 (Policy & Practice). Geneva, WHO.

Lock, K., M. Gabrijelcic-Blenkus, M. Martuzzi, P. Otorepec, P. Wallace, C. Dora, A. Robertson and M. Zakotnic Jozica (2003). "Health impact assessment of agriculture and food policies: lessons learnt from the Republic of Slovenia." *Bulletin of the World Health Organization* **81**(6): 391–398.

Lock, K. and M. McKee (2005). "Health impact assessment: assessing opportunities and barriers to intersectoral health improvement in an expanded European Union." *Journal of Epidemiology and Community Health* **59**: 356–360.

Mahoney, M., S. Simpson, E. Harris, R. Aldrich and J. Stewart Williams (2004). *Equity Focused Health Impact Assessment Framework*. Newcastle, NSW, The Australian Collaboration for Health Equity Impact Assessment (ACHEIA).

Marmot, M., J. Allen, R. Bell, E. Bloomer, P. Goldblatt and Consortium for the European Review of Social Determinants of Health and the Health Divide (2012). "WHO European review of social determinants of health and the health divide." *The Lancet* **380**(9846): 1011–1029.

Milner, S. J. (2004). "Using HIA in local government." In *Health Impact Assessment: Concepts, theory, techniques and applications*. J. Kemm, J. Parry and S. Palmer, Eds. Oxford, Oxford University Press.

Mindell, J., J. Biddulph, L. Taylor, K. Lock, A. Boaz, M. Joffe and S. Curtis (2010). "Improving the use of evidence in health impact assessment." *Bulletin of the World Health Organization* **88**: 543–550.

Mindell, J., L. Reynolds, D. Cohen and M. McKee (2012). "All in this together: the corporate capture of public health." *British Medical Journal* **345**: e8082.

National Institute for Clinical Excellence (NICE) (2005). *Clarifying Approaches to: Health Needs Assessment, Health Impact Assessment, Integrated Impact Assessment, Health Equity Audit, and Race Equality Impact Assessment*. London, NHS Health Development Agency.

NHS Health Development Agency (2002). *Introducing Health Impact Assessment (HIA): Informing the decision-making process*. London, NHS Health Development Agency.

NHS Health Development Agency (2003). *Clarifying Health Impact Assessment, Integrated Impact Assessment and Health Needs Assessment*. London, NHS Health Development Agency.

Nottingham City Council (NCC) (2011). *Integrated Impact Assessment*. Nottingham, NCC.

Public Health Advisory Committee (PHAC) (2007) *An Idea whose Time has Come: New opportunities for health impact assessment in New Zealand public policy and planning.* Wellington, NZ, PHAC.

Put, G. V., L. d. Broeder, M. Penris and E. W. R. Abbin (2001). *Experience with HIA at National Policy Level in the Netherlands: A case study.* Copenhagen, WHO Regional Office for Europe.

Rainer, F. and O. Mekel (2010). *Health Impact Assessment (HIA) in Germany.* NRW Institute of Health and Work (LIGA.NRW). Düsseldorf/Bielefeld, WHO Collaborating Centre for Regional Health Policy and Public Health.

Salay, R. and P. Lincoln (2009). "Increasing the use of health impact assessments: is the environment a model?" *Eurohealth* **15**(2): 20–22.

Smith, K., G. Fooks, J. Collin, H. Weishaar, S. Mandal and A. Gilmore (2010). " 'Working the system' – British American tobacco's influence on the European union treaty and its implications for policy: an analysis of internal tobacco industry documents." *PLoS Medicine* **7**(1): e1000202.

Sparrow, A. (2012). "Cameron hits out at 'bureaucratic rubbish' holding back UK economy." *The Guardian* [http://www.guardian.co.uk/politics/2012/nov/19/cameron-bureacratic-rubbish-uk-economy, accessed 17 May 2013].

St.-Pierre, L., G. Hamel, G. Lapointe, D. McQueen and M. Wismar (2009). *Governance Tools and Framework for Health in All Policies* [http://rvz.net/uploads/docs/Achtergrondstudie_-_Governance_tools_and_framework.pdf, accessed 30 July 2013]. Montréal, National Collaborating Centre for Healthy Public Policy.

Ståhl, T. (2010). "Is the increasing policy use of impact assessment in Europe likely to undermine efforts to achieve healthy public policy?" *Journal of Epidemiology and Community Health* **64**(6): 476.

Ståhl, T. and K. Perttilä (2010). "Health in All Policies at the local level in Finland." *Public Health Bulletin SA* **7**(2): 24–27.

Ståhl, T., M. Wismar, E. Ollila, E. Lahtinen and K. Leppo, Eds. (2006). *Health in All Policies: Prospects and potentials.* Helsinki, Ministry of Social Affairs and Health.

The Marmot Review Team (2010). *Fair Society, Healthy Lives: Strategic review of health inequalities in England post 2010.* London, Marmot Review.

United Nations (UN)/Regional Environmental Center for Central and Eastern Europe (2006). *Resource Manual to Support Application of the Protocol on SEA* [http://www.unece.org/fileadmin/DAM/env/eia/sea_manual/welcome.html, accessed 30 July 2013]. Geneva, UN/Regional Environmental Center for Central and Eastern Europe.

Wismar, M., J. Blau, K. Ernst and J. Figueras, Eds. (2007). *The Effectiveness of Health Impact Assessment: Scope and limitations of supporting decision making in Europe.* Copenhagen, WHO Regional Office for Europe on behalf of the European Observatory on Health Systems and Policies.

World Health Organization (WHO) European Centre for Health Policy (2001). "Health impact assessment: main concepts and suggested approach." Gothenburg consensus paper, December 1999. In *Health Impact Assessment: From theory to practice.* V. Diwan, M. Douglas, I. Karlberg, J. Lehto, G. Magnusson and A. Ritsatakis, Eds. Göteborg, Nordic School of Public Health: 89–103.

World Health Organization (WHO) Regional Office for Europe (2011). *Health Impact Assessment – Policy: Including health in environmental assessments.* [http://www.euro.who.int/en/what-we-do/health-topics/environmental-health/health-impact-assessment/policy]. Copenhagen, WHO Regional Office for Europe.

Wright, J., J. Parry and E. Scully (2005). "Institutionalizing policy-level health impact assessment in Europe: is coupling health impact assessment with strategic environmental assessment the next step forward? *Bulletin of the World Health Organization* **83**: 472–477.

chapter fourteen

Organization and financing of public health

Bernd Rechel, Helmut Brand, Martin McKee

Introduction

Assuring sustainable organizational structures and financing has been identified as one of the ten essential public health operations (EPHOs) in the European Action Plan for Strengthening Public Health Capacities and Services (see Chapter 1, "Facets of public health in Europe: an introduction"). This chapter explores the great diversity that exists in the organization and financing of public health in Europe. To begin with, understandings of public health vary among European countries (Kaiser and Mackenbach 2008; Tragakes, Brigis et al. 2008), with major ramifications for the organization and financing of public health activities. Countries also differ in the balance between centralized and decentralized public health operations, consistent with their constitutional and governmental arrangements (Saltman, Bankauskaite et al. 2007). There is also diversity with regard to how countries address the vertical and horizontal integration of public health activities across different programmes, sectors, and levels of care. The financing of public health, on the other hand, has been described as a "black box" (Duran and Kutzin 2010). Yet, several key dimensions can be distinguished, including the share of total health expenditure devoted to public health and the mechanisms in place for raising revenues for public health activities. Just as with health financing generally, models in Europe differ greatly and there tends to be a mix of financing sources, with growing interest by health ministries in taxes earmarked for public health purposes, although finance ministries have long been much less enthusiastic (Rechel, Brand et al. 2013).

This chapter, building on earlier work (Rechel and McKee 2012) informing WHO's 2012 European Action Plan for Strengthening Public Health Capacities and Services, aims to provide an overview of the organization and financing of public health activities in Europe. We start by examining the historical context and current reform initiatives with regard to the organization of public health in Europe. We then explore how far responsibility for public health has been devolved to sub-national levels, which we found to be one of the main ways in which countries across Europe differ with regard to the organization and delivery of public health operations. We then examine the vertical and horizontal integration of public health activities and the administrative set-up of public health services in Europe. Next, we review mechanisms for the financing of public health in Europe, exploring such issues as the share of total health expenditure spent on public health and the sources of funds. We conclude that a more systematic examination of the organization and financing of public health in Europe is urgently required.

Organization

Public health is a very broad area of societal action, involving many actors (see Chapter 1, "Facets of public health in Europe: an introduction"). Tobacco control efforts, for example, include action that goes far beyond the traditional health sector and involves agriculture, trade, education, fiscal policy, and law enforcement, at the local, national, and global level (Allin, Mossialos et al. 2004). Given the variety of public health operations and functions, they are generally not performed by a single entity. Instead, the provision of public health activities in Europe is characterized by a multitude of actors from both the public and private sectors, including dedicated public health agencies, institutes of public health, other state agencies working on public health, state organizations outside the health system, healthcare providers, and non-governmental organizations (NGOs).

Historical context and current reform initiatives

While recognizing that there are marked differences across countries, in general the scope of public health in Europe has slowly evolved in recent decades, from a focus on sanitary supervision and communicable disease control to one on "new" public health – concerned with health promotion, disease prevention, and intersectoral action – increasingly emphasizing interventions outside the health system. These developments are in line with major international initiatives to move beyond a medical model of public health, including the 1977 World Health Assembly resolution on Health for All, the Declaration of Alma-Ata (WHO 1978), WHO's 1981 Health for All strategy, and the Ottawa Charter for Health Promotion (WHO 1986). The Tallinn Charter, Health Systems for Health and Wealth, recognized in 2008 that "health systems are more than health care and include disease prevention, health promotion and efforts to influence other sectors to address health concerns in their policies" (WHO 2008).

However, as a concept "public health" is still characterized by a huge diversity of terminologies and interpretations. Across Europe there is not even a consensus on the meaning of public health (Kaiser and Mackenbach 2008) or what it should do (Weil and McKee 1998). Consequently, there are different understandings among European countries on the tasks and limits of public health services, and there are wide differences in the extent to which public health features on national agendas (Aluttis, Chiotan et al. 2013).

A number of countries are currently reforming their systems for delivering public health services or operations. Although reforms of public health services in central and eastern Europe have lagged behind those in other parts of the health system, particularly in some of the former Soviet countries (Maier, Palm et al. 2009), this area of Europe has witnessed some of the most significant changes to the organization of public health services over the last two decades. In the communist period, public health services in central and eastern Europe were organized in ways similar to the model of sanitary-epidemiological (SANEPID) services established in the Soviet Union. These services were highly centralized and hierarchical and represented at all administrative levels. They were charged with health protection, mainly the control and surveillance of communicable diseases, the monitoring of environmental conditions, and the enforcement of sanitary-hygienic regulations (Rechel and McKee 2006; WHO 2009b; Maier and Martin-Moreno 2011). Although the SANEPID services initially made great progress in the fight against communicable diseases, setting up comprehensive childhood vaccination programmes and contributing to the decline of many communicable diseases, they were much less effective in the areas of non-communicable diseases, occupational health, and environmental health, while health promotion and intersectoral action were largely neglected (WHO 2009b; Maier and Martin-Moreno 2011). The prevention of infectious diseases through vaccination was one of the main strengths of the SANEPID services and this, after some disruptions in the early 1990s, has to a large degree been maintained, with very high vaccination rates persisting (Maier, Palm et al. 2009; Maier and Martin-Moreno 2011). However, there continue to be great problems in addressing more complex communicable diseases, most notably HIV/AIDS and TB, with poorly integrated vertical structures, whereas in western European countries services are more often integrated into mainstream healthcare provision.

Many of the countries of central and eastern Europe have embarked on reforms after the collapse of communism, usually involving some degree of deconcentration, with the transfer of responsibilities from the centre to the periphery (Gotsadze, Chikovani et al. 2010). Reforms were typically less extensive in the countries of the former Soviet Union. In those countries, some (including Azerbaijan, Belarus, the Russian Federation, and Ukraine) have largely preserved the SANEPID structure inherited from the Soviet period (Popovich, Potapchik et al. 2011), some (including Kazakhstan, Kyrgyzstan, Moldova, and Uzbekistan) have built additional structures, and others (in particular Georgia) have set up new public health infrastructures. In Georgia, the high speed of reforms, the privatization of some public health functions, and the unclear lines of responsibility following decentralization of public health services led to problems in communicable disease control (Armenian, Crape et al. 2009; Maier and Martin-Moreno 2011). However, an understanding of "new" public health, as concerned with the main threats to population health, is still underdeveloped in both central and eastern Europe and the former Soviet countries. Instead, public health services in many countries of the region are more concerned with hygiene, sanitation, and communicable disease control, and less with health promotion and intersectoral action for health (Rechel and McKee 2006; Armenian, Crape et al. 2009; WHO 2009b). Indeed, many post-communist countries struggled with the very concept of "public health", as the term was difficult to translate into national languages (Tragakes, Brigis et al. 2008).

The situation is slightly different in countries of the former Yugoslavia, as they had a long-standing public health tradition under the leadership of the Andrija Štampar School of Public Health (Rechel and McKee 2006). There are historically well-developed public health institutions in the form of the institutes of public health and there has traditionally been a comprehensive and high-quality network of public health laboratories. However, the public health structures have in many cases been allowed to deteriorate, suffering from under-investment and the failure to adjust to new public health threats (WHO 2009b).

It should also be noted that in several western European countries too, public health services were for a long time limited to sanitary supervision and communicable disease control and only more recently have efforts been made to make health promotion and disease prevention more prominent (Hofmarcher and Rack 2006). This can be explained in part by the historical context of public health in some of these countries. The discipline of public health emerged in the eighteenth century based on the sanitary movement, complemented later by a focus on hygiene. However, the emphasis on "genetic" or "racial hygiene" in the 1930s in Nazi Germany and, after it joined with Germany in 1938, in Austria, led to it being discredited in these countries in the post-war period (McKee and Pomerleau 2005). Some other western European countries, such as Greece, also still have very weak public health systems (Economou 2010).

In western Europe, countries where health financing is based on social insurance have traditionally had weak public health services, detached from health care and with difficulty attracting talented staff. Several countries, such as Austria and Switzerland, have established new foundations for health promotion (Saltman, Allin et al. 2012). In Austria, there is now a national centre for health promotion, the Fund for a Healthy Austria. However, the provision of health promotion in these countries tends to be outsourced to external institutions such as non-governmental organizations (NGOs) or foundations (Ladurner, Gerger et al. 2011). In Switzerland, there is a range of small-scale health promotion programmes, many undertaken by NGOs and foundations (OECD/WHO 2011). Some of the most successful health promotion activities have been implemented in the Nordic countries (Glenngård, Hjalte et al. 2005). In Finland, health promotion and disease prevention have been at the centre of health policy for decades, following the example of the often-cited North Karelia Project and after having been a pilot country for the 1984 Health for All strategy of the WHO Regional Office for Europe (Vuorenkoski, Mladovsky et al. 2008). In Denmark, however, despite a strong tradition of public health research, health policy, especially where it challenged vested interests such as the food, alcohol, and tobacco industries, has been weak until recently. Although there has been less progress against hazardous alcohol consumption and smoking, the government introduced the world's first tax on foods containing saturated fats in 2011, a tax that was dropped again in 2012 (Strandberg-Larsen, Nielsen et al. 2007; Olejaz, Juul Nielsen et al. 2012).

Overall legal framework

In most countries in Europe, there is an overall legal framework defining responsibilities for many public health services and operations. In a study on public health capacity in the EU, 26 of 27 countries reported having legislation fully or partially in place that defined responsibilities for setting up structures to protect and promote the health of the population (Aluttis, Chiotan et al. 2013). However, the authors of the study could identify no clearly defined modern public health structure in Austria; nor could they identify a national priority-setting process or national health targets (Ladurner, Gerger et al. 2011). Yet, even where formal responsibilities have been designated, this does not automatically imply a well-functioning system, as implementation may be incomplete. In addition, while many countries have clear responsibilities with regards to traditional public health issues such as communicable disease control, hygiene, and immunization, responsibilities were less clearly established for many of the "new" aspects of public health, such as behavioural and social determinants of health and health inequalities (Aluttis, Chiotan et al. 2013).

Level of decentralization

Throughout Europe, countries generally have a basic infrastructure in place for public health service delivery at national, regional, and local level, maintaining relevant public health activities and formally granting virtually universal access to the population. However, there is great diversity in the ways in which public health operations are organized and delivered. One of the main ways in which they differ is how far responsibility has been devolved to sub-national levels, which is in large part due to the size of each country and its population, and the underlying constitutional, political, and administrative framework.

While all countries have some national public health capacity, such as reference laboratories and statistical offices, in federal or highly decentralized systems, the majority of public health services are often the responsibility of regional or even local administrative tiers. Examples are Belgium, Denmark, Finland, Italy (Box 14.1), Spain, Sweden, Switzerland, and the United Kingdom (Allin, Mossialos et al. 2004; Glenngård, Hjalte et al. 2005; Vuorenkoski, Mladovsky et al. 2008; Lo Scalzo, Donatini et al. 2009; García-Armesto, Abadía-Taira et al. 2010; Gerkens and Merkur 2010; Boyle 2011; OECD/WHO 2011; Anell, Glenngård et al. 2012; Olejaz, Juul Nielsen et al. 2012). In Austria and Germany, the Länder (states) have almost complete autonomy in most aspects of public health, but they delegate some tasks to local authorities and regional health insurance funds (Allin, Mossialos et al. 2004; Busse and Riesberg 2004; Hofmarcher and Rack 2006).

Box 14.1   Regional differences in public health structures in Italy

As Italian regions have exercised their autonomy very differently, northern regions have been more successful in establishing effective structures for public health, programme delivery, and health monitoring than regions in the south. Regional variations reflect differences in contextual, political, economic, and cultural factors, as well as differences between regional health systems.

Source: Aluttis, Chiotan et al. (2013)

In contrast, in the remaining European countries, national authorities are predominantly responsible for planning and organizing public health services, although administration and implementation is often delegated to lower levels of administration. The health system in Ireland used to be characterized by a degree of decentralization, but has been recentralized, including its public health services (McDaid, Wiley et al. 2009).

Even in federal or decentralized systems, the Ministry of Health or another umbrella public health body usually provides an overall strategic framework, and is responsible for drawing up legislation and regulations on the various aspects of public health, as well as for monitoring population health and coordinating activities between national and local level (Allin, Mossialos et al. 2004; Armenian, Crape et al. 2009; Lo Scalzo, Donatini et al. 2009). There are also national agencies in charge of research, public health expertise, surveillance, and health promotion. In all European countries, communicable disease surveillance and control is vested at the national level, reflecting responsibilities under the International Health Regulations. International cooperation is crucial in communicable disease control (Rowe and Rechel 2006), and WHO and the European Centre for Disease Prevention and Control, established by the EU in 2004, support epidemiological surveillance activities at the European level, and run an early warning and response system (see Chapter 4, "The health security framework in Europe"). However, few countries in Europe have a single national body to review screening practice and policy, and population registers for call and re-call and follow-up of patients are also comparatively rare (Holland, Stewart et al. 2006).

National coordination and leadership of public health activities can pose a major challenge for decentralized health systems, as was noted for example in Switzerland, where cantons have a high degree of autonomy (OECD/WHO 2011). Decentralization can also have implications for the coordination of health information systems, illustrated by the long delays involved in publishing national mortality data from Belgium (see Chapter 3, "Monitoring the health of the population").

Vertical and horizontal integration

The many actors involved in the delivery of public health activities make horizontal and vertical integration pivotal (Mays, Scutchfield et al. 2010). The horizontal integration of services is a particular challenge in countries where separate vertical public health structures are in place, such as for HIV/AIDS, tuberculosis, and substance abuse in many countries of central and eastern Europe (Koppel, Kahur et al. 2008; Koppel, Leventhal et al. 2009; Duran and Kutzin 2010; Gotsadze, Chikovani et al. 2010). Poor integration of public health activities was noted as a particular problem in Armenia, where more than half a dozen government ministries and many state agencies have a substantial role in public health, while the Ministry of Health covers only some public health services. In addition, some public health activities are provided by international organizations and national NGOs. There is no overriding central state authority responsible for the integration, coordination, and oversight of all public health authorities in Armenia (Armenian, Crape et al. 2009). Integration of public health services can sometimes be easier at a regional level (Koppel, Leventhal et al. 2009). In Spain, for example, following political decentralization, the integration of different inspectorates and administrations was achieved at the regional level (García-Armesto, Abadía-Taira et al. 2010).

The vertical integration of public health services across different administrative tiers is another challenge, as public health services are partly integrated with curative services and partly organized as separate activities by special institutions. In many European countries, primary care physicians or specialists are increasingly involved in providing preventive services, such as immunizations, health check-ups or screening, and are also responsible for the notification of communicable diseases (Saltman, Allin et al. 2012). There is, however, considerable variation in how far these physicians provide health promotion and advice on unhealthy lifestyles (Aluttis, Chiotan et al. 2013), an activity particularly lacking in south-east Europe (Rechel and McKee 2006; WHO 2009b). Yet, most preventive services, such as immunizations and screening, are provided within primary health care. In Croatia and Slovenia, for example, childhood and adolescent immunizations are administered by primary care paediatricians (public and private), family physicians or GPs (private and public), and school health physicians (WHO 2007b). In Germany, the administration of preventive services by office-based physicians has even been described as a cause of the low profile of public health services (Busse and Riesberg 2004). Primary health care reforms in some countries in central and eastern Europe have also diminished the role of primary health care in public health. In some countries of the region, a decline in home visits and preventive check-ups has been noted, as these were not incentivized for newly independent primary healthcare providers (Rechel, Bozikov et al. 2012). In Croatia, following the partial replacement of medical centres by independent GPs, some of the public health functions previously provided were taken over by Institutes of Public Health, such as epidemiological services and school health services (WHO 2007b). Countries that seem to have achieved a better integration of public health services into primary care include Denmark, Estonia, Finland, Portugal, Spain, and Sweden (Glenngård, Hjalte et al. 2005; Barros and de Almeida Simoes 2007; Strandberg-Larsen, Nielsen et al. 2007; Vuorenkoski, Mladovsky et al. 2008; Koppel, Leventhal et al. 2009; García-Armesto, Abadía-Taira et al. 2010; Anell, Glenngård et al. 2012; Olejaz, Juul Nielsen et al. 2012). Those in secondary care increasingly recognize their role in public health, as exemplified by the Health-Promoting Hospital initiative (Whitehead 2004).

Irrespective of these examples, the vertical and horizontal integration of public health activities remains a major challenge in many European countries. It requires careful planning, as well as aligning strategic goals and priorities with available resources (see Chapter 16, "Developing public health leadership").

Administrative set-up

Another way in which public health services differ across Europe is their administrative set-up. In several countries, such as the Netherlands and Germany, many core public health services are subordinated to local government, while in Scotland, Wales, and Northern Ireland they report to health ministries. In England, the delivery of public health services underwent a major shift in April 2013, when the responsibility for public health at the local level was transferred from primary care trusts (PCTs) and, by extension, the National Health Service (NHS), to local government authorities. Although it is too early to draw conclusions on the impact of this transition, concerns have been raised about increasing fragmentation, budgetary shortfalls, and the disruption to service delivery that this shake-up could entail (McKee, Hurst et al. 2011). In the countries of the former Yugoslavia, national and regional public health institutes play a key role in the planning and provision of public health operations (WHO 2007c, 2007d).

Financing

As noted above, the financing of public health activities has been described as a "black box" (Duran and Kutzin 2010). Many actors and sectors are involved, some costs fall on private enterprises and are unaccounted for, and even the definition of what public health activities are differs from one country to the next (Allin, Mossialos et al. 2004; Sensenig 2007). Some definitions include personal health services delivered by public health agencies, while others only include population-based services (Sensenig 2007). Only in 2011 was a global standard of health accounts published (OECD, Eurostat/WHO 2011). According to this standard, prevention and public health services are defined as "services designed to enhance the health status of the population as distinct from curative services, which repair health dysfunction" (OECD, Eurostat/ WHO 2011). Sub-components include maternal and child health, school health services, prevention of communicable or non-communicable diseases, and occupational health care.

While this clarifies the boundaries considerably, and explicitly includes areas such as environmental surveillance for public health purposes, there are many areas that fall under a more "upstream" and "whole-of-society" understanding of public health, such as strategies to improve health through active transport programmes, that are not captured by the system of health accounts as expenditure on prevention and public health (de Bekker-Grob, Polder et al. 2007).

What share of the overall health budget is devoted to public health?

Health accounts data provide the best available estimates of expenditure on prevention and public health for most countries of the WHO European Region (Table 14.1). They are based on national reporting and published in the WHO Global Health Expenditure database. Where adjustments or estimates are required, these are validated by national ministries of health prior to publication (WHO 2012).

Table 14.1 Expenditure on prevention and public health as a percentage of total health expenditure, WHO European Region, 2003–2011

	2003	*2004*	*2005*	*2006*	*2007*	*2008*	*2009*	*2010*	*2011*
Albania	1.57	—	—	—	5.48	3.21	2.90	3.28	—
Armenia	0.61	0.90	3.86	5.15	3.90	4.47	4.69	—	—
Austria	1.67	1.93	1.90	1.90	1.89	1.78	1.72	1.69	1.69
Belarus	—	—	—	—	—	—	—	3.81	3.93
Belgium	1.88	1.84	2.44	2.09	2.15	2.53	2.48	1.97	1.97
Bosnia and Herzegovina	—	2.70	2.80	2.89	2.65	3.06	1.10	1.07	0.96
Bulgaria	3.45	3.86	3.01	3.45	3.86	4.09	3.46	4.20	—
Croatia	—	—	—	0.58	0.62	0.76	1.21	1.21	—
Cyprus	0.58	0.55	0.55	0.61	0.64	0.55	0.55	0.53	0.53
Czech Republic	1.68	1.96	1.67	2.08	2.19	2.59	2.60	2.41	2.41
Denmark	2.26	2.20	2.12	2.02	2.06	2.08	2.16	2.22	2.22
Estonia	2.47	2.23	2.31	2.53	2.67	2.67	2.24	2.72	2.71
Finland	4.81	4.89	5.05	5.10	5.40	5.43	5.25	5.18	5.21
France	2.02	2.04	1.97	1.95	1.98	2.07	2.26	1.96	1.93
Georgia	2.20	2.27	1.80	1.12	1.15	0.64	1.20	1.61	—
Germany	3.20	3.23	3.21	3.28	3.50	3.56	3.52	3.13	3.13
Greece	—	—	—	—	—	—	—	—	1.34
Hungary	4.81	4.36	4.34	4.12	4.07	4.03	4.34	4.35	4.35
Iceland	1.39	1.45	1.54	1.52	1.62	1.55	1.45	1.48	1.45
Ireland	2.32	2.96	2.96	3.01	2.98	2.98	3.12	2.99	2.99
Israel	0.92	0.85	0.77	0.71	0.65	0.63	0.68	0.70	0.70
Italy	0.71	0.62	0.56	0.56	0.60	—	—	—	—
Kyrgyzstan	—	2.20	—	2.27	2.84	4.44	3.84	3.63	2.87
Latvia	2.73	0.98	—	2.86	1.39	1.43	2.83	2.82	—
Lithuania	—	1.72	1.69	1.18	1.74	1.17	1.13	1.13	—

(continued)

Table 14.1 Expenditure on prevention and public health as a percentage of total health expenditure, WHO European Region, 2003–2011 (*continued*)

	2003	*2004*	*2005*	*2006*	*2007*	*2008*	*2009*	*2010*	*2011*
Luxembourg	1.77	1.47	2.06	1.68	1.90	1.72	1.90	1.74	1.74
Malta	1.58	1.55	1.44	1.31	1.44	1.13	1.32	1.55	—
Montenegro	—	0.57	0.56	0.68	—	—	—	—	—
Netherlands	4.89	4.49	4.33	4.58	4.48	4.10	4.50	4.44	3.61
Norway	1.93	1.94	1.91	1.90	1.99	2.00	—	2.42	2.43
Poland	3.30	1.68	2.28	2.31	2.26	2.23	2.18	1.93	1.92
Portugal	1.97	1.89	1.94	1.66	1.66	1.74	1.95	2.02	2.02
Republic of Moldova	—	—	—	—	—	—	4.35	7.56	—
Romania	6.16	6.63	6.73	5.24	6.51	5.72	8.10	6.03	—
Serbia	8.70	8.02	7.43	7.33	7.05	6.68	7.49	6.33	6.33
Slovakia	1.64	2.73	2.28	4.29	4.71	4.61	4.62	5.04	—
Slovenia	3.41	3.65	3.57	3.58	3.70	3.56	3.50	3.64	—
Spain	2.30	2.31	2.34	2.36	2.45	2.30	2.67	2.25	—
Sweden	3.10	3.06	3.29	3.07	3.34	3.45	3.65	3.41	3.41
Switzerland	2.28	2.20	2.18	2.16	2.32	2.43	2.50	2.36	2.36
Tajikistan	0.94	0.92	1.32	—	2.19	3.03	2.78	2.84	5.06
Turkey	4.67	5.11	4.97	4.91	5.38	5.57	5.63	5.62	5.62
Ukraine	3.68	3.68	3.47	3.65	3.50	3.39	3.08	3.18	2.83

Note: No data available for Andorra, Azerbaijan, Kazakhstan, Monaco, the Russian Federation, San Marino, the former Yugoslav Republic of Macedonia, Turkmenistan, the United Kingdom, and Uzbekistan.
Source: WHO (2013)

According to the data available, expenditure on prevention and public health varied in 2011 from 0.53% of total health expenditure in Cyprus to 6.33% in Serbia (WHO 2013). Although these data are at best estimates, they allow some tentative conclusions. The first is that they are improbably low for some countries (such as Cyprus), raising serious concerns about the reliability of expenditure data. A second conclusion is that spending on prevention and public health only constitutes a fairly minor share of total health expenditure in most European countries, indicating considerable room for increased financial allocations to public health. Unsurprisingly, in the study on public health capacity in the EU, the lack of adequate resource provision was identified as often the most significant barrier to the effective implementation of public health programmes and interventions (Aluttis, Chiotan et al. 2013). Third, national reporting is incomplete. A number of countries in Europe, including Andorra, Azerbaijan, Kazakhstan, Monaco, the Russian Federation, San Marino, the former Yugoslav Republic of Macedonia, Turkmenistan, the United

Kingdom, and Uzbekistan, have failed to report expenditure data on prevention and public health altogether, while for other countries expenditure data are only available for selected years.

An attempt to fill some of these gaps and to quantify expenditure on prevention and public health in England, based on the OECD System of Health Accounts, found that it amounted to 4.0% of total health expenditure in 2006–2007, which was above the OECD average of 2.8% (Butterfield, Henderson et al. 2009). However, attempts to quantify expenditure on prevention and public health in England seem to have remained limited to the years 1999–2000 and 2006–2007 (Butterfield, Henderson et al. 2009).

Apart from the major variations across European countries, there are also large variations within countries. In Italy, absolute and relative expenditure on public health varies considerably across regions. Although there is guidance from the national Ministry of Health that 5% of regional health expenditure should be allocated to public health, regions are free to vary this (Lo Scalzo, Donatini et al. 2009).

Who pays for public health?

A breakdown of budgets for prevention and public health by financing agent reveals that public funds are the main source of financing in most European countries for which data exist (Table 14.2). There are also major gaps, with no reporting for 2010 by Greece, Ireland, Luxembourg, Turkey, and the United Kingdom.

In some countries, there has been a deliberate policy to increase the role of private sources of funding, especially in the countries of central and eastern Europe, south-east Europe, and the former Soviet Union, where laboratories derive additional income from commercial activities (WHO 2009b; Duran and Kutzin 2010; Gotsadze, Chikovani et al. 2010). In Slovenia, for example, fees for services diverted attention from core activities of institutes of public health (WHO 2009a). The Ministry of Health decided in 2012 to address this situation by separating all laboratories from public health institutes and merging them to create a national Laboratory for Health, Environment and Food. In several former Soviet countries, including Armenia and Kyrgyzstan, charges have been introduced for public health inspections, with uncertain consequences (Duran and Kutzin 2010). These examples illustrate the potential pitfalls that can arise when basing expenditure for public health on private sources of funding.

With regard to the public financing of those aspects of public health activities linked to the health system, countries differ in terms of funding sources (with the main divide between taxation and social insurance-based financing) and (when tax-based) which administrative level pays for public health activities (see Table 14.2). Countries with social health insurance systems have traditionally had less comprehensive public health activities than those with tax-based systems, due to the more population-oriented approach of the latter systems (Allin, Mossialos et al. 2004). However, the situation now is more complex than this dichotomy would suggest, and also differs for various types of public health activity (see Box 14.2).

Table 14.2 Expenditure on prevention and public health as a percentage of total health expenditure by financing agent, European OECD member states, 2010

	General government (excl. social security) = Territorial government	Social security funds	Private insurance	Private households out-of-pocket expenditure	Non-profit institutions serving households	Corporations (other than health insurance)	Rest of the world	Total expenditure on prevention and public health
Austria	0.80	0.72	—	0.11	0.04	0.12	—	1.79
Belgium	1.88	0.08	0.00	0.00	—	0.00	—	1.97
Czech Republic	0.49	1.66	—	—	—	0.33	—	2.47
Denmark	2.24	0.00	0.00	0.00	0.07	0.00	—	2.31
Estonia	1.49	0.86	0.00	0.00	0.01	0.14	0.24	2.74
Finland	1.29	1.82	—	—	—	2.33	—	5.44
France	1.03	0.43	—	—	—	0.66	—	2.12
Germany	0.73	2.03	0.05	0.02	0.17	0.25	—	3.25
Greece	—	—	—	—	—	—	—	—
Hungary	1.60	0.90	0.05	0.20	0.38	1.35	—	4.48
Iceland	1.48	0.00	—	—	—	—	—	1.48
Ireland	—	—	—	—	—	—	—	—
Italy	—	—	—	—	—	—	—	0.46
Luxembourg	—	—	—	—	—	—	—	—
Netherlands	1.79	1.27	0.00	0.13	0.32	1.29	0.00	4.79
Norway	2.18	0.02	—	—	—	—	—	2.51
Poland	1.16	0.40	—	—	0.05	0.47	—	2.07
Portugal	1.46	0.00	0.05	0.08	0.01	0.54	—	2.14

Slovak Republic	1.98	0.00	0.00	0.00	0.00	3.37	0.00	5.34
Slovenia	0.52	2.36	0.04	0.00	0.03	0.86	0.00	3.80
Spain	2.25	0.02	0.00	0.00	0.04	—	—	2.31
Sweden	2.79	—	—	0.10	—	0.70	—	3.60
Switzerland	1.00	0.55	—	0.38	0.44	—	—	2.37
Turkey	—	—	—	—	—	—	—	—
United Kingdom	—	—	—	—	—	—	—	—

Source: OECD (2012)

Box 14.2 Funding streams for public health in Estonia

In Estonia, services and programmes for public health are financed through budgetary allocations to the Ministry of Social Affairs, the national health insurance fund, as well as other ministries and municipal and private sources. The Estonian Health Insurance Fund pays for health checks tailored to various risk groups, both as part of specially targeted disease prevention projects and within the health system generally. National strategies are mostly financed through state budget allocations, but some cross-sectoral public health strategies are financed largely by other ministries. For example, the National Strategy for Prevention of Cardiovascular Diseases 2005–2020 has been co-financed by the Ministry of Education and Research. In addition to the nationally organized services, the larger municipalities finance some preventive services according to local needs. Some funding for public health also comes from the European Social Fund, as well as international agencies, such as the Global Fund to Fight AIDS, Tuberculosis and Malaria.

Systematic health promotion activities were launched in Estonia in 1993, when the Ministry of Social Affairs decided to create a system for financing national and community-based health promotion projects. The demand-driven system was financed from an earmarked share of the budget of the Estonian Health Insurance Fund and managed by a committee of experts making funding decisions and coordinating evaluation. The objective was to create demand for health promotion at the national and county level, and to help to build capacity and competence in health promotion. Applications for health promotion projects are submitted once a year on a competitive basis. Since 2002, project applications need to include outcome measurements.

The principal weakness of disease prevention programmes could be said to be the structure of their financing. Each programme or strategy is allocated funds on an annual basis, leaving them potentially open to being undermined by short-term budgetary considerations. This form of funding also impedes longer-term planning, a significant weakness in the financial framework for disease prevention. Another challenge is that some services are not funded or subsidized for the uninsured, such as some screening programmes and general health counselling from GPs, with potential implications for inequalities in health. Some types of services also have high co-payments for groups of the population who may have major difficulty paying, such as some drug addiction services (from providers who do not have contracts with the National Institute for Health Development) and all alcohol addiction services.

Source: Koppel, Leventhal et al. (2009)

In some countries, such as France (Sandier, Paris et al. 2004), the multiplicity of funding sources was noted as a weakness of disease prevention and health promotion activities. The lack of stable funding for these activities was also noted in several countries of south-east Europe, where funding is often allocated on an ad hoc basis and in some cases relies largely on international agencies, leading to haphazard planning and a lack of overall strategies. The financing mechanisms for disease prevention and health promotion activities are separate from the rest of the health system (WHO 2009b). Lack of output-based financing of public health services has been identified as another weakness (WHO 2009a).

In countries with health insurance systems, public financing for public health activities can come from insurance funds, taxation or a mix of the two. In Germany, most preventive measures aimed at individuals, such as immunizations, screening programmes, and health check-ups are carried out by office-based physicians and paid from the sickness funds' benefit package, while population-based health promotion activities are also paid for by the sickness funds (Busse and Riesberg 2004). In Croatia and Slovenia, too, the national vaccination programme is completely covered by the Health Insurance Institute (WHO 2007b, 2009a).

In contrast, the Netherlands, which like Germany largely relies on health insurance to pay for curative health services, finances prevention activities through general taxation (Schäfer, Kroneman et al. 2010). The countries of central and eastern Europe and the former Soviet Union also use taxation-based budgetary funding from the central level to fund public health services (Gotsadze, Chikovani et al. 2010), with no significant reforms since the fall of communism (Duran and Kutzin 2010). However, even in these countries a mix of public financing sources seems to be common, such as in the Czech Republic, where preventive services provided by GPs (vaccinations and screening) are covered by the benefits package of the health insurance fund, but the Ministry of Health provides direct, tax-based funding to public health services, such as specialized health programmes (Bryndova, Pavlokova et al. 2009). Austria also relies on a mix of financing sources; two-thirds of the cost of vaccines is borne by the federal government, and a sixth each by the Länder (regions) and the social health insurance institutions. The Länder cover the costs of administration, distribution, and administering the vaccines. The financing of health promotion activities also draws on a mix of federal and Länder funds (Hofmarcher and Rack 2006).

In some European countries (including Austria, the Netherlands, Denmark, the Czech Republic, and the United Kingdom), payment of primary healthcare providers involves a mixed system, based on the number of registered patients (capitation), fee-for-service, payment for implementation of certain programmes, and payment for performance (Fujisawa and Lafortune 2008; Katic, Jurkovic et al. 2012; Olejaz, Juul Nielsen et al. 2012). Performance or programme-based payment usually involves targets, some of which are related to public health activities. In Sweden, for example, some county councils use a small performance-based element of payment (2–3% of the total payment) that is partly dependent on the provision of preventive services (Anell, Glenngård et al. 2012). In Estonia, GPs receive specific incentives to offer preventive services, including counselling patients on medical and behavioural risks. Since 2006, preventive check-ups have been linked with the GPs' bonus system, which includes criteria for coverage of certain age groups (people aged 40–60 years) (Koppel, Kahur et al. 2008). In south-east Europe, several countries have adopted such combined payment systems (Rechel, Bozikov et al. 2012). In Montenegro, 10% of the earnings of primary healthcare teams are directly related to implementing prevention programmes (Ostojic and Andric 2012). One model that has attracted much interest is the Quality and Outcomes Framework introduced for family medicine in the United Kingdom in 2004 (Katic, Jurkovic et al. 2012). This pays extra funds to GPs for meeting a range of targets, some of which relate to disease prevention (Boyle 2011).

While in many countries preventive services are covered by the main public financing body, such as the national health insurance fund in Estonia (Koppel, Leventhal et al. 2009), in others, such as Armenia (Armenian, Crape et al. 2009), a lack of incentives to practise preventive medicine among physicians has been noted, as well as the existence of out-of-pocket costs to consumers. The challenge of putting health promotion activities on a sustainable financial basis has been noted in several countries. The problem is particularly acute where funding mechanisms are not linked to the general health financing system, but are ad hoc or based on external funding (Bayarsaikhan and Muiser 2007; WHO 2009b). To address this issue, in Estonia a system of financing health promotion projects was established (Box 14.2).

Earmarked taxes for public health

Some European countries have introduced earmarked taxes for public health activities. The most prominent example is the earmarking of tobacco tax revenues for national tobacco control programmes. By 2007, 13 countries in the WHO European Region (Austria, Belarus, Bulgaria, Estonia, Finland, France, Greece, Iceland, Poland, Romania, Serbia and Montenegro, Switzerland, the United Kingdom) had established mechanisms for the earmarking of tobacco tax. Some of these countries (including Finland, Iceland, Poland, Serbia and Montenegro, and Switzerland) used the earmarked funds for tobacco control and health promotion. Poland, Finland, and Iceland earmarked 0.5%, 0.75%, and 0.9% of tobacco tax for this purpose (WHO 2007a). Crucially, public support for increases in tobacco tax (an effective way of reducing tobacco consumption) seems to be greater when increases are earmarked for health promotion and tobacco control (Vardavas, Filippidis et al. 2012).

Earmarking of alcohol tax for public health activities is also done in several European countries. One example is Poland, where licensing fees for retail sales of alcoholic beverages are paid to municipal councils and earmarked for the implementation of municipal programmes for the prevention of alcohol-related problems.

With the exception of taxes on tobacco and alcohol, however, the use of fiscal instruments for public health is not yet widespread, although some countries have attempted to introduce taxes on foods containing saturated fats (see

Chapter 7, "Food security and healthier food choices"). One of the potential challenges for earmarked taxes for public health is that they might aim to merge conflicting goals by basing funds for public health on the consumption of unhealthy goods.

Level of government

European countries also differ with regard to which level of government provides tax-based funding for public health activities. In general, sub-national levels play an important financing role in federal or decentralized systems. In Finland, for example, municipalities are responsible for funding immunizations (Vuorenkoski, Mladovsky et al. 2008). They are also the main funders of health promotion activities, but they are supplemented by central budgetary allocations (Vuorenkoski, Mladovsky et al. 2008). In Denmark, vaccination programmes are financed by the regions (Strandberg-Larsen, Nielsen et al. 2007; Olejaz, Juul Nielsen et al. 2012), while in Belgium two-thirds of vaccination costs are borne by the federal government and one-third by the communities (Gerkens and Merkur 2010). In almost all countries of central and eastern Europe and the former Soviet Union, tax-based funding comes from the central government, but there are exceptions, such as Poland, which has introduced co-funding from the local government (Gotsadze, Chikovani et al. 2010).

Impact of the economic crisis

As a result of the current economic crisis, the financing of public health is in danger in many countries, as the long-term benefits of public health interventions are often overlooked (Martin-Moreno, Anttila et al. 2012). Many structures for delivering public health operations in Europe are already facing substantial cutbacks and public health programmes and interventions in several countries, including Bulgaria, Latvia, and the United Kingdom, have been scaled down (Aluttis, Chiotan et al. 2013).

Conclusion

This chapter has provided a tentative overview of the organization and financing of public health in Europe. If policy-makers in Europe are serious about implementing WHO's European Action Plan for Strengthening Public Health Capacities and Services, they will need to invest significant resources simply to maintain what currently exists. Ultimately, the organization and financing of public health activities in Europe will have to be assessed against the improvements of population outcomes they achieve (Brand, Schroder et al. 2006). However, it is exactly this information that seems to be almost entirely missing. Not only are there very few assessments of the effectiveness of disease prevention programmes in the medium term, as was noted in Estonia (Koppel, Leventhal et al. 2009), but broader evaluations of organizational reforms are generally lacking (Maier and Martin-Moreno 2011). More systematic research seems to have been undertaken in the United States, where a National Public Health Performance Standards Program has been developed by the Centers for Disease Control and Prevention, but there, too, a lack of research to guide public health practice has been noted (Scutchfield, Bhandari et al. 2009). Crucially, empirical evidence on the effectiveness or efficiency of different public health structures is so far lacking, with uncertainties surrounding the impact, effectiveness, and efficiency of different governing structures and financing arrangements (Mays, Smith et al. 2009).

The material presented in this chapter nevertheless allows some conclusions to be drawn. The first is that basic institutional structures for delivering essential public health operations are not yet present in all countries of the WHO European Region. In the context of the current economic crisis, it will be a major challenge even to maintain existing structures. Furthermore, it needs to be emphasized that institutional models alone are insufficient to bring about improvements in the absence of sufficient funding and political will.

Another key conclusion that emerges from this review is the wide diversity that exists in public health operations across Europe, especially with regard to organization and financing. Our review suggests, for example, that some of the federal or decentralized systems of public health face problems in ensuring equity across regions. However, decentralization can also help to make public health services more responsive to local needs (Mays, Smith et al. 2009). While recognizing that the degree of decentralization reflects the wider political and administrative context of the country in question, a more systematic comparison and evaluation of public health structures in Europe is needed to identify which organizational structures and financing arrangements work best and why. At the same time, it is important to realize that the structures for the organization and financing of public health that have emerged in the different European countries can have a large degree of inertia and might be difficult to change in the short run, even if there was compelling evidence of best practices.

This review of the financing of public health has shown that existing data only provide an approximation of real expenditure levels and are improbable for some countries. They also suggest that expenditure on prevention and public health constitutes only a very small share of total health expenditure – despite the proven cost benefits of public health interventions. Under-financing seems to present one of the main challenges to public health in Europe, in particular in the current economic circumstances, but better information on the effectiveness and efficiency of public health structures is also needed to make sure that available resources are used to maximum effect.

References

Allin, S., E. Mossialos, M. McKee and W. Holland (2004). *Making Decisions on Public Health: A review of eight countries*. Copenhagen, WHO on behalf of the European Observatory on Health Systems and Policies.

Aluttis, C., C. Chiotan, K. Michelsen, C. Costongs and H. Brand (2013). *Review of Public Health Capacity in the EU*. Luxembourg, European Commission Directorate General for Health and Consumers.

Anell, A., A. Glenngård and S. Merkur (2012). "Sweden: health system review." *Health Systems in Transition* **14**(5): 1–159.

Armenian, H. K., B. Crape, R. Grigoryan, H. Martirosyan, V. Petrosyan and N. Truzyan (2009). *Analysis of Public Health Services in Armenia.* Yerevan, American University of Armenia.

Barros, P. P. and J. de Almeida Simoes (2007). "Portugal: health system review." *Health Systems in Transition* **9**(5): 1–142.

Bayarsaikhan, D. and J. Muiser (2007). *Financing Health Promotion.* Geneva, WHO.

Boyle, S. (2011). "United Kingdom (England): health system review." *Health Systems in Transition* **13**(1): 1–486.

Brand, H., P. Schroder, J. Davies, I. Escamilla, C. Hall, K. Hickey, E. Jelastopulu, R. Mechtler, W. Yared, J. Volf and B. Weihrauch (2006). "Reference frameworks for the health management of measles, breast cancer and diabetes (type II)." *Central European Journal of Public Health* **14**(1): 39–45.

Bryndova, L., K. Pavlokova, M. Rokosova, M. Gaskins and E. Ginneken (2009). "Czech Republic: health system review." *Health Systems in Transition* **11**(1): 1–122.

Busse, R. and A. Riesberg (2004). *Health Care Systems in Transition: Germany.* Copenhagen, WHO Regional Office for Europe on behalf of the European Observatory on Health Systems and Policies.

Butterfield, R., J. Henderson and R. Scott (2009). *Public Health and Prevention Expenditure in England.* London, Department of Health.

de Bekker-Grob, E., J. Polder, J. P. Mackenbach and W. Meerding (2007). "Towards a comprehensive estimate of national spending on prevention." *BMC Public Health* **7**: 252.

Duran, A. and J. Kutzin (2010). "Financing of public health services and programmes: time to look into the black box." In *Implementing Health Financing Reform: Lessons from countries in transition.* J. Kutzin, C. Cashin and M. Jakab, Eds. Copenhagen, WHO on behalf of the European Observatory on Health Systems and Policies: 247–268.

Economou, C. (2010). "Greece: health system review." *Health Systems in Transition* **12**(7): 1–180.

Fujisawa, R. and G. Lafortune (2008). *The Remuneration of General Practitioners and Specialists in 14 OECD Countries: What are the factors influencing variations across countries?* Paris, OECD.

García-Armesto, S., M. Abadía-Taira, A. Durán, C. Hernández-Quevedo and E. Bernal-Delgado (2010). "Spain: health system review." *Health Systems in Transition* **12**(4): 1–295.

Gerkens, S. and S. Merkur (2010). "Belgium: health system review." *Health Systems in Transition* **12**(5): 1–266.

Glenngård, A., F. Hjalte, M. Svensson, A. Anell and V. Bankauskaite (2005). *Health Systems in Transition: Sweden.* Copenhagen, WHO Regional Office for Europe on behalf of the European Observatory on Health Systems and Policies.

Gotsadze, G., I. Chikovani, K. Goguadze, D. Balabanova and M. McKee (2010). "Reforming sanitary-epidemiological service in Central and Eastern Europe and the former Soviet Union: an exploratory study." *BMC Public Health* **10**: 440.

Hofmarcher, M. and H.-M. Rack (2006). "Austria: health system review." *Health Systems in Transition* **8**(3): 1–247.

Holland, W., S. Stewart and C. Masseria (2006). *Screening in Europe.* Policy Brief. Copenhagen, WHO on behalf of the European Observatory on Health Systems and Policies.

Kaiser, S. and J. Mackenbach (2008). "Public health in eight European countries: an international comparison of terminology." *Public Health* **122**(2): 211–216.

Katic, M., D. Jurkovic and V. Juresa (2012). "The combined way of paying family medicine in Croatia." In *Health Reforms in South East Europe*. W. Bartlett, J. Bozikov and B. Rechel, Eds. Basingstoke, Palgrave Macmillan: 193–206.

Koppel, A., K. Kahur, T. Habicht, P. Saar, J. Habicht and E. van Ginneken (2008). "Estonia: health system review." *Health Systems in Transition* **10**(1): 1–230.

Koppel, A., A. Leventhal and M. Sedgley, Eds. (2009). *Public Health in Estonia 2008: An analysis of public health operations, services and activities*. Copenhagen, WHO Regional Office for Europe.

Ladurner, J., M. Gerger, W. Holland, E. Mossialos, S. Merkur, S. Stewart, R. Irwin and J. Soffried, Eds. (2011). *Public Health in Austria: An analysis of the status of public health*. Copenhagen, WHO on behalf of the European Observatory on Health Systems and Policies.

Lo Scalzo, A., A. Donatini, L. Orzella, S. Profili, A. Cicchetti, l. S. Profi and A. Maresso (2009). "Italy: health system review." *Health Systems in Transition* **11**(6): 1–216.

Maier, C., W. Palm, J. M. Martin-Moreno, D. Mircheva and M. Haralanova (2009). *The Reform of Public Health and the Role of the Sanitary-Epidemiological Services (sanepid) in the Newly Independent States*. Meeting report, Bishkek, Kyrgyzstan, 10–12 November 2008. Copenhagen, WHO Regional Office for Europe.

Maier, C. B. and J. M. Martin-Moreno (2011). "Quo vadis SANEPID? A cross-country analysis of public health reforms in 10 post-Soviet states." *Health Policy* **102**(1): 18–25.

Martin-Moreno, J. M., A. Anttila, L. von Karsa, J. L. Alfonso-Sanchez and L. Gorgojo (2012). "Cancer screening and health system resilience: keys to protecting and bolstering preventive services during a financial crisis." *European Journal of Cancer* **48**(14): 2212–2218.

Mays, G. P., F. Scutchfield, M. Bhandari and S. A. Smith (2010). "Understanding the organization of public health delivery systems: an empirical typology." *The Milbank Quarterly* **88**(1): 81–111.

Mays, G. P., S. A. Smith, R. C. Ingram, L. J. Racster, C. D. Lamberth and E. S. Lovely (2009). "Public health delivery systems." *American Journal of Preventive Medicine* **36**(3): 256–265.

McDaid, D., M. Wiley, A. Maresso and E. Mossialos (2009). "Ireland: health system review." *Health Systems in Transition* **11**(4): 1–268.

McKee, M., L. Hurst, R. W. Aldridge, R. Raine, J. S. Mindell, I. Wolfe and W. Holland (2011). "Public health in England: an option for the way forward?" *The Lancet* 378: 536–539.

McKee, M. and J. Pomerleau (2005). "The emergency of public health and the centrality of values." In *Issues in Public Health: Understanding public health*. J. Pomerleau and M. McKee. Maidenhead, Open University Press: 5–23.

OECD (2012). *Health Data 2012* [stats.oecd.org, accessed 8 December 2012]. Paris, OECD.

OECD/Eurostat/WHO (2011). *A System of Health Accounts*, 2011 edition [http://www.who.int/nha/sha_revision/sha_2011_final1.pdf, accessed 28 January 2013]. Paris, OECD.

OECD/WHO (2011). *OECD Reviews of Health Systems: Switzerland*. Paris, OECD Publishing.

Olejaz, M., A. Juul Nielsen, A. Rudkjøbing, H. Okkels Birk, A. Krasnik and C. Hernández-Quevedo (2012). "Denmark: health system review." *Health Systems in Transition* **14**(2): 1–192.

Ostojic, D. and R. Andric (2012). "Reforms of the organization and financing of primary health care in Montenegro." In *Health Reforms in South East Europe*. W. Bartlett, J. Bozikov and B. Rechel, Eds. Basingstoke, Palgrave Macmillan: 207–217.

Popovich, L., E. Potapchik, S. Shishkin, E. Richardson, A. Vacroux and B. Mathivet (2011). "Russian Federation: health system review." *Health Systems in Transition* **13**(7): 1–190.

Rechel, B., J. Bozikov and W. Bartlett (2012). "Lessons from two decades of health reforms in South East Europe." In *Health Reforms in South East Europe*. W. Bartlett, J. Bozikov and B. Rechel, Eds. Basingstoke, Palgrave Macmillan: 229–239.

Rechel, B., H. Brand and M. McKee (2013). "Financing public health in Europe." *Gesundheitswesen* 75: e28–e33.

Rechel, B. and M. McKee (2006). "Health systems and policies in South-Eastern Europe." In *Health and Economic Development in South-Eastern Europe*. WHO, Ed. Paris, WHO: 43–69.

Rechel, B. and M. McKee (2012). *Preliminary Review of Institutional Models for Delivering Essential Public Health Operations in Europe*. Copenhagen, WHO Regional Office for Europe.

Rowe, L. and B. Rechel (2006). "Fighting tuberculosis and HIV/AIDS in Northeast Europe: sustainable collaboration or political rhetoric?" *European Journal of Public Health* **16**(6): 609–614.

Saltman, R., S. Allin, E. Mossialos, M. Wismar and E. van Ginneken (2012). "Assessing health reform trends in Europe." In *Health Systems, Health, Wealth and Societal Well-being*. J. Figueras and M. McKee, Eds. Maidenhead, Open University Press: 209–246.

Saltman, R. B., V. Bankauskaite and K. Vrangbaek, Eds. (2007). *Decentralization in Health Care: Strategies and outcomes*. Maidenhead, Open University Press.

Sandier, S., V. Paris and D. Polton (2004). *Health Care Systems in Transition: France*. Copenhagen, WHO Regional Office for Europe on behalf of the European Observatory on Health Systems and Policies.

Schäfer, W., M. Kroneman, W. Boerma, M. van den Berg, G. Westert, W. Deville and E. Van Ginneken (2010). "The Netherlands: health system review." *Health Systems in Transition* **12**(1) 1–228.

Scutchfield, F., M. Bhandari, N. Lawhorn, C. Lamberth and R. Ingram (2009). "Public health performance." *American Journal of Preventive Medicine* **36**(3): 266–272.

Sensenig, A. L. (2007). "Refining estimates of public health spending as measured in national health expenditures accounts: the United States experience." *Journal of Public Health Management and Practice* **13**(2): 103–114.

Strandberg-Larsen, M., M. Nielsen, S. Vallgårda, A. Krasnik, K. Vrangbæk and E. Mossialos (2007). "Denmark: health system review." *Health Systems in Transition* **9**(6): 1–164.

Tragakes, E., G. Brigis, J. Karaskevica, A. Rurane, A. Stuburs, E. Zusmane, O. Avdeeva and M. Schäfer (2008). "Latvia: health system review." *Health Systems in Transition* **10**(2): 1–253.

Vardavas, C., F. Filippidis, I. Agaku, V. Mytaras, M. Bertic, G. Connolly, Y. Tountas and P. Behrakis (2012). "Tobacco taxation: the importance of earmarking the revenue to health care and tobacco control." *Tobacco Induced Diseases* **10**(1): 21.

Vuorenkoski, L., P. Mladovsky and E. Mossialos (2008). "Finland: health system review." *Health Systems in Transition* **10**(4): 1–168.

Weil, O. and M. McKee (1998). "Setting priorities for health in Europe: are we speaking the same language?" *European Journal of Public Health* **8**: 256–258.

Whitehead, D. (2004). "The European Health Promoting Hospitals (HPH) project: how far on?" *Health Promotion International* **19**(2): 259–267.

World Health Organization (WHO) (1978). *Declaration of Alma-Ata* [http://www.who.int/publications/almaata_declaration_en.pdf].

World Health Organization (WHO) (1986). *The Ottawa Charter for Health Promotion* [http://www.who.int/healthpromotion/conferences/previous/ottawa/en/index4.html]. Geneva, WHO.

World Health Organization (WHO) (2007a). *European Tobacco Control Report 2007.* Copenhagen, WHO Regional Office for Europe.

World Health Organization (WHO) (2007b). *Evaluation of Public Health Services in South-eastern Europe: Croatia.* Draft National Report. Copenhagen, WHO Regional Office for Europe.

World Health Organization (WHO) (2007c). *Evaluation of Public Health Services in South-eastern Europe: Federation of Bosnia and Herzegovina.* Draft National Report. Copenhagen, WHO Regional Office for Europe.

World Health Organization (WHO) (2007d). *Evaluation of Public Health Services in South-eastern Europe: Republika Srpska.* Draft National Report. Copenhagen, WHO Regional Office for Europe.

World Health Organization (WHO) (2008). *The Tallinn Charter: Health systems for health and wealth.* Copenhagen, WHO Regional Office for Europe.

World Health Organization (WHO) (2009a). *Evaluation of Public Health Services in Slovenia.* Copenhagen, WHO Regional Office for Europe.

World Health Organization (WHO) (2009b). *Evaluation of Public Health Services in South-eastern Europe.* Copenhagen, WHO Regional Office for Europe.

World Health Organization (WHO) (2012). *General Statistical Procedures Used to Construct WHO Health Expenditure Database* [http://apps.who.int/nha/database/ResourcesPage.aspx, accessed 28 January 2013]. Geneva, WHO.

World Health Organization (WHO) (2013). *Global Health Expenditure Database* [http://apps.who.int/nha/database/DataExplorer.aspx?ws=0&d=1, accessed 17 May 2013]. Geneva, WHO.

chapter fifteen

Developing the public health workforce

*Christoph Aluttis, Claudia Bettina Maier,
Stephan Van den Broucke,
Katarzyna Czabanowska*

Introduction

Assuring a sufficient and competent public health workforce has been defined by the WHO Regional Office for Europe as one of the essential public health operations (EPHOs; see Chapter 1, "Facets of public health in Europe: an introduction"). Health systems require a sufficient number of well-trained people to deliver high-quality services. This applies equally to public health as to health care. Increasing antimicrobial resistance in many countries, the emergence of multidrug-resistant tuberculosis (MDR-TB) in the eastern part of the WHO European Region, the epidemic of non-communicable diseases (NCDs), and widening health inequalities within and across European countries all illustrate the need for effective public health action, based on a strong and sustainable public health workforce (WHO 2000; PAHO/WHO 2002; Tilson and Gebbie 2004; Paccaud 2011).

European health systems are still largely focused on treatment, cure, and care (Beaglehole and Dal Poz 2003), despite the fact that substantial health improvements can be achieved by changes in exposure to the causes of diseases, through health protection, health promotion, and disease prevention (Foldspang 2008). As governments across Europe grapple with the problem of maximizing the return on health spending, there is a strong case for arguing that public health should play a larger role in health systems across Europe. This will require the availability and adequate distribution of a highly skilled public health workforce, but also a clear understanding of existing training capacities, career opportunities, and the role of professional organizations in Europe (Whitfield 2004).

This chapter provides an overview of key issues relevant to the public health workforce in Europe. It starts by exploring existing definitions and common characteristics of the public health workforce in Europe. It then describes the current status of this workforce and argues for the importance of quantifying it. The chapter concludes by outlining existing systems of education and professional development for public health in Europe and the measures needed for their further development.

Defining and conceptualizing the public health workforce

Unlike the medical workforce with its clearly established professions and pathways, describing the workforce for public health is more difficult. This is exemplified by the existence of a variety of definitions. For instance, Rotem and colleagues (Rotem, Walters et al. 1995) define the public health workforce as "people who are involved in protecting, promoting and/or restoring the collective health of whole or specific populations (as distinct from activities directed to the care of individuals)". This definition distinguishes between public health and medical practices, and stresses the societal perspective of public health workers. In a similar vein, Beaglehole and Dal Poz (2003) define the public health workforce as "a diverse workforce whose prime responsibility is the provision of core public health activities, irrespective of their organizational base", highlighting that the public health workforce can be located both inside and outside the health sector.

Increasingly, conceptualizations of public health also consider the role of the "wider" workforce, referring to workers who are indirectly involved in public health activities, but whose work can contribute to improving population health (Sim, Lock et al. 2007). Examples of this wider workforce include teachers, welfare workers, fitness instructors, and housing planners (Gebbie, Merrill et al. 2002). However, while this wider workforce has an enormous potential to contribute to positive health outcomes, it remains important to have an education system in place for formally recognized public health professionals, in order to safeguard a scientific and evidence-based approach to public health interventions. This is emphasized by the US Institute of Medicine (2002), which includes an educational component in its definition of the public health workforce, characterizing them as "persons educated in public health or a related discipline who are employed to improve health through a population focus".

In general, the definitions presented, while setting some boundaries and providing some inclusion and exclusion criteria, remain ambiguous about who actually belongs to the public health workforce. This does not make these definitions very useful when it comes to describing in detail the public health workforce of a particular country or region. This task is further complicated by the substantial differences in the terminology and conceptualizations of public health that exist across European countries (see Chapter 14, "Organization and financing of public health"). Differences in culture, language, and the historical developments of health systems have led to variations in the understanding of public health (Kaiser and Mackenbach 2008), which in turn is reflected in the definition and scope of the public health workforce in different countries.

Whitfield (2004) presented a theoretical conceptualization of public health activities and the related workforce that can be applied regardless of the national context. According to this concept, the public health workforce can be divided into three groups: (1) "public health specialists", (2) "people indirectly involved

Table 15.1 Three categories of public health workers

(1) Public health specialists	*(2) Partial public health role*	*(3) Awareness of public health issues*
Health professionals with specialization in public health	Physicians	Police
	Nurses	Architects
Health policy-makers	Dentists	Urban planners
Epidemiologists	Pharmacists	Teachers
Environmental health experts	Midwives	Journalists
Health economists	Food inspectors	etc.
Health promotion specialists	Nutritionists	
etc.	Fitness instructors	
	Psychologists	
	Social workers	
	etc.	

Source: Authors' compilation, based on Whitfield (2004)

in public health activities through their work"; and (3) "people who should be aware of public health implications in their professional life" (Table 15.1).

The category of public health specialists has been traditionally involved in public health matters and their public health function is largely undisputed. It includes professionals who are primarily occupied with public health in their daily work, such as public health specialists, epidemiologists, and researchers whose work is primarily focused on public health issues.

The second category includes those professionals whose work is not primarily concerned with public health, but does have an important contribution to public health. It includes, for instance, general practitioners providing counselling on disease prevention, nutritionists giving advice on proper nutrition, and fitness instructors helping people to remain physically active.

The third category refers to professionals who do not work directly on public health issues, but whose awareness of public health in their daily work can contribute to positive population health outcomes. Examples in this category include scientists who design products that are safer, urban planners who take health considerations into account when designing urban environments, and teachers advising pupils on health-related issues as part of their daily work. Professionals in this category tend not to perceive themselves as being part of the public health workforce, but can have a significant impact on health outcomes. They tend to be situated outside the health system as it is traditionally understood.

Distinguishing between these three categories of the public health workforce clarifies the different roles of public health workers and also emphasizes the multidisciplinary and diverse character of public health itself. While countries need a professionalized public health workforce, acknowledging and explicitly addressing the role of the wider workforce for population health is a necessary step to dealing with the multidisciplinary nature of contemporary public health challenges.

Differences across countries

All countries in Europe have a public health workforce, albeit of differing degrees of effectiveness and following different organizational patterns (Porter 1994). Despite many differences among countries, medical doctors tend to dominate the professional public health workforce in Europe, although there has been a shift towards more multidisciplinary teams since the 1990s and 2000s, with Finland, Ireland, and the United Kingdom among the first countries in Europe to educate professionals with different backgrounds in public health. However, the delivery of preventive services, health education, and patient counselling is to a large extent still performed by health workers in primary care or hospitals (Vuorenkoski, Mladovsky et al. 2008; McDaid, Wiley et al. 2009; Boyle 2011). In some countries of central and eastern Europe, in particular, public health is still dominated by medical professionals specializing in public health. This is partly a legacy of the sanitary-epidemiological services of the Soviet period, which have been retained in many former Soviet countries, with a strong medical orientation and a focus on just a few public health functions, such as hygiene or immunization programmes (Goodman, Overall et al. 2008; Gotsadze, Chikovani et al. 2010; Maier and Martin-Moreno 2010).

As outlined above, the public health workforce not only comprises individuals who are specialized in the field, but also the large group of workers who deliver public health services but who are not specialists and have received only limited or no training in public health. In Kyrgyzstan and Tajikistan, for example, community health workers and health promotion workers with diverse disciplinary backgrounds work in communities on relevant public health issues, such as maternal and child health, education on hygiene and nutrition, and disease prevention (Khodjamurodov and Rechel 2010; Maier and Martin-Moreno 2010; Ibrahimova, Akkazieva et al. 2011). With only minimal training in public health, these people are the front-line public health workers at the community level. In addition to helping to improve the health of the population, their work contributes to raising awareness and competences for public health, health promotion, disease prevention, and health protection at the community level (Ibrahimova, Akkazieva et al. 2011). However, very little is known about the size, scope, and effectiveness of this wider public health workforce across the WHO European Region.

Quantifying the public health workforce in Europe

It is common wisdom that what you cannot measure, you cannot change. Determining the quantity and quality of the public health workforce in the countries of the WHO European Region is of vital importance for the planning and governance of health systems. While this has been acknowledged widely among policy-makers and health professionals, factual knowledge about the public health workforce in Europe is, at best, limited. Unlike the generally well-established data on medical personnel, registries of public health specialists and practitioners are rare, and subject to definitional issues (a rare example is the United Kingdom voluntary register of those who have completed an appropriate course of training; see Sim, Lock et al. 2007). This creates gaps in information on the number and distribution of the public health workforce in a given country, ultimately limiting the ability of policy-makers to address shortages. As the previous sections of this chapter have shown, assessing the size of the public health workforce is complicated by the fact that it is neither homogeneous nor an entirely regulated profession; the public health workforce is highly diverse in terms of educational background and training, areas of work, job positions, and qualifications.

One of the most elaborate attempts to quantify the public health workforce for planning purposes was undertaken in the United Kingdom, where in 2001 the Department of Health acknowledged that "public health workforce development can only be achieved on the basis of good knowledge of how many public health workers are out there, what they are doing, and where they are located" (Department of Health 2001). Walters and colleagues tried to obtain data on the available public health workforce in the area of Greater London, distinguishing between similar categories of professionals as described in Whitfield's model outlined above, with the goal of quantifying these groups and performing an analysis of supply and demand (Walters, Sim et al. 2002). In total, the public health workforce was estimated to comprise at least 250,000 people, of which 98% belonged in the "wider workforce" category (Sim, Schiller et al. 2002). This large number of potential advocates for public health offers much potential for improving population health, if properly trained and empowered (Sim, Lock et al. 2007).

Other examples to map or quantify the workforce for public health in European countries can be found at the national and sub-national level, including in Switzerland (Frank, Weihofen et al. 2013), the Netherlands (Jambroes, Essink-Bot et al. 2012), and Wales (Barley 2010). Mapping initiatives outside Europe can be found in the United States, Australia, and Canada. Increased communication between researchers and institutes of different countries could help in the sharing of knowledge and experiences, possibly leading to the identification of best practices and ultimately benefiting public health workforce planning.

One potential way forward might be to quantify not all three categories of public health workers identified above (see Table 15.1), but only those in the first two categories. This could then be complemented through a mapping of available positions, in order to determine whether employment opportunities match the current and future supply of public health workers. In addition to absolute numbers of workers in each category, an appropriate mix will be needed, allowing the collaboration of "generalists" (such as policy-makers and health planners) and "specialists" (such as nutritionists and experts in anti-smoking measures).

Developing the public health workforce in Europe

Ensuring the existence of a well-trained workforce for public health has been identified as one of ten essential public health functions or "operations", as proposed by the Pan American Health Organization (PAHO/WHO 2002) and later by the WHO Regional Office for Europe (2011). Developing and strengthening the public health workforce requires not only a clear understanding of public health, but also adequate educational facilities and a clear set of competencies for public health workers. However, in a project assessing the public health capacities of EU member states (EAHC 2009), 14 countries reported not having a strategy to develop the public health workforce and ten countries reported only having one partially in place, mostly as part of general health workforce strategies (Aluttis, Chiotan et al., 2013).

Education of the public health workforce in Europe

Across the WHO European Region, the training and education of health professionals is still strongly focused on medical and clinical aspects, with medical schools dominating the field. While the availability of a sufficiently large and well-trained medical workforce is crucial for the effective functioning of health systems, it has been argued that there is a risk of an "over-medicalization" of health (Tulchinsky and Varavikova 2009). In many European countries, the imbalance between the medical field and public health is also reflected in salary differentials and vastly diverging training and research agendas.

A central element of education and training, and thus the supply of the public health workforce in Europe, is the Schools of Public Health. While the same definitional issues that beset workforce planning preclude specifying the number of educational institutes providing public health training in Europe, the Association of Schools of Public Health in the European Region (ASPHER) currently counts over 80 institutional members, located throughout 42 member states of the WHO European Region (ASPHER 2011). In addition, other academic institutions dealing with hygiene, epidemiology, social medicine, and other related disciplines contribute to education and training of the public health workforce in Europe.

In western Europe, the United Kingdom and the Nordic countries were among the first to introduce education in public health based on a broad curriculum, covering essential public health areas and core competences, and following a multidisciplinary approach (Johnsen 2006; Strandberg-Larsen, Nielsen et al. 2007; Boyle 2011). In other countries, both in western and eastern Europe, education and training for public health continues to evolve, with the Schools of Public Health in the United Kingdom and the United States often serving as role models. For instance, France has set up the French School of Advanced Studies in Public Health, which includes an English-taught Master of Public Health, based on the "Anglo-Saxon" model of public health education (Enserink 2008).

Other countries are following this example, and there are an increasing number of programmes that apply a multidisciplinary lens to their public health education. Despite these developments, education for public health still differs widely across Europe. A medical orientation of public health can still be observed in many countries of the former Soviet Union, such as Azerbaijan, Belarus, Kyrgyzstan, Tajikistan, and Georgia (Goodman, Overall et al. 2008; Richardson, Malakhova et al. 2008; Ibraimov, Ibrahimova et al. 2010; Khodjamurodov and Rechel 2010; Ibrahimova, Akkazieva et al., 2011). Recognizing this, a public health workforce capacity-building project under the leadership of ASPHER has been implemented in 20 countries of central and eastern Europe, with the aim of supporting capacity building and improving public health education through new training models, updated curricula, and the introduction of educational standards and quality criteria (Goodman, Overall et al. 2008). Since many post-Soviet countries face high mortality rates from preventable diseases, as well as underperforming health systems (Tulchinsky 2002), strengthening public health research and education will be crucial to address these challenges.

One challenge is that, in central and eastern European countries, the training of public health professionals has been traditionally divided into social medicine, hygiene, and epidemiology, which has affected the organization of public health and the professional development of the public health workforce. However, there is a move towards a unified specialty of public health, facilitated by institutions such as the Andrija Štampar School of Public Health in Croatia. Accession to the European Union (EU) has also given rise to increased international cooperation in the new EU member states, increasing demand for a well-educated public health workforce, and improving exchange of knowledge and access to renowned Schools of Public Health in western European countries. However, there is still a challenge to recruit highly skilled professionals and a shortage of well-paid positions once they graduate (Müller-Nordhorn, Holmberg et al. 2012).

It is not only the availability of public health education that is important; it is also its quality. Until recently, no widely accepted quality assurance mechanism or accreditation system was in place for public health training programmes in Europe. Recognizing this, and in light of the Bologna process which aims to harmonize higher education in Europe, a consortium of European organizations involved in public health, including ASPHER, the European Public Health Association (EUPHA), the European Public Health Alliance (EPHA), the European Health Management Association (EHMA), and EuroHealthNet, has established the Agency for Accreditation of Public Health Education in Europe (APHEA), which has started to accredit Master of Public Health programmes or their equivalent (Otok, Levin et al. 2011). The creation of this agency represents an important milestone for developing public health education in Europe, as it aims to facilitate quality improvements and help institutions to raise their profile (Otok, Levin et al. 2011).

Other important areas include the increasing information exchange across borders, the internationalization of public health, and the emergence of new technologies, allowing distance learning and new forms of networking for public health professionals.

Core competencies for public health

Public health is an evolving subject, requiring public health professionals constantly to acquire new competencies over their entire working life (Biesma,

Pavlova et al. 2008). A list of core competencies for public health has been developed by ASPHER, setting out what should be attained by graduates from European Schools of Public Health. The list is comprehensive, including skills in scientific methods for public health, knowledge on the social, biological, chemical, and physical environments and health, skills related to health policy, organization, management, economics, health promotion, and disease prevention, as well as further cross-disciplinary themes, such as strategy development or ethics for public health (Birt and Foldspang 2011).

Other competency systems are also being developed, often with a view of facilitating the accreditation of the public health workforce. For instance, for health promotion, the CompHP project funded by the European Commission developed competency-based standards, as well as an accreditation system for health promotion practice, education, and training. It is hoped that these will strengthen the capacity of the workforce to deliver public health improvements in Europe (Dempsey, Battel-Kirk et al. 2011). Another example is the "Public Health Skills and Career Framework" that has been developed in the United Kingdom, defining competencies at nine levels of the public health career (Rao 2008). This framework serves as a tool for describing the skills and knowledge the workforce should acquire at different career levels.

While required competencies are often related specifically to public health, more generic competencies should not be disregarded. In their study on what competencies employers would like to see public health graduates attain, Biesma and colleagues (Biesma, Pavlova et al. 2007) found that generic competencies (e.g. teamwork and communication skills) were often valued as more important than competencies specific to public health. The inclusion of generic competencies should therefore be considered in the design and implementation of competency frameworks.

Conclusion

Despite the fact that a specification of the boundaries and quantity of the workforce for public health in Europe is difficult, its importance to society is clear to see. Public health professionals, as well as the wider public health workforce, contribute significantly to the functioning of health systems and to population health. Their role should therefore be more formally acknowledged and supported by decision-makers in the governance of health systems. Since most European countries still follow a medical paradigm, focusing on treating rather than preventing diseases, health systems would benefit from a stronger public health focus and a better-developed public health workforce, which could advocate for a shift in thinking towards tackling the causes of the disease. Particularly with regard to the social determinants of health (see Chapter 11, "Tackling the social determinants of health"), there is a need for a multidisciplinary approach to population health that acknowledges the role of the wider workforce for public health.

To be able to include the public health workforce effectively in future strategies for health (such as the Health 2020 strategy of the WHO Regional Office for Europe), several key questions need to be addressed by the European public health community. These include: Who belongs to the public health workforce? How do these people contribute to health outcomes? Where are they located and do they have the relevant resources and competencies to perform in an effective manner? The European public health community has so far struggled to find satisfactory answers to these and related questions. Attempts to enumerate the public health workforce in Europe have faced a series of methodological difficulties in providing reliable estimates of size and scope. Furthermore, different understandings and terminologies across Europe with regard to the role and meaning of "public health" create ambiguities, making it difficult to establish a European consensus.

Despite these difficulties in conceptualizing the public health workforce, Europe has also seen encouraging developments in this field. Education for public health has been further institutionalized, with Schools of Public Health being established across the WHO European Region, open to non-medical personnel and following a multidisciplinary approach in their research and educational activities. In addition, the creation of the Agency for Accreditation of Public Health Education in Europe can be expected to lead to a further professionalization of public health institutions (www.aphea.net). This can help the public health profession as a whole to strengthen its visibility and credibility. Furthermore, various processes have been initiated to develop formal sets of competencies for professionals in public health and health promotion, with the aim not only to strengthen the skills of public health workers, but also to improve their chances on the labour market. There seems to be a growing consensus among the public health community that public health workforce mapping and development should become a more central element in health policy and planning. What is needed is an increased focus on developing the capacities of public health workers at the national and supranational level. The new European health policy of the WHO Regional Office for Europe, "Health 2020", has already taken up this challenge, arguing that it is necessary to strengthen the capacity of the public health workforce in order to strengthen public health as a whole. This could serve as a stimulus for member states and the public health community to focus more prominently on the prerequisites and methodologies for the effective appraisal and development of the public health workforce in Europe. The next step could be a mapping exercise of the existing public health workforce in the WHO European Region, including an appraisal of such issues as skills mix, training capacities, job positions, and current and future need, followed by actions at country levels to strengthen and sustain the public health workforce.

References

Aluttis. C. A., C. Chiotan, M. Michelsen, C. Costongs and H. Brand on behalf of the Public Health Capacity Consortium (2013). *Review of Public Health Capacity in the EU.* Luxembourg, European Commission Directorate General for Health and Consumers.

Association of Schools of Public Health in the European Region (ASPHER) (2011). *About Aspher* [http://www.aspher.org/index.php?site=about_aspher, accessed 28 May 2011].

Barley, C. (2010). *Public Health Workforce Mapping* [http://www.wales.nhs.uk/sitesplus/888/page/44414, accessed 29 May 2013]. Cardiff, Public Health Wales.

Beaglehole, R. and M. Dal Poz (2003). "Public health workforce: challenges and policy issues." *Human Resources for Health* 1(1): 4.

Biesma, R. G., M. Pavlova, G. G. van Merode and W. Groot (2007). "Using conjoint analysis to estimate employers' preferences for key competences of master level Dutch graduates entering the public health field." *Economics of Education Review* 26: 375–386.

Biesma, R. G., M. Pavlova, R. Vaatstra, G. van Merode, K. Czabanowska, T. Smith and W. Groot (2008). "Generic versus specific competencies of entry-level public health graduates: employers' perceptions in Poland, the UK, and the Netherlands." *Advances in Health Sciences Education* 13(3): 325–343.

Birt, C. and A. Foldspang (2011). *European Core Competencies for Public Health Professionals (ECCPHP)*. ASPHER Publication No. 5 [http://2011.aspher.org/pg/file/read/597/european-core-competences-for-public-health-professionals-eccphp, accessed 27 May 2013].

Boyle, S. (2011). "United Kingdom (England): health system review." *Health Systems in Transition* 13(1): 1–486.

Dempsey, C., B. Battel-Kirk and M. M. Barry (2011). *The CompHP Core Competencies Framework for Health Promotion Handbook*. Paris, International Union of Health Promotion and Education.

Department of Health (2001). *Report of the Chief Medical Officer's Project to Strengthen the Public Health Function*. London: Department of Health.

Enserink, M. (2008). "Education: France launches public health school a l'Anglo-Saxonne." *Science* 319(5862): 397.

Executive Agency for Health and Consumers (EAHC) (2009). Call for tender n° EAHC/2009/Health/05 concerning developing public health capacity [http://ec.europa.eu/eahc/documents/health/tenders/EAHC_H_05_TenderSpecificationsPublicHealthCapacity_EN.pdf, accessed 30 May 2011].

Foldspang, A. (2008). "Editorial: Developing the public health workforce in Europe: Association of Schools of Public Health in European Region (ASPHER)." *Journal of Public Health Policy* 1: 143–146.

Frank, M., A. Weihofen, M. Duetz Schmucki and F. Paccaud (2013). *Public Health Workforce in Switzerland: A national census* [http://www.ssphplus.ch/IMG/pdf_public_health_february_2013b-4-2.pdf, accessed 29 May 2013].

Gebbie, K., J. Merrill and H. Tilson (2002). "The public health workforce." *Health Affairs* 21(6): 57–67.

Goodman, J., J. Overall and T. Tulchinsky (2008). *Public Health Workforce Capacity Building: Lessons learned from "quality development of public health teaching programmes in Central and Eastern Europe"*. ASPHER Publication No. 3 [http://www.aspher.org/pliki/pdf/ASPHER_BOOK_FINAL_04.04.08.pdf, accessed 27 June 2011]. Open Society Institute and ASPHER.

Gotsadze, G., I. Chikovani, K. Goguadze, D. Balabanova and M. McKee (2010). "Reforming sanitary-epidemiological service in Central and Eastern Europe and the former Soviet Union: an exploratory study." *BMC Public Health* 10: 440.

Ibrahimova, A., B. Akkazieva, A. Ibraimov, E. Manzhieva and B. Rechel (2011). "Kyrgyzstan: health system review." *Health Systems in Transition* 13(3): 1–152.

Ibraimov, F., A. Ibrahimova, J. Kehler and E. Richardson (2010). "Azerbaijan: health system review." *Health Systems in Transition* 12(3): 1–117.

Institute of Medicine (IOM) (2002). *Shaping the Future: Who will keep the public healthy? Educating public health professionals for the 21st century* [http://www.nap.edu/openbook.php?record_id=10542&page=R1, accessed 15 May 2011].

Jambroes, M., M. L. Essink-Bot, T. Plochg and K. Stronks (2012). "Public healthcare occupations – insight into size and composition is limited." *Nederlands Tijdschrift voor Geneeskunde* **156**(31): A4529.

Johnsen, J. R. (2006). *Health Systems in Transition: Norway.* Copenhagen, WHO Regional Office for Europe on behalf of the European Observatory on Health Systems and Policies.

Kaiser, S. and J. P. Mackenbach (2008). "Public health in eight European countries: an international comparison of terminology." *Public Health* **122**(2): 211–216.

Khodjamurodov, G. and B. Rechel (2010). "Tajikistan: health system review." *Health Systems in Transition* **12**(2): 1–154.

Maier, C. B. and J. M. M. Martin-Moreno (2010). "Quo vadis SANEPID? A cross-country analysis of public health reforms in 10 post-Soviet states." *Health Policy* **102**(1): 18–25.

McDaid, D., M. Wiley, A. Maresso and E. Mossialos (2009). "Ireland: health system review." *Health Systems in Transition* **11**(4): 1–268.

Müller-Nordhorn, J., C. Holmberg, K. G. Dokova, N. Milevska-Kostova, G. Chicin, T. Ulrichs, B. Rechel, S. N. Willich, J. Powles and P. Tinnemann (2012). "Perceived challenges to public health in Central and Eastern Europe: a qualitative analysis." *BMC Public Health* **12**: 311.

Otok, R., I. Levin, S. Sitko and A. Flahault (2011). "European accreditation of public health education." *Public Health Reviews* **33**: 30–38.

Paccaud, F. (2011). "Editorial: Educating and training the public health workforce." *European Journal of Public Health* **21**(2): 137.

PAHO/WHO (2002). *Public Health in the Americas: Conceptual renewal, performance assessment, and bases for action.* Washington, D.C., PAHO/WHO.

Porter, D., Ed. (1994). *The History of Public Health and the Modern State.* Amsterdam: Editions Rodopi BV.

Rao, M. (2008). *Public Health Skills and Career Framework* [http://www.sph.nhs.uk/what-we-do/public-health-workforce/outcomes/public-health-skills-and-career-framework, accessed 27 June 2011]. London, Department of Health.

Richardson, E., I. Malakhova, I. Novik and A. Famenka (2008). "Belarus: health system review." *Health Systems in Transition* **10**(6): 1–118.

Rotem, A., J. Walters and J. Dewdney (1995). "Editorial: The public health workforce education and training study." *Australian Journal of Public Health* **19**(5): 437–438.

Sim, F., K. Lock and M. McKee (2007). "Maximizing the contribution of the public health workforce: the English experience." *Bulletin of the World Health Organization* **85**(12): 935–940.

Sim, F., G. Schiller and R. Walters (2002). *Public Health Workforce Planning for London: Mapping the public health function in London.* A Report to the DHSC London [http://www.lho.org.uk/Download/Public/8772/1/phwfreport_3.pdf, accessed 20 November 2011]. London, Department of Health and Social Care.

Strandberg-Larsen, M., M. B. Nielsen, S. Vallgårda, A. Krasnik, K. Vrangbæk and E. Mossialos (2007). "Denmark: health system review." *Health Systems in Transition* **9**(6): 1–164.

Tilson, H. and K M. Gebbie (2004). "The public health workforce." *Annual Review of Public Health* **25**(1): 341–356.

Tulchinsky, T. H. (2002). "Developing schools of public health in countries of Eastern Europe and the Commonwealth of Independent States." *Public Health Review* **30**: 179–200.

Tulchinsky, T. H. and E. A. Varavikova (2009). *The New Public Health,* 2nd edition. London, Elsevier Academic Press.

Vuorenkoski, L., P. Mladovsky and E. Mossialos (2008). "Finland: health system review." *Health Systems in Transition* **10**(4): 1–168.

Walters, R., F. Sim and G. Schiller (2002). "Mapping the public health workforce I: a tool for classifying the public health workforce." *Public Health* **116**: 201–206.

Whitfield, M. (2004). "Public health job market." In *Employment in Public Health in Europe* [*Zatrudnienie w Zdrowiu Publicznym w Europie*]. K. Czabanowska and C. Włodarczyk, Eds. Kraków, Jagiellonian University Press.

World Health Organization (WHO) (2000). *The World Health Report, 2000* [http://www.who.int/whr/2000/en/>, accessed 20 May 2011]. Geneva, WHO.

WHO Regional Office for Europe (2011). *Strengthening Public Health Capacities and Services in Europe: A framework for action* [http://www.euro.who.int/__data/assets/pdf_file/0008/147914/wd10E_StrengtheningPublicHealth_111348.pdf, accessed 23 November 2011]. Copenhagen, WHO Regional Office for Europe.

chapter sixteen

Developing public health leadership

Elke Jakubowski, Liam Donaldson, Jose M. Martin-Moreno

Introduction

Assuring governance for health and well-being is one of the ten essential public health operations (EPHOs) identified by the WHO Regional Office for Europe (see Chapter 1, "Facets of public health: an introduction"). Public health leadership is one crucial aspect of successful governance for health and well-being (Kickbusch and Gleicher 2012). However, our understanding of public health leadership has evolved over time, in line with the scope and objectives of public health. Previously associated with a single person, position or institution, leadership in public health is now dispersed among local governments and communities, as well as other stakeholders connected globally through the Internet and other modern means of communication. Those leading on public health today include national and regional ministers advocating for health protection legislation, local communities adopting health promotion policies, and the World Health Organization (WHO) coordinating standards and policies to protect and promote health. They can also include prime ministers and presidents, non-governmental organizations (NGOs), philanthropic bodies, and industrial enterprises drawing attention to public health concerns (WHO 2012).

So what does public health leadership entail and what forms can it take? How is leadership organized, and how can it be strengthened and developed? This chapter addresses these questions from a European perspective.

What is public health leadership?

A reflection on historical public health leaders who catalysed profound progress and instilled fundamental values and norms in the public health movement can identify key characteristics of public health leadership. Public health icons are often associated with innovative thinking or outstanding courage in the face of adversity, savage opposition, and the absence of any systematically organized public health system. Florence Nightingale (1820–1910), for instance, helped to establish the concept of professional nursing and hospital hygiene, as well as being a pioneering statistician. She made the case for a fundamental reform of healthcare provision. Albert Schweitzer (1875–1965), a doctor of theology and medicine, led the fight against leprosy in Africa, drawing attention to the social dimension of medicine; this achievement led to him being awarded the Nobel Peace Prize in 1952. Scientific leaders in public health such as Louis Pasteur (1822–1895) and Robert Koch (1843–1910) advanced the discipline of microbiology, in particular bacteriology, immunization, and sterilization. Rudolph Virchow (1821–1892) made seminal contributions to pathology before founding the discipline of social medicine, famously noting that "medicine is a social science, and politics is nothing else but medicine on a large scale" and that the advancement of a population required "full and unlimited democracy" and "education, freedom and prosperity" (Brown and Fee 2006). Archie Cochrane (1909–1988) provided the basis for the evidence-based medicine movement, which emphasized the importance of using evidence for medical and public health practice and promoted the "gold standard" of randomized controlled trials. Halfdan Mahler (born in 1923) served three terms as Director General of the World Health Organization, leading the organization into the modern era and paving the way for a modern understanding of public health, as expressed in the 1978 Alma Ata Declaration and the Health for All strategy.

Leadership in public health in nineteenth- and twentieth-century Europe corresponded with scientific discoveries, breakthroughs in knowledge, and wider political changes. Since then, organized public health systems have emerged, with ever more elaborate administrative and service infrastructures. This evolution of public health systems has also triggered new thoughts on public health leadership. Among recent conceptualizations, Rowitz (2009) associates public health leadership with a commitment to the community and values, the fortitude and flexibility necessary to put vision into action, and the ability to work with others and follow someone else who is a better lead. In a similar vein, Goodwin (2007) defines public health leadership as a dynamic, relationship-based process that creates an agenda for change using a strong vision and builds a strong implementation network to get things done through other people. Extending these notions, Gray (2009) argues that, in the twenty-first century, public health leadership also has to shape culture.

Other definitions of leadership have emerged from different sectors. Religious literature highlights the ability to attract followers and exert influence over others, while the business world emphasizes the ability to unite people in achieving common goals. A crucial distinction of relevance to public health is between leadership and management. Leadership is about vision and inspiration, setting the agenda, innovating, and challenging the status quo. In contrast, management tends to deal more with administration and effective implementation (Table 16.1).

Political leadership requires both management skills and leadership. Politicians operate within a formal mandate and are accountable to their electorates. They are typically aligned to the values of specific political parties. Whether they become leaders or not can be determined by the specific historical circumstances surrounding their mandate.

Table 16.1 Leadership versus management

Leaders	*Managers*
• innovate	• administrate
• focus on people	• focus on systems and structures
• inspire trust	• focus on control
• see the big picture	• laser in on the details
• ask what and why	• ask how and when
• have eyes on the horizon	• have eyes on the bottom line
• challenge the status quo	• accept the status quo
• do the right thing	• do things right
• guide others	• guide employees

Finally, in the context of health systems, leadership can be conceptualized as a form of health system stewardship – defined as the careful and responsible management of the resources that promote people's well-being (Travis, Egger et al. 2002). Travis and colleagues have broken down health system stewardship into six functional domains, all of which are integral to effective leadership: formulating strategic health policies, exerting influence through formal mechanisms, collecting and using intelligence, building coalitions and communicating effectively, seeking a fit between strategy and structure, and ensuring transparency and accountability.

However, while all these conceptualizations of leadership contain useful insights, there is no single, generally accepted definition of public health leadership (Gill 2006). For the purpose of this chapter, we define public health leadership as the deliberate process of driving fundamental progress in public health. This is in no way limited to the public health community, as public health leadership can operate in many other settings, including civil society, politics, environment, industry, philanthropy or the media, using various means and tools.

Functions of public health leadership

In line with the domains identified by Travis (Travis, Egger et al. 2002), the functions of public health leadership typically include decision-making and problem-solving, forecasting and visioning, strategy and policy development, communicating and advocating for health, and coalition-building and networking. We will now consider these functions in turn.

Decision-making and problem-solving

Public health leadership is about thinking and acting in imaginative and inspiring ways, often in difficult situations that require immediate solutions to population health problems. This calls for systems thinking, organizational

Box 16.1   Selected policy measures of European countries in response to the economic crisis

> ***A social protection plan to support vulnerable population groups in Italy***
>
> In Italy, the economic crisis accelerated the adoption of a social protection plan in 2009, targeted at low-income families and individuals. Measures included the creation of a guarantee fund for couples with newborn children, a family bonus, and subsidies for purchasing milk and diapers for infants; rental subsidies; a halt to the planned increase in regional train tariffs; and a freeze on increases in motorway tolls for low-income households.
>
> ***Compensating for food price inflation in Kyrgyzstan***
>
> In Kyrgyzstan in 2009, the government responded to the economic crisis by introducing nutritional supplements and cash transfer programmes for the poor and other vulnerable groups, including pregnant women and children under five years of age. This was in recognition of substantial food price inflation in Kyrgyzstan in the past, amounting to 32% in 2007, the highest value in the WHO European Region.
>
> *Source*: WHO (2009)

insight, and the capacity to analyse the environment for public health risks and opportunities. It is particularly important that public health leaders understand the wider economic, political, and social contexts and the implications they might have for the immediate local situation. For instance, the global financial and economic crisis that began to unfold in 2008 prompted some European governments – albeit only on a small scale – to attempt to protect their populations from the implications of the economic turmoil (Box 16.1).

There are also many examples of leadership deficits. Some governments have failed to monitor the consequences of the current financial crisis for the health of their populations and, worse, sought to deflect attention from reports that show the scale of the problem. Measles continues to be a global tragedy, killing people despite the availability of a safe, effective vaccine that was discovered and made widely available more than 40 years ago (Foege 2002). Another example of a collective weakness in public health leadership is the continuing global epidemic of premature deaths and morbidity from cardiovascular disease, despite overwhelming evidence on the benefits of prevention (Beaglehole 2001). In many European countries, alcohol policies are also poorly developed, failing to address the affordability, accessibility, and cultural acceptance of alcohol consumption, although, as was argued in the United Kingdom (Nutt, King et al. 2010), alcohol can have greater negative impacts on society than the consumption of heroin, crack cocaine or tobacco. This case illustrates how a major killer can be left unaddressed due to the interests of other government departments, such as those responsible for commerce and industry. Public health leadership in these cases requires not only overcoming the resistance of multinational corporations, but also that of other government departments (see Chapter 12, "Intersectoral working").

To the public, leadership in public health is often most visible during times of crisis, although, ironically, high-quality leadership consists in preventing crises, by necessity an invisible role. In those cases in which a crisis cannot be avoided, leadership is required to resolve it and prevent a full-blown catastrophe. However, public health crises are often characterized by uncertainties regarding health risks, the scale of the problem, and the potential impact on the population. In such situations, decision-making requires the careful interpretation of available information, including that on appropriate avenues for action.

Forecasting and visioning

Population health problems are often multifaceted and deep-rooted, requiring a strong health policy mandate to tackle them. However, clear-sighted vision, supported by forecasting, and the ability to translate this into appropriate and timely action, is an inherently challenging aspect of public health leadership, as the future always holds some degree of unpredictability. Furthermore, change, especially when disrupting a status quo that is comfortable or profitable to some, can face resistance from many social actors. Effective forecasting requires drawing lessons from the past, gaining widespread societal support, and minimizing unknowns by the best possible use of available data and forecasting tools.

Sometimes, failures to forecast public health challenges have given lead to measures to recreate strong public health leadership. One example is the heat wave in 2003, which resulted in approximately 30,000 excess deaths across Europe. While Portugal was well prepared and managed to avert the worst consequences, other European countries, such as France, were not. This experience galvanized preparedness planning for extreme weather events across Europe, demonstrating a willingness to learn from past failures in public health leadership (Box 16.2).

Box 16.2   Examples of managing extreme heat in 2003

France

In August 2003, most areas of France experienced record temperatures for over two weeks. Between 1 and 20 August, 15,000 excess deaths were recorded, many among elderly patients living in long-term care nursing institutions and psychiatric hospitals. As the media started blaming and shaming the relevant authorities, a political crisis unfolded, and the then Director General for Health was asked to resign. His retrospective analysis identified a series of errors in public health leadership:

1. Surprise: The authorities took five days to realize that the extreme heat caused excess morbidity and mortality.
2. Lack of alert: Most newspapers failed to disseminate warnings of high night temperatures, and the national surveillance authorities failed to report excess deaths in a timely way, due to a lack of preparation for extreme weather events.
3. Risk unawareness: Extreme weather events were not identified during a nationwide consultation on health risks, conducted shortly before the summer, illustrating that heat was not recognized as a potential health threat.
4. Lack of effective response measures: Most public institutions did not have air-conditioning and there were no systematic efforts to train health professionals and advise the public on hydration and cooling. Since the authorities were unprepared for a heat wave, public health services, hospitals, general practitioners, the military, and NGOs had no clearly defined roles for dealing with this eventuality.
5. Miscommunication: Many health officials were on holiday at the time, and there were few direct interventions in the mass media to offer information and advice.

Portugal

The situation was very different in Portugal, which had already had an indicator for emergency health alerts in place since 1998. Three heat alerts were issued in 2003, leading to an official report within 24 hours that was issued to regional health authorities and a network of health professionals. Information for health professionals and the public was also provided online, and a public health emergency telephone line was in operation 24 hours a day. There was also a monitoring system in place for daily rates of emergency consultations in hospitals and deaths. This showed that, between 1 June and 30 September 2003, emergency consultations increased by 40% and the overall number of deaths by 6%, especially among those above 75 years of age. The increase in mortality triggered the development of a collaborative preparedness plan for health authorities, health and social services, and civil protection. New initiatives also included a sentinel screening system for daily emergencies, an improved national monitoring of mortality, and a simplified and quicker exchange of information.

Source: WHO (2004a)

Failures to address major public health problems and forecast the damage they can bring are often due to a failure to overcome powerful countervailing forces, such as the strong vested interests of multinational companies. The history of tobacco control provides ample examples for this. The detrimental effect of smoking on health was massively underestimated in the 1950s and 1960s. An employee of the US National Cancer Institute still claimed in 1954 that, "if excessive smoking actually plays a role in the production of lung cancer, it seems to be a minor one" (Foege 2002), while a surgeon even told *Newsweek* in 1963 that for the "majority of people, smoking has a beneficial effect" (Foege 2002). After the risks of smoking became apparent to the medical community, the tobacco industry invested massive energy and resources into misleading the public, hiding facts, and pressuring governments, giving dire predictions of the economic distress that anti-tobacco legislation would cause (Diethelm and McKee 2009). It took decades of persistent lobbying by health professionals and NGOs, supported by irrefutable scientific evidence on the harms of tobacco, for governments to pass increasingly restrictive measures to protect population health. However, many European countries are still far behind the world leaders, such as Australia, which has now introduced plain packs, so there is still a long way to go.

The case of tobacco illustrates that sometimes evidence is available but is not acted upon. Other examples include the deaths of the elderly poor in England who cannot afford to pay for heating or older people across Europe who die from largely preventable falls. Public health leadership in these cases will need to build on notions of solidarity and inclusion.

The technical capacity of forecasting methods has made enormous progress. Clinical data can be linked with population-based data and risk factor surveillance, enabling predictions of the future morbidity and mortality attributable to the major diseases (Foege 2002). Weather forecasts, traffic monitors, and pollution forecasts can be used to predict short-term health risks, and personal movements can be tracked through data on public transportation, car and air travel, making it possible to anticipate the spread of infectious disease. These tools have enormous potential to assist leaders in forecasting future health needs, but they have also added complexity and make it ever more crucial to use information effectively and wisely (see Chapter 3, "Monitoring the health of the population").

Creating a vision for the future is also integral to effective leadership in public health. It requires excellent personal communication and must be based on trust, reliable information, and a common set of values. Passion and clarity will help to motivate, engage, and inspire people, and to create a common cause in pursuing public health goals, even those plagued by obstacles and uncertainties. Through a careful analysis of past experiences, as well as current risks, opportunities, and options, public health leaders can formulate sound responses to future health needs and be better prepared to react quickly to unexpected challenges (Goodwin 2007).

Developing strategy and policy

Developing strategy and policy involves a core set of public health activities, including assessing population health needs, defining priorities on the basis of available resources and capacities to address those needs, defending public health against demands from other priorities, and contributing to health policies and legislation. Defining the strategic direction for health systems as a whole is one of the most important leadership responsibilities in the new era of public health (Beaglehole, Bonita et al. 2004). It involves intersectoral working that demonstrates to other sectors the advantages of promoting health and well-being (see Chapter 12, "Intersectoral working").

Health strategies are essential tools for committing stakeholders to common strategic health goals, objectives, and targets. They can establish the objective of improving population health, formulate financial and technical commitments to health and health system objectives, and establish accountability for these commitments. Public health leadership is demonstrated in formulating ambitious but achievable strategic goals, objectives, and targets. The new health policy developed by the WHO Regional Office for Europe, Health 2020, provides an overall strategic framework for the WHO European Region. Some examples of national health strategies in selected European countries are given in Box 16.3.

Box 16.3 Examples of national health strategies in selected European countries

---

The National Strategy to Reduce Social Inequalities in Health in Norway

This strategy was adopted in 2007. It formed part of a comprehensive government policy to reduce social inequalities, improve inclusion, and combat poverty. The strategy had four priority areas: reducing social inequalities that contribute to inequalities in health; reducing social inequalities in health behaviour and use of health services; targeted initiatives to promote social inclusion; and developing knowledge and cross-sectoral tools.

The Estonian National Health Plan 2009 to 2020

The Estonian National Health Plan 2009 to 2020 is a comprehensive national health strategy with the overall goal of increasing healthy life expectancy to 65 years for females and 60 years for males, and life expectancy to 84 years for females and 75 years for males. The plan defines actions in five different fields: social cohesion, children's and young people's health, the environment, healthy lifestyles, and health care. To monitor progress, performance indicators have been identified and targets defined for consecutive four-year cycles, leading up to 2020. The plan provides a common framework for various pre-existing population health strategies and programmes and sets out a number of new activities to achieve specified targets.

The Portuguese National Health Plan 2004 to 2010

The Portuguese National Health Plan 2004 to 2010 set out key principles and strategies to contribute to improvements in health outcomes in Portugal in this period. The plan's core strategic goal was to achieve health gains, with an emphasis on health promotion, disease prevention, and the integrated management of diseases. The plan gave priority to four national health programmes (cardiovascular disease, cancer, HIV/AIDS, and mental health) and aimed to integrate the other 18 national health programmes by better managing chronic diseases and promoting health in specific settings, such as schools, the workplace, and prisons.

A health equity strategy in Finland

Finland adopted a cross-governmental health equity strategy and action plan in 2007. The strategy was developed by the intersectoral national public health committee, the institutions subordinate to the Ministry of Health, and in close collaboration with the municipalities, which play a major part in health service provision in Finland's decentralized health system. The health equity strategy built on a central theme of Finland's EU presidency in the second half of 2006, the Health in All Policy agenda (WHO 2007).

National health policies in England

England has used national health strategies and policies since the early 1990s. The first of these was "The Health of the Nation – A Strategy for England", published in 1992, following WHO's "Health for All by the Year 2000" policy. It contained a national framework for five priority areas (coronary heart disease and stroke, cancer, mental health, HIV/AIDS and sexual health, and accidents) and 27 associated targets for achieving health gains. The policy was the central guide for health services planning in the English National Health Service (NHS).

This policy was succeeded in 1999 by "Our Healthier Nation", a government action plan with the aim of improving health, with particular attention to those worst off in society. A number of targets were set, aimed at the four main causes of death in England: cancer, coronary heart disease and stroke, accidents, and poor mental health.

A subsequent national health policy, "Choosing Health: Making Healthy Choices Easier", was launched in 2004. It applied a twin-pillar approach of improving health and tackling health inequities through helping people to make healthier choices, protecting people's health from the actions of others, and recognizing the particular needs and the emotional and physical development of the young.

Communication and advocacy for health

Communication bridges scientific evidence, public health practice, and people, and is thus one of the most important leadership functions. Building on the goal of improving population health through disease prevention and health promotion, effective communication in public health cuts to the heart of people's personal interest, helping them to come to terms with what can be difficult messages or bad news (Gray 2009).

In public health emergencies, communication must capture and distil key information needed to bolster public confidence, shape personal actions, and influence the evolution of events. Transparency is absolutely essential; the slightest suspicion that information is being withheld puts public health leaders at risk of losing credibility and public authority (WHO 2004b). Unfortunately, being transparent and providing appropriate information is often easier said than done, especially in rapidly evolving health emergencies, when solid evidence is scarce and misinformation spreads rapidly. The influenza H1N1 outbreak in 2009 exposed many of the shortcomings that still exist in twenty-first-century public health communication strategies. A sensationalist 24-hour news cycle, combined with a profusion of misinformation on the Internet and in social media, contributed to widely conflicting perceptions of the situation, ranging from panic to denial (Henrich and Holmes 2011).

Clearly, public health communication must draw lessons from this experience. It will be essential to engage key stakeholders (including primary healthcare workers, industry, and the mass and online media), come up with comprehensive and coherent messages, and develop innovative health communication tools that address modern public health needs. This not only applies to public health emergencies arising from communicable diseases, but also to more slowly evolving threats to public health, such as in the epidemic of chronic diseases.

Coalition-building and networking

Effective public health leaders must not only work across their own organizations, but also reach out to foster and develop networks across sectors, resolving conflicts of interests where they arise. The scope of this coalition-building and networking can be wide, involving sectors such as retail, manufacturing, education, tourism, health and social care. The ultimate aim is to mobilize financial, intellectual or human resources for public health, including through action in other sectors.

The introduction of legislation securing smoke-free public places and workplaces in Ireland in 2004 (Box 16.4) is an example of public health leadership that operated through a strong coalition between different political and professional actors, including politicians, the public, and the media, against powerful opposition from the hospitality sector and the tobacco industry.

Box 16.4 Smoke-free workplaces in Ireland

On 29 March 2004, Ireland was one of the first European countries to adopt legislation to ban smoking in the workplace. Two national strategy papers, one on a tobacco-free society (2000) and one on the harmful effect of second-hand smoking (2003), paved the way for this law. The strategy papers were made widely available and discussed intensively in academic, civil, and political circles. The health minister made tobacco a priority and engaged passionately in the debate. The legislative initiative to ban smoking in workplaces gained support from the general public, the political parties represented in parliament, and NGOs. This effective alliance of advocates was supported by and facilitated a mass media campaign in favour of a tobacco ban in workplaces. Preparation of the draft legislation created a cascade of support and gradually watered down opponents, mainly from the hospitality sector and the tobacco industry. An important success factor in passing the legislation was the consistency of the message that argued that employees should be protected from second-hand smoke. The progress made in Ireland had important repercussions for tobacco control beyond its national borders, as it demonstrated what was possible to achieve.

Source: WHO (2005)

Building coalitions, alliances, and networks is a vital prerequisite for achieving public health targets, but it will often require trade-offs. One is related to questions of resource allocation. Health leaders in high-level positions often have considerable control over resources within their own service, resources needed to achieve fundamental change. Some of this autonomy will need to be given up, as coalitions make joint decisions on policies and related resource allocations (Goodwin 2007). A particular challenge will be to achieve an appropriate balance in ownership, resource allocation, accountability, and implementation.

Forms of public health leadership

Several forms of public health leadership can be distinguished. Ultimately, the different forms of public health leadership are not exclusive, and mixed forms will prevail, such as when an organizational and administrative apparatus backs their chief health officer, or when healthy cities form an international collaborative network. Leadership at the national or intergovernmental level in Europe also attests to the prevalence of mixed leadership forms.

Individual leadership

Individual leadership is associated with a specific person; its success depends on the right blend of personal qualities and professional skills and experience. Individual leaders actively and intentionally initiate developments in public health. While each will deploy their own leadership style and techniques, some working principles and skills seem to be common elements of success. These include passion, integrity, and dedication to values and public health principles, underpinned by the solid yet pragmatic knowledge of public health practice. Foresight, creativity, and openness to innovative solutions will help to establish a vision of future public health challenges and the tools required to tackle them. Finally, experience, wisdom, courage, and people skills help public health leaders to engage and empower others in carrying out a common mission (Rowitz 2009).

Organizational leadership

Organizational leadership also relies on the effectiveness of processes and relationships. However, in contrast to individual leadership, it is embedded in and based on an organization. Sometimes, organizational leadership involves leadership teams, operating effectively across organizational boundaries. This involves developing and maintaining interpersonal relationships within and outside organizational boundaries, clarifying the agenda for change, and building credibility (Goodwin 2007).

Community-led leadership

Community-led leadership is heavily dependent on being able to discern, represent, and act on the views and needs of local people and institutions. It refers to local-level leadership models that often include an intersectoral and sometimes even an integrated approach to local policies and services. Their appeal lies in the proximity to the needs and interests of people they serve. The global healthy cities movement is an example of community-led public health leadership, tackling urban health problems such as traffic pollution, noise, violence, social isolation, injuries, alcohol and substance abuse. In the WHO European Region, national healthy cities networks comprise more than 1400 cities and towns.

Collaborative leadership

Collaborative leadership models rely on more formally organized networks and partnerships. Depending on the nature of their commitment, they may provide access to information and resources, but might also be sources of constraints. Successful collaborative leadership will lead to increased resources and reduction of constraints through networking and collaboration (Goodwin 2007). A study of health authorities in the United Kingdom found that collaborative leadership requires similar interpersonal skills as with organizational leadership, including effective communication and listening, persuasion, and the capacity to build long-term relationships (Ferlie and Pettigrew 1996).

It is also important to note that collaborative and organizational leadership are often most successful when there is no visible face related to a given initiative. Rather, different organizations work together behind the scenes towards a common goal, without being identified with any particular individual, which might even be counterproductive. One example of such a collaborative or organizational initiative is text4baby (www.text4baby.org) in the United States, which, since its launch in 2010, has brought together more than 500 private and public partners to provide informative, free text messages to expectant mothers.

The organization of public health leadership in Europe

National level

The diversity of health systems in Europe extends to their arrangements for public health leadership at the national level (see Chapter 14, "Organization and financing of public health"). Politicians determine the priority of health within government and the organizational division of responsibilities between sectors. This responsibility is often diffused. There is a trade-off between political engagement and independence; there are benefits for public health institutions having close links to ministers, making it possible to have a voice in cabinet. However, there are also drawbacks, such as the political prioritization of vested interests (e.g. the tobacco and alcohol industry), especially where they are political donors. For this reason, NGOs and the media can play an important role, promoting transparency and holding governments to account.

Another important leadership role (both in political and technical terms) is the position of the chief medical officer or director general for health. This role is most developed in the four countries of the United Kingdom. In England, the Chief Medical Officer is the government's principal medical adviser and the professional head of the medical profession. In most other European Union (EU) countries, the chief medical officer or equivalent has a rather different profile (Jakubowski, Martin-Moreno et al. 2010). The variety of organizational settings and mandates in Europe means that responsibilities and roles of these posts differ greatly. They can be limited to the surveillance of communicable diseases, such as in Austria and Germany, or extend to the control of communicable and non-communicable diseases, epidemic and crisis response, and the implementation of the International Health Regulations. A common challenge is the medical focus of these posts, which can distract from upstream determinants of health.

International level

The landscape of international public health leadership has changed dramatically in recent years. Humanitarian concerns for the health of the poor, fear of the spread of pandemics, and the recognition of health as a key determinant of economic growth has put health higher on the international political agenda than ever before. The increased recognition of health has brought many opportunities as well as challenges. Globally and in Europe, many new and diverse partners in public health have emerged over the past four decades in addition to WHO, including: the institutions of the EU, in particular the European Commission and the European Centre for Disease Control (ECDC); UN institutions such as the United Nations Children's Fund (UNICEF), the Joint United Nations Programme on HIV/AIDS (UNAIDS), and the United Nations

Development Programme (UNDP); and, more recently, the Organisation for Economic Co-operation and Development (OECD), GAVI Alliance, and the Global Fund to Fight AIDS, Tuberculosis and Malaria. Several EU presidencies have moved the public health agenda in Europe forward, and fora such as the European Health Forum in Gastein have helped to shape priorities. There are also European networks that facilitate information exchange on public health leadership, such as the High Level Groups led by the European Commission (on Health Services and Medical Care and on Nutrition and Physical Activity) or the Alcohol Policy Network in Europe [http://alcoholpolicynetwork.eu/]. The roles of the private sector and civil society have also increased. Because funding comes from many different, often uncoordinated, sources, it has been distributed unevenly among health priorities and countries, greatly increasing the need for leadership and coordination (see Chapter 14, "Organization and financing of public health"). While health has gained more attention, international collaboration in health has become more fragmented, posing new demands on international public health leadership.

Exerting, strengthening, and developing public health leadership

Effectively exerting, strengthening, and developing leadership to realize a strong vision of public health requires many barriers be overcome. Despite the fact that many public health leaders emerge from public health services, these institutions often fail to recruit or retain the most talented leaders, partly because of low levels of pay. Training schemes often fail to develop leadership (McKee 2013). Public health leadership might also be restrained by hierarchical settings, regulations, and organizational rules. Furthermore, there is the increasing need to develop leadership across organizational boundaries and constituencies.

Public health leadership has to negotiate powerful ministries and other stakeholders, which are often motivated by strong self-interest. Political leadership in public health might be constrained by the wish of politicians to be re-elected, to conform to the agendas of their political parties, and to please the electorate's short-term wishes, which can clash with long-term population health interests. Relying only on political leadership for public health is therefore risky, particularly in view of the short-term nature of political posts.

Strengthening public health leadership requires a more systematic approach, such as including leadership training in the training of public health professionals (Rowitz 2009). Such training should focus on interpersonal leadership skills and on network and system-based strategies (Goodwin 2007). Learning will need to be experience-based and involve professionals who work across and beyond health, and at the local, national, and international level. It should cover inter-organizational team building, local strategy development, and individual and team coaching, and involve public health leaders (Goodwin 2007). Training and skills development can also make better use of existing fora, such as WHO's Futures Forum, the European Health Forum in Gastein, and the Summer School of the European Observatory on Health Systems and Policies.

A range of additional options exists for strengthening public health leadership in Europe (Table 16.2).

Table 16.2 Policy options for strengthening public health leadership

Subject field (and main actors)	Policy options
Promoting public health leadership practice at national and European level (WHO, EU, national governments, NGOs)	Establishing networks of public health leadership within and between countries
	Reviewing the effect of institutional policies and legislation on encouraging or discouraging leadership
	Introducing leadership reviews, including in other sectors
	Defining leadership roles and models to incentivize performance
	Promoting successful leadership practices
Mobilizing human and financial resources (national governments, ministries of health)	Setting up a sponsoring scheme and network
	Establishing a pool of public health leaders
	Reviewing recruitment practices, especially in the public sector
Improving leadership requisites within organizations (national governments, organizations in the public and private sector)	Clarifying management, leadership, political, and administrative roles
	Reviewing organizational rules in terms of whether they constrain or encourage leadership
	Promoting strategies to recruit the best leaders
Promoting policy research (WHO, EU, national governments, ministries of health, public health institutes, professional associations)	Improving the evidence base on public health leadership
	Fostering and sharing understanding of leadership behaviour
Education (ministries of health, ministries of education, universities)	Including public health leadership modules in under- and postgraduate curricula of health professionals
Training (WHO, EU, national governments, public health organizations)	Fostering joint learning of political and administrative leaders, and developing modules for learning across sectors
	Utilizing taught, mentoring, and coaching practices involving experienced leaders

Conclusion

There is huge potential to apply lessons learned from public health leadership worldwide, in order to spark progress in public health and avoid repeating past mistakes. However, it is clear that there are no "one-size-fits-all" solutions in achieving good public health leadership, and sometimes we do not know why leadership has worked in one and not in another setting. Is it about the right people in charge? Or do we underestimate the role of the right momentum? How important is mandate?

We have argued that people matter for a health leadership culture; so does good timing to gain momentum and support, as well as an appropriate organizational set-up and mandate. However, in an increasingly interconnected, mobile, and diffused global world, traditional public health governance and leadership structures need to be re-imagined beyond hierarchical, vertical, and geographical constituencies. Public health leadership now requires working both vertically and horizontally, and in networks. Success in stimulating developments in public health will increasingly depend on the capacity of public health leaders to reach out to others, influence those that work beyond their control, and build coalitions and alliances. This will require leadership competences and skills, such as the ability to mobilize, inspire, convince, and engage people, and the capacity to mediate conflicts of interests. There is also more room for leadership choices, such as whether to act visibly or behind the scenes; within a political party, community setting, academia, or an NGO; at local, national, or international level; and whether to leap on the right moment or plant the seeds for future change.

References

Beaglehole, R. (2001). "Global cardiovascular disease prevention: time to get serious." *The Lancet* **358**(9282): 661–663.

Beaglehole, R., R. Bonita, R. Horton, O. Adams and M. McKee (2004). "Public health in the new era: improving health through collective action." *The Lancet* **363**(9426): 2084–2086.

Brown, T. M. and E. Fee (2006). "Rudolf Carl Virchow." *American Journal of Public Health* **96**(12): 2104–2105.

Diethelm, P. and M. McKee (2009). "Denialism: what it is and how should scientists respond?" *European Journal of Public Health* **19**(1): 2–4.

Ferlie, E. and A. Pettigrew (1996). "Managing through networks: some issues and implications for the NHS." *British Journal of Management* **7**(Suppl. S1): S81–S99.

Foege, W. H (2002). "Challenges to public health leadership." In *Oxford Textbook of Public Health, Vol. I: The scope of public health*, 4th edition. New York, Oxford University Press: 401–414.

Gill, R. (2006). *Theory and Practice of Leadership*. London, Sage.

Goodwin, N. (2007). "Leadership in public health." In *New Perspectives in Public Health*, 2nd edition. S. Griffith and D. J. Hunter, Eds. Oxford, Radcliffe Publishing: 330–337.

Gray, M. (2009). "Public health leadership: creating the culture for the twenty-first century." *Journal of Public Health* **31**(2): 208–209.

Henrich, N. and B. Holmes (2011). "What the public was saying about the H1N1 vaccine: perceptions and issues discussed in on-line comments during the 2009 H1N1 pandemic." *PLoS One* **6**(4): e18479.

Jakubowski, E., J. M. Martin-Moreno and M. McKee (2010). "The governments' doctors: the roles and responsibilities of chief medical officers in the European Union." *Clinical Medicine* **10**(6): 560–562.

Kickbusch, I. and D. Gleicher (2012). *Governance for Health in the 21st Century*. Copenhagen: World Health Organization Regional Office for Europe.

McKee, M. (2013). "Seven goals for public health training in the 21st century." *European Journal of Public Health* **23**(2): 186–187.

Nutt, D. J., L. A. King and L. D. Phillips, on behalf of the Independent Scientific Committee on Drugs (2010). "Drug harms in the UK: a multicriteria decision analysis." *The Lancet* **376**(9752): 1558–1565.

Rowitz, L. (2009). *Public Health Leadership: Putting principles into practice*, 2nd edition. Sudbury, MA, Jones & Bartlett.

Travis, P., D. Egger, P. Davies and A. Mechbal (2002). *Towards Better Stewardship: Concepts and critical issues*. Discussion Paper 02.48 [http://www.who.int/healthinfo/paper48.pdf, accessed 1 August 2011]. Geneva, WHO.

World Health Organization (WHO) (2004a). *Fifth Futures Forum on Rapid Response Decision-making Tools* [http://www.euro.who.int/__data/assets/pdf_file/0006/98304/E83347.pdf]. Copenhagen, WHO Regional Office for Europe.

World Health Organization (WHO) (2004b). *Sixth Futures Forum on Crisis Communication* [http://www.euro.who.int/en/what-we-publish/abstracts/sixth-futures-forum-on-crisis-communication]. Copenhagen, WHO Regional Office for Europe.

World Health Organization (WHO) (2005). *Seventh Futures Forum on Unpopular Decisions in Public Health* [http://www.euro.who.int/en/what-we-publish/abstracts/seventh-futures-forum-on-unpopular-decisions-in-public-health]. Copenhagen, WHO Regional Office for Europe.

World Health Organization (WHO) (2009) *Health in times of global economic crisis: Implications for the WHO European Region, Regional Committee for Europe*, Fifty-ninth session, Copenhagen, 14–17 September 2009 [http://www.euro.who.int/__data/assets/pdf_file/0006/66957/RC59_edoc07.pdf, accessed 14 February 2014].

World Health Organization (WHO) (2012). *Health 2020: A European policy framework supporting action across government and society for health and well-being* [http://www.euro.who.int/en/who-we-are/governance/regional-committee-for-europe/sixty-second-session/documentation/working-documents/eurrc629-health-2020-a-european-policy-framework-supporting-action-across-government-and-society-for-health-and-well-being]. Copenhagen, WHO Regional Office for Europe.

chapter seventeen

Public health research

*Stefania Boccia, Ilmo Keskimäki,
Walter Ricciardi*

Introduction

Advancing public health research has been identified as one of the essential
public health operations (see Chapter 1, "Facets of public health in Europe:
an introduction"). Public health research aims to improve population health
through inputs to policy-making and public health practice. According to a
recent definition (McCarthy, Harvey et al. 2009), public health research is the

> organized quest for new knowledge to protect, promote and improve
> people's health. It is undertaken at population or health services level [. . .].
> It is usually goal-oriented, addressing questions of policy relevance, and
> may be published in either academic journals or reports. It uses a range of
> observational methods, including surveys, registers, data sets, case studies
> and statistical modelling, and draws on disciplines including epidemiology,
> sociology, psychology and economics, and interdisciplinary fields of
> environmental health, health promotion, disease prevention, health care
> management, health services research and health systems research.

Given the dearth of information on public health research in the eastern part of
the WHO European Region, this chapter focuses primarily on the situation in
the European Union (EU). It begins by reviewing EU-level structures to support
public health research, followed by a discussion of recent EU-funded research
projects that aimed to map public health research in the EU. The chapter then
turns to a discussion of national structures to support public health research
in Europe, with case studies of Italy, Finland, Poland, and Estonia. It argues
that there is a need for national strategies for public health research, improved
coordination between ministries of science, health, and finance, improved
coordination across different research and innovation programmes within the
EU, and better engagement with public health researchers, users, and partners,
including civil society organizations.

EU-level structures to support public health research

The EU began operating technological programmes in the 1950s and launched its First Framework Programme for Research and Technological Development in 1984. The EU's role in research policy has evolved considerably since 1987, when the Single European Act revised the 1957 Treaty of Rome with the objective of establishing a single market. This brought science and technology within the competence of the European Community. Since the late 1980s, a succession of Framework programmes has been put in place. While the First Framework Programme, covering the years 1984–1987, had a budget of €3.25 billion, the Seventh Framework Programme was allocated €53 billion for research and technological development for 2008–2013. The latest framework programme for research and innovation, Horizon 2020, has an anticipated budget of approximately €80 billion for 2014–2020. Since the 2000s, the number of financing instruments has also increased, and some evaluations suggest too rapidly (European Commission 2010).

Although the starting point of EU research programmes lay in technology development, funding for health research was already present in the early framework programmes, such as for BIOMED I and II within the Third and Fourth Framework Programmes. Since then, health research has become much more prominent, being second to research on information and communication technology in terms of annual funding in the Seventh Framework Programme and comprising around 20% of the overall budget. While the general aim of the framework programmes is to support research that makes Europe more competitive in economic terms, the focus has recently broadened to include areas such as health services research.

In the 2000s, at both the EU and national level, there were increasing attempts to strengthen the role of research and technological innovations as a means to boost competitiveness and economic growth. This has led to increased funding for research and development through EU-wide collaborative initiatives under the umbrella of the European Research Area (ERA). The ERA aims to facilitate transnational cooperation across national and institutional boundaries. It includes initiatives such as ERA-Nets, aiming to facilitate the development of European research infrastructure. Funded from the Seventh Framework Programme, the EU has also established the European Research Council (ERC) to support researcher-driven science. The ERC is the first European funding body set up to support investigator-driven, bottom-up frontier research, with the main aim of stimulating scientific excellence. The ERC complements other funding activities in Europe, such as those of national funding agencies. It allows researchers to identify new opportunities and directions in any field of research, rather than being led by priorities set by politicians. Although the ERC does not set funds aside specifically for public health research, many projects in this area are being financed. ERC funding offers Starting Independent Researcher Grants to support up-and-coming research leaders in Europe who are about to establish or consolidate a research team and start conducting independent research, and Advanced Investigator Grants targeting researchers who have already established themselves as independent research leaders. Of 566 starting grant proposals accepted in 2012, 209 (37%) were in the area of life sciences, and many of those focused on diagnostic tools, therapies, and public health (European Research Council 2012).

Nevertheless, public health research itself has remained marginalized in the development of the EU's research funding instruments. This can largely be explained by economic competitiveness being the main driver for EU research policies, but there are also other reasons, such as the EU's limited mandate in the area of health. Public health research to date has accounted for only a small proportion of EU research funding, amounting to 5% of the total funding allocated for health research in the Seventh Framework Programme. Until the 1990s, the EU's mandate only covered such health issues as occupational health and safety and the protection of the population from ionizing radiation, but new health threats emerging in the late 1980s and early 1990s, such as bovine spongiform encephalopathy (BSE) and severe acute respiratory syndrome (SARS), illustrated the need for EU-level public health policies and actions. The 1992 Maastricht Treaty introduced wider health-related considerations into the constitutional framework of the EU, which were subsequently extended in the 1997 Amsterdam Treaty; the first by requiring public health protection, the second through its emphasis on human health safety (Mossialos, Permanand et al. 2010). In the early 2000s, these provisions gave rise to the EU's first public health programme. However, this programme and its successor, the Health Programme 2008–2013, were oriented towards public health action and did not support research-focused proposals.

The Health Programme 2008–2013, which is managed by the Executive Agency for Health and Consumers (EAHC, formerly the Public Health Executive Agency), has three main objectives: to improve health security, promote health (including the reduction of health inequalities), and generate and disseminate health information and knowledge. The public health programme finances four main types of actions: projects, conferences, joint actions, and operation grants. The programme is not intended to fund research projects in public health, but rather to support implementation activities and the sharing of good practices in public health. Actions need to have a European dimension, with involvement of partners from different European countries. With the exception of tendered projects, the core principle of the programme is co-financing, and reimbursement is usually capped at 60% of total project costs.

Within the EU, member states are responsible for their health and research policies, including training and capacity planning. In principle, the actions of the EU should provide added value to national or sub-national activities. Accordingly, the European Commission has recently increased its collaboration with WHO and OECD, such as in the field of publishing health indicators (OECD 2012). However, tensions can arise between the European Commission and member states over the competencies of the Commission in these policy areas; comprehensive integrated health policy programmes are somewhat outside the remit of the Commission. For instance, developing a policy like the WHO's Health for All and Health 21 – Health for All in the 21st Century, which also set out research priorities and the request for strategic health research planning by WHO member states, would be difficult to achieve in the EU.

There are, however, some potentially promising developments in EU research policy. In 2008, the European Commission proposed a new coordination initiative, joint programming, designed to promote collaborative research programmes organized and funded by member states (European Commission 2008). The initiative may help to advance public health research in Europe, as it responds to the observation that EU research instruments have failed to address major societal challenges common to member states. About 85% of public research funding in the EU is allocated by national research programmes, but these are not coordinated and may involve a significant degree of duplication. The joint programming initiative seeks to make better use of European research resources to tackle societal challenges, including demographic and climate change, urbanization, and environmental sustainability. The process is voluntary for member states, which can choose topics they want to be involved in. However, the aim is to build up joint research programmes among countries with a commonly agreed focus. In the preparation of Joint Programme Initiatives (JPI), public health topics have been relatively well addressed. Public-health-related programmes currently in preparation include "A healthy diet for a healthy life", "More years, better life", and "Antimicrobial resistance". In addition, public health is also linked with other themes, such as "Connecting climate knowledge for Europe", "Urban Europe", and "Agriculture, food security and climate change". There are still unresolved issues in joint programming and the process has been slower than anticipated, but the initiative could help to bring societal issues such as public health closer to the centre of EU research policy, on a level with competitiveness and technological innovations.

As mentioned earlier, a promising development is the proposed new EU framework programme on research and innovation, Horizon 2020. This includes several technical improvements, such as simplifying bureaucratic rules and procedures in managing EU research funding. If its budget is approved, the programme will also bring 50% more EU resources for research per year. The new programme is anticipated to include major structural reform, bringing together all funding for research, development, and innovation that has so far been channelled through separate programmes. In addition, Horizon 2020 would allow the use of Structural Funds for research activities. To boost the quality of research in the EU, funding for the ERC is anticipated to be doubled. As in the initiative on joint programming, the research themes in Horizon 2020 relate to societal challenges, which also include public-health-related issues.

In 2013, calls were made for an increased share of funding to research in health systems, public health, and health policy (Browne and Sorensen 2013; Walshe, McKee et al. 2013a, 2013b). While the initiatives on joint programming and Horizon 2020 are promising developments that might enhance EU support to public health research, it remains to be seen whether they can realize this potential. So far, in their reactions to the Horizon 2020 health research agenda, public health researchers have expressed disappointment for the lack of public health focus (Joint Statement 2013). The draft work programme for the 2014–2015 health, demographic change, and well-being strand of Horizon 2020, circulated in September 2013, concentrated heavily on research on biotechnology and personalized therapeutic innovations. However, at the time of writing (November 2013) the final document has not yet been published. Furthermore, the draft work programme only covers the first two years of the programme, and subsequent work programmes may better balance priorities in terms of public health and health systems research.

Mapping public health research in Europe: the SPHERE and STEPS projects

The EU-funded projects SPHERE (www.ucl.ac.uk/public-health/sphere) and STEPS (www.steps-ph.eu), both coordinated by University College London, provide insights into the state of public health research in EU member states.

SPHERE was established in 2005 to collect information on the state of public health research in Europe. The project had 18 partners from 12 European countries, and collaborated with the European Public Health Association (EUPHA). A questionnaire was sent to the ministries of health and ministries of science of the then 25 EU member states, as well as Iceland, Norway, and Switzerland. Replies from 42 of 56 ministries in 25 countries indicated that the majority of countries did not have formal priorities for public health research, although three areas of public health research were described by at least one ministry for 18 countries: disease control, health promotion and health services, and methods (epidemiology) (Conceição, Leandro et al. 2009).

Another questionnaire on national and international priorities for public health research was sent to national public health associations (McCarthy, Harvey et al. 2009). Replies were received from 22 countries, identifying research priorities in most areas (Table 17.1), although with noticeable differences across countries. At the national level, the most important priorities in northern European countries were health services and patient safety; southern European countries gave priority to infectious diseases, health services, and cardiovascular diseases, while eastern European countries prioritized food safety and nutrition, environmental health, and occupational health. At the international level, northern European countries prioritized infectious diseases, cardiovascular diseases, and cancer research; southern European countries gave most priority to health services, cancer research, drug addiction, food safety and nutrition, health technology assessment, and mental health, while eastern European countries identified cardiovascular diseases and mental health as priorities.

Finally, 80 civil society health organizations provided information on their perspectives on the needs for public health research (McCarthy, Harvey et al. 2009). General areas, such as public health or the environment and health were most frequently reported. In the middle range were topics linked to behavioural determinants of health, while specific diseases, organizational aspects of health care, and professional needs were least frequently mentioned.

The STEPS Project built on the results of SPHERE, aiming to convene civil society organizations, researchers, and national ministries to debate and develop a European strategy for public health research. STEPS was a collaboration from January 2009 to June 2011 between University College London, EUPHA, Assocation Skalbes, and 12 country partners (STEPS 2011). The project described public health research systems in all EU member states, promoted workshops in the 12 new EU member states to share experience on public health research systems, and investigated the use of Structural Funds for public health

Table 17.1 Priorities for public health research according to respondents from national public health associations in 22 countries of the European Economic Area

Overall theme	Sub-theme	National N (%)	International N (%)
Disease control	Cardiovascular diseases	18 (78)	7 (30)
	Cancer	16 (70)	8 (35)
	Infection diseases	17 (75)	7 (30)
	Mental health	15 (65)	—
	Migrant health	8 (35)	3 (13)
Health promotion	Environmental health	17 (74)	—
	Occupational medicine	15 (65)	—
	Bioterrorism	12 (53)	3 (13)
	Food safety and nutrition	18 (78)	
	Health education and promotion	15 (65)	5 (22)
	Drug addiction	13 (56)	6 (26)
Health services	Health services research	18 (78)	5 (22)
	Patient safety	15 (65)	—
	Health technology assessment	13 (56)	5 (22)
	Health management	14 (61)	4 (17)
	Use of medicines	13 (56)	4 (17)
Methods	Epidemiology	15 (65)	4 (17)

Source: Adapted from McCarthy, Harvey et al. (2009)

research. The workshops discussed how the public health research system functions in each country, and how it could be developed through European contacts and the contribution of civil society organizations. Drawing on the work of the STEPS Project, the next section describes national structures in place to support public health research in selected European countries.

National structures to support public health research

The STEPS Project found that ministries of health or of science usually commission public health research in EU member states, except in Austria, Belgium, Denmark, Lithuania, and the United Kingdom, where regions play a major role in allocating funds. Private foundations sponsoring research are to some extent present in most of the countries, but are particularly important in Austria, France, Germany, Ireland, Poland, Portugal, Slovakia, Sweden, and the United Kingdom. Almost all EU member states have state institutes (Austria being an exception – see below) and universities that carry out public health research, while in only eight countries, especially in northern and eastern Europe, healthcare delivery organizations were reported to be involved in public health research. In Austria, there is no national research strategy for public health research and public funding is difficult to obtain; there is no defined public budget for public health research (Ladurner, Gerger et al. 2011).

In a study of public health capacities in the EU, respondent countries reported capacities for public health research to be relatively well established. However, according to this study, funding priorities for health research in EU member states were in general dominated by a medical approach, with a weak public health agenda. This may reflect a lack of coordination between ministries of health and ministries of science to agree on health research strategies. The extent of governmental support for public health research varied substantially across the EU. In five of 27 countries (Greece, Austria, Latvia, Italy, Slovakia), it was reported that there was no government support for public health research (Aluttis, Chiotan et al. 2012). In several countries, the national experts in this study indicated a poorly developed capacity for communicating effectively research results to policy-makers.

Self-assessments of public health capacities and services undertaken by WHO member states, supported by the WHO Regional Office for Europe and using a self-assessment tool structured around the 10 essential public health operations (EPHOs), provide some additional insights into capacities for public health research. In Estonia, a lack of applied research in public health was noted (Koppel, Leventhal et al. 2009). In Uzbekistan, the overall directions for epidemiological and scientific research are determined by the Main Department for Science and Educational Institutions of the Ministry of Health. However, priority-setting takes insufficient account of the practical needs of the health system, much research is not applied in practice, there is insufficient state funding, and a lack of cost-effectiveness studies (Ministry of Health of the Republic of Uzbekistan 2011). In the countries of south-east Europe, public health research is still limited and the use of health information to support policy and strategy is not yet common, although most countries incorporate research evidence in some areas and to some extent. There are few examples of concrete evidence that research has been used directly to inform strategies and programmes for health promotion and disease prevention (WHO 2009b). In Slovenia, it is reported that public health research is fragmented, although most is co-financed by the Slovenian Research Agency, the Ministry of Health, and other ministries (WHO 2009a). In the former Yugoslav Republic of Macedonia, research activities are planned by the Republican Institute for Health Protection, the Institute for Occupational Health or by public health departments in the medical faculty. The government does not play an important role in planning public health research, but contributes as a funding agency (WHO 2007c). In Bulgaria, priorities for public health research are defined by the Ministry of Health in the National Health Strategy (WHO 2007a). In Bosnia and Herzegovina, epidemiological and public health research is sporadic, mainly due to the limited amount of public funding (WHO 2007b).

Public health research in Italy

Research programmes and funders

Research in Italy's health sector is under the control of the Ministry of Education, University, and Research, and the Ministry of Health. The budget of the Ministry of Education, University, and Research is set out annually in the National Budget Law and provides resource to the National Research Council and the universities (Figure 17.1). The research funding of the Ministry of

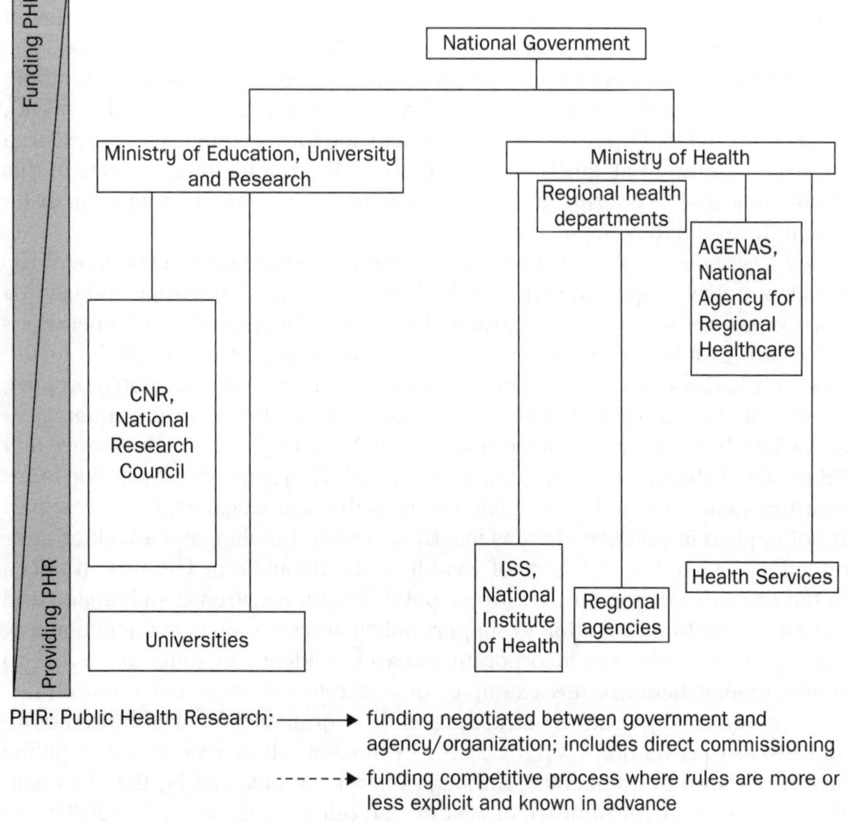

PHR: Public Health Research: ⟶ funding negotiated between government and agency/organization; includes direct commissioning

⤍ funding competitive process where rules are more or less explicit and known in advance

Figure 17.1 Funding flows for public health research in Italy

Source: STEPS [https://www.ucl.ac.uk/public-health/STEPS_folder/Italy_STEPS_countryprofile_5oct10.pdf, accessed 9 July 2012]

Health is part of the budget of the country's National Health Service (NHS). The ministry defines the general strategies for health research in the NHS every three years, and launches annual calls for funding. According to the latest programme of research of the Ministry of Health (covering the period 2013–2015), two main areas are funded: clinical-biomedical research, oriented to support both clinical research and the development of new technologies, and organizational-management research, which supports research on health determinants, as well as health management and policy.

Research bodies

The National Institute of Health is the leading technical and scientific public body of the Italian NHS. Its activities include research, monitoring, training, and consultation in the interest of public health protection. The institute conducts scientific research in a wide variety of fields, from molecular and genetic research to population-based studies of risk factors for disease and disability. Research priorities are based on those set out in the National Health Plan. The institute is supervised by the General Directorate for Scientific and Technological Research under the Ministry of Health.

The National Agency for Regional Health Care Services carries out its activities in close collaboration with the Ministry of Health and the regions and participates in research programmes funded by the Ministry of Health. Activities include health technology assessment, patient safety, and clinical and organizational guidelines. In addition, there are regional agencies that undertake public health research. For example, the Agency for Regional Health Care Services in the Emilia Romagna region provides technical and regulatory support for the health region of Emilia Romagna. It aims to integrate assistance, research, and training. Another example from the same region is the Centre for Health Service Effectiveness Evaluation.

Public health research in Finland

Research programmes and funders

In Finland, the overall coordinating body of the government's research policy is the Research and Innovation Council chaired by the Prime Minister (Figure 17.2). Its tasks include reviewing national and international developments, coordinating government activities, and drawing up a research and innovation strategy (Research and Innovation Council of Finland 2010). Academic public health research is mainly funded by the Research Council for Health of the Academy of Finland, which falls under the administration of the Ministry of Education and Culture. The most important funding instruments of the Academy of Finland are researcher-driven. Research programmes funded by the Academy often address public health topics, such as the recent programmes on "Responding to Public Health Challenges", "Health and Welfare of Children and Young People", "Climate Change", and "Nutrition, Food and Health". The Finnish Funding Agency for Technology and Innovation (TEKES) has started to fund research and development programmes on public services, including health services. The Academy of Finland and TEKES coordinate international research collaboration and EU research programmes in Finland. In the 2000s, the role of the Ministry of Social Affairs and Health in funding research and development activities has increased, but a large part of its funding is restricted to developing health and social services. The ministry also funds health promotion projects, including research proposals, and allocates funding for research carried out in the health system.

Currently, the operational environment of public health research in Finland is changing. In 2013, the Finnish Government decided to cut the budget frameworks of the research institutes under the Ministry of Social Affairs and Health by €30 million. In addition, the government decided to reorganize its funding for research mainly carried out by government research institutes. It plans to establish gradually in 2015–2017 a new funding system for strategic

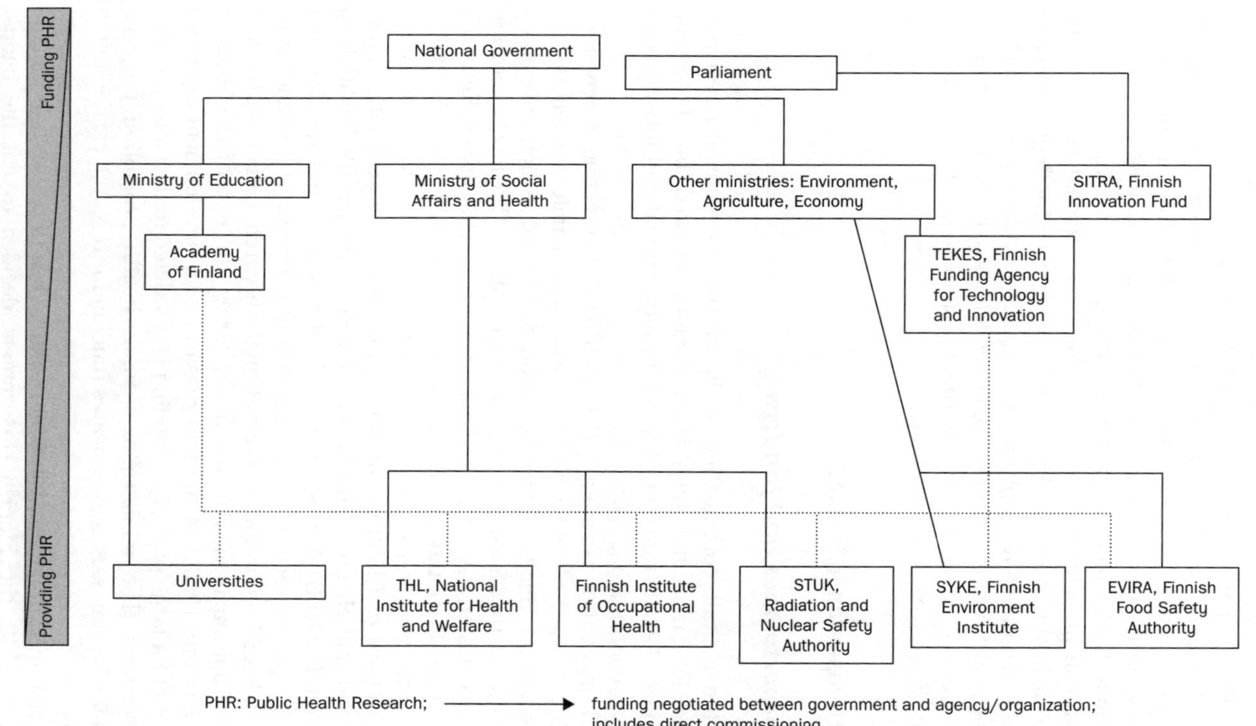

Figure 17.2 Funding flows for public health research in Finland

Source: STEPS [https://www.ucl.ac.uk/public-health/STEPS_folder/Finland_STEPS_countryprofile_2oct10.pdf, accessed 9 July 2012]

research supporting political decision-making. Funding will be collected from the budgets of government research institutes and the research funding of the Academy of Finland and the Finnish Funding Agency for Technology and Innovation. Together, these decisions will result in funding cuts corresponding to a redundancy of approximately 900 persons in government research institutes in the field of public health research. However, these institutes may gain part of the funding back through competition for grants from the new funding instrument.

Research bodies

Much public health research in Finland is currently carried out by "sector research institutes", administered by the Ministry of Social Affairs and Health. These institutes are the National Institute for Health and Welfare (1200 staff), the Finnish Institute for Occupational Health (800 staff), the Finnish Food Safety Authority (750 staff), the Centre for Health Promotion Research (60 staff), the Radiation and Nuclear Safety Authority (360 staff), and the Finnish Environment Institute (590 staff). Most of these institutes have some administrative and supervisory tasks, but also conduct public health research. The institutes are mainly funded from the state budget and also receive competitive research funding from various sources, including the Academy of Finland, TEKES, and EU programmes.

The country's higher education system also conducts public health research. It consists of two complementary sectors: 15 universities and 27 polytechnics. Since 2010, universities have operated as independent corporations under public law or as foundations under private law. The universities conduct scientific research and provide undergraduate and postgraduate education. Public health research is mainly carried out in the five universities providing medical training and in universities hosting institutes related to health sciences. The universities receive basic funding from the state budget, but are dependent on competitive or commissioned funding for research activities. The Finnish system of polytechnics is relatively new. The first polytechnics started to operate on a trial basis in 1991–1992 and some were made permanent in 1996. Polytechnics train professionals in response to specific needs of the labour market. They also conduct small-scale research with the aim of promoting regional development. In the area of health, these projects are often carried out in collaboration with local healthcare authorities and municipalities.

Public health research in Poland

Research programmes and funders

The share of research and development expenditure in Poland dropped from 0.96% of GDP in 1991 to 0.56% in 2003. The 2015 Science Strategy aims to increase it to 1.7%. The Ministry of Health, the Ministry of Science and Higher Education, and private foundations finance research in the health sector (Figure 17.3). The

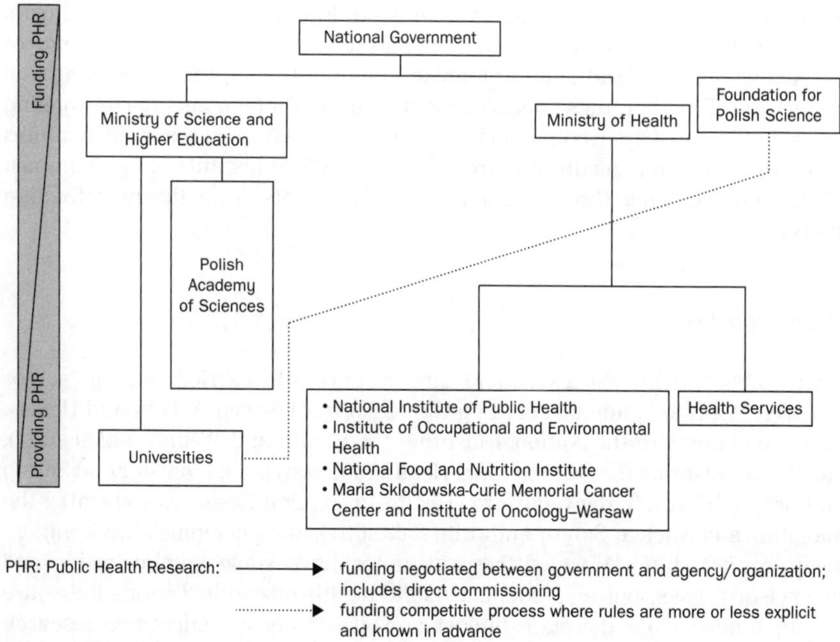

Figure 17.3   Funding flows for public health research in Poland

Source: STEPS [https://www.ucl.ac.uk/public-health/STEPS_folder/Poland_STEPS_countryprofile_8oct10.pdf, accessed 9 July 2012]

State Committee for Scientific Research, chaired by the Minister of Science, presents to the government and the parliament draft guidelines on the national science policy, and also distributes funds. The Foundation for Polish Science is an independent fund established in 1991 through a levy on state privatizations. Its funding is fully competitive, with emphasis on support for individual researchers. The foundation is the largest non-governmental source of funding for science in Poland. The 2005 National Framework Programme for Research outlined nine strategic research areas, three of which were directly related to public health: epidemiology, molecular foundation of risk factors affecting the ageing processes; epidemiology, pathogenesis, genetics, and immunology of cancer; and environmental conditions and their impact on health threats.

Research bodies

There are about 200 research and development institutes subordinate to different ministries. The National Centre for Research and Development represents and coordinates these institutes, 17 of which are funded by the Ministry of Health. There are 18 universities (11 with medical faculties) and 95 higher schools of economics.

Public health research in Estonia

Research programmes and funders

The Estonian Parliament has adopted two national strategies for research and development: Knowledge-Based Estonia I: Research and Development Strategy for 2003–2006, and Knowledge-Based Estonia II: Research, Development and Innovation Strategy for 2007–2013. The 2007–2013 round of the EU's Structural Funds in Estonia supports research and development in several ways. The Operational Programme "Economic Environment" includes the priority axis "Improving the competitiveness of Estonian research and development through the research programmes and modernisation of higher education and research and development institutions". In the Operational Programme "Human Resource Development", the second priority is "Developing human resources for research and development".

Health research is under the control of the Ministry of Social Affairs and the Ministry of Education and Research (Figure 17.4). The Ministry of Social Affairs is responsible for health, labour policy, and social affairs. The Health Board, established in 2010, provides leadership, surveillance, and enforcement in the areas of health care, communicable disease monitoring and control,

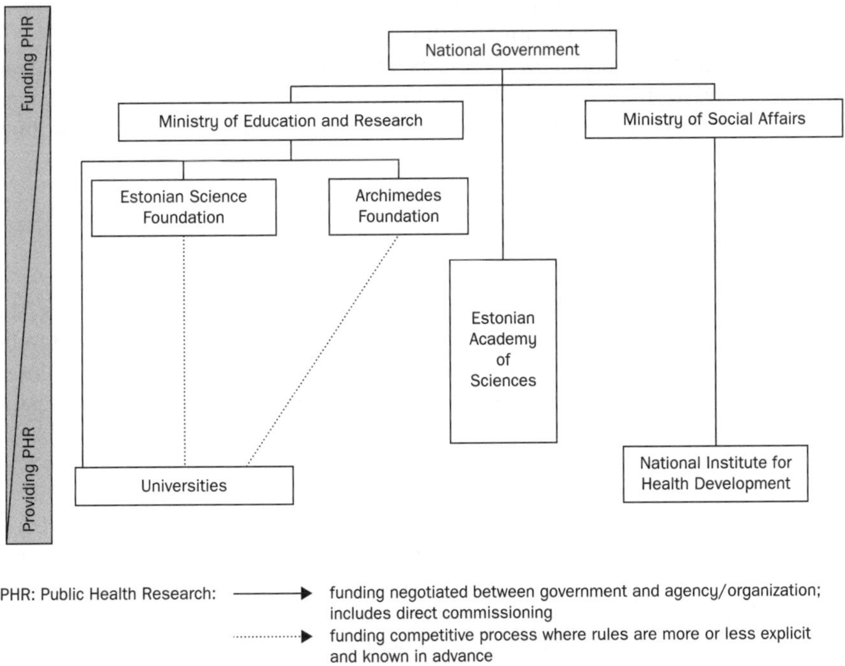

Figure 17.4   Funding flows for public health research in Estonia

Source: STEPS [https://www.ucl.ac.uk/public-health/STEPS_folder/Estonia_STEPS_countryprofile_13oct10.pdf, accessed 9 July 2012]

environmental health, chemical safety, and medical devices. The Ministry of Education and Research draws up national research and education policies, organizes the financing and evaluation of research institutes, and coordinates international cooperation in research. The country's universities and research organizations receive annual core funding on the basis of their research and development performance, amounting to approximately €83 million in 2009. Lastly, the Estonian Science Foundation (www.etf.ee) allocates over €8 million per year to "high-level" research, equivalent to about one-fifth of total government research funding in Estonia.

Research bodies

The National Institute for Health Development was established in 2003 as a governmental body under the Ministry of Social Affairs. Its main activities include: fundamental, applied, and evaluation research on public health and life quality (including biomedicine, epidemiology, biostatistics, health economics, occupational health and behaviour, measurement of the health status of the population, and assessing health hazards related to the outdoor environment); creation and maintenance of databases needed for assessing the performance of research, development, and management of health and social protection; collection of data for research and analysis; making policy proposals; preparing forecasts and development plans; and participating in the implementation of policies within the administration of the Ministry of Social Affairs.

The Estonian Academy of Sciences is a scientific association involved in the formulation of science policy and planning. It has 73 domestic and 19 foreign members, and an annual budget of €1.5 million from the national government.

Conclusions

When reviewing public health research in Europe, it is apparent that the importance of health in EU policies has gradually increased. Health used to be rather marginal to EU policies and has only recently assumed a more prominent role, due to changes in EU treaties, deepening economic integration, increasing migration, and newly emerging public health threats, such as BSE and SARS. These factors have led to an increasing recognition of the importance of EU-level collaboration on health.

EU joint programming initiatives have progressed slowly and it is still too early to judge whether they will develop into a substantial new form of collaboration between European research funders or simply follow the networking approach used in ERA-Nets. Among the existing joint programming initiatives, public health research has a relatively strong position.

It is evident that biomedical and clinical research is necessary to improve the population's health, but, without research-based public health knowledge, biomedical or clinical innovations cannot be implemented effectively. At the national level, many European governments have also begun to see research as a tool for economic growth and competitiveness, although this has come under threat as a result of the austerity programmes that some governments have chosen to – or in some cases been compelled to – adopt. This also applies to health research, which has become ever more oriented towards potential economic and commercial interests. In Finland, for example, there is a governmental initiative called Strategic Centres for Science, Technology, and Innovation, covering joint ventures of private companies, universities, and research institutes, supported by public research funding. The aim of this initiative is to direct research to where it can yield quick economic benefits. In health research, the rapid development of biomedical research has contributed to such expectations.

The STEPS Project developed five recommendations for supporting public health research in Europe. The first – rather ambitious – recommendation was to increase funding for public health research considerably, to reach a minimum of 25% of all health research funding in the EU and its member states. Other recommendations concerned research strategy, leadership, and coordination. In particular, the project recommended the following: development of national strategies for public health research; improved coordination between ministries of science, health, and finance; improved coordination across the different research and innovation programmes within the EU; and better engagement with public health researchers, users, and partners, including civil society organizations. Many of these recommendations remain valid.

References

Aluttis, C. A., C. Chiotan, M. Michelsen, C. Costongs and H. Brand, on behalf of the Public Health Capacity Consortium (2012). *Reviewing Public Health Capacity in the EU.* Maastricht, Maastricht University.

Browne, J. and T. I. A. Sørensen (2013). "Editorial: European public health research in Horizon 2020." *European Journal of Public Health* **23**: 722.

Conceição, C., A. Leandro and M. McCarthy (2009). "National support to public health research: a survey of European ministries." *BMC Public Health* **9**: 203.

European Commission (2008). *Towards Joint Programming in Research: Working together to tackle common challenges more effectively.* Brussels, European Commission.

European Commission (2010). *Interim Evaluation of the Seventh Framework Programme: Report of the Expert Group.* Brussels, European Commission.

European Research Council (ERC) (2012). *Statistics* [http://erc.europa.eu/project-and-results/statistics, accessed 8 July 2012]. Brussels, ERCl.

Joint Statement of the Public Health Associations of Europe (IEA, ISEE, EUPHA) on the health research programme 2014–2015 (Horizon 2020) proposed by the European Commission, 30 September 2013.

Koppel, A., A. Leventhal and M. Sedgley, Eds. (2009). *Public Health in Estonia 2008: An analysis of public health operations, services and activities.* Copenhagen, WHO Regional Office for Europe.

Ladurner, J., M. Gerger, W. Holland, E. Mossialos, S. Merkur, S. Stewart, R. Irwin and J. Soffried, Eds. (2011). *Public Health in Austria: An analysis of the status of public health.* Copenhagen, WHO on behalf of the European Observatory on Health Systems and Policies.

McCarthy, M., G. Harvey, C. Conceição, G. l. Torre and G. Gulis (2009). "Comparing public-health research priorities in Europe." *Health Research Policy and Systems* **7**: 17.

Ministry of Health of the Republic of Uzbekistan (2011). *Self-Assessment of Public Health Services in the Republic of Uzbekistan.* Technical report. Copenhagen, WHO Regional Office for Europe.

Mossialos, E., G. Permanand, R. Baeten and T. Hervey (2010). "Health systems governance in Europe: the role of European Union law and policy." In *Health Systems Governance in Europe: The role of EU law and policy.* E. Mossialos, G. Permanand, R. Baeten and T. Hervey, Eds. Cambridge, Cambridge University Press: 1–83.

OECD (2012). *Health at a Glance: Europe 2012.* Paris, OECD Publishing.

Research and Innovation Council of Finland (2010). *Research and Innovation Policy Guidelines for 2011–2015.* Helsinki: Research and Innovation Council of Finland.

STEPS (2011). *Strengthening Engagement in Public Health Research Final Report* [http://www.steps-ph.eu/wp-content/uploads/STEPS_Report.pdf, accessed 5 December 2011].

Walshe, K., M. McKee, P. Groenewegen, J. Hansen, J. Figueras, S. Boccia and W. Ricciardi (2013a). "Editorial: Reshaping the agenda of the European Commission for the health systems and policy research in Europe within Horizon 2020." *Epidemiology, Biostatistics, and Public Health* **10**(2): e8951.

Walshe, K., M. McKee, M. McCarthy, P. Groenewegen, J. Hansen, J. Figueras and W. Ricciardi (2013b). "Editorial: Health systems and policy research in Europe: Horizon 2020." *The Lancet* **382**(9893): 668–669.

World Health Organization (WHO) (2007a). *Evaluation of Public Health Services in Bulgaria.* Draft National Report. Copenhagen, WHO Regional Office for Europe.

World Health Organization (WHO) (2007b). *Evaluation of Public Health Services in South-eastern Europe: Federation of Bosnia and Herzegovina.* Draft National Report. Copenhagen, WHO Regional Office for Europe.

World Health Organization (WHO) (2007c). *Evaluation of Public Health Services in South-eastern Europe: The former Yugoslav Republic of Macedonia.* Draft National Report. Copenhagen, WHO Regional Office for Europe.

World Health Organization (WHO) (2009a). *Evaluation of Public Health Services in Slovenia.* Copenhagen, WHO Regional Office for Europe.

World Health Organization (WHO) (2009b). *Evaluation of Public Health Services in South-eastern Europe.* Copenhagen, WHO Regional Office for Europe.

chapter eighteen

Knowledge brokering in public health

Cristina Catallo, John N. Lavis, and the BRIDGE Study Team[1]

Introduction

Knowledge translation of public health information is a dynamic and iterative process that includes synthesis, dissemination, and exchange, but, most importantly, the application of information in decision-making. While a great deal of information is produced by public health systems, it is not always used in public health policy and practice, resulting in potentially ineffective, inequitable, and costly public health strategies and programmes. Knowledge brokering, a component of knowledge translation, can help to address the gap between knowledge on the one hand and policy and practice on the other through an emphasis on innovative information-packaging and interactive knowledge-sharing mechanisms.

This chapter aims to encourage a discussion of the ways in which public health information is packaged for and interactively shared among public health policy-makers and stakeholders in Europe. We draw on findings of the European Union (EU) funded research project "BRIDGE" (Brokering knowledge and Research Information to support the Development and Governance of health systems in Europe) that was carried out in 2009–2011. The project explored efforts to broker information for policy and to bridge the information–action gap in European health systems. The project defined health information as both data (on performance and outcomes, among other topics) and research evidence (about policy and programme options to improve performance or achieve better outcomes, among other topics).

Knowledge brokering in public health

Public health policy-making is complex and requires a variety of decisions by policy-makers and stakeholders. To make informed decisions, these groups need access to high-quality information that is easy to understand (Lavis, Permanand et al. 2013a, 2013b). Meeting this need is made challenging by the many other factors that policy-makers must consider when making decisions, such as institutional constraints, competing interests such as lobby groups, prevailing beliefs and values, and factors beyond the control of local policy-makers, such as the current global economic crisis (Lavis, Ross et al. 2002; Oxman, Lavis et al. 2009).

When policy decisions are made without consideration of sound health information, intended goals may not be achieved. Public health programmes and services may, for example, not target the right problem, or be ineffective, inefficient or inequitable (Oxman, Lavis et al. 2009). Such consequences, both real and potential, have led the World Health Organization (WHO), among others, to highlight the need for using reliable health information in public health policy-making (WHO 2004). This need extends to how influential organizations, such as the World Bank and WHO, identify and report the use of health information in their recommendations (Oxman, Lavis et al. 2007; Hoffman, Lavis et al. 2009).

These concerns centre on the continuing gaps in the processes by which health information is identified, disseminated, and used for decision-making. Understanding how to address and resolve these gaps is key to knowledge translation.

Knowledge translation in the health sector is the systematic process of harnessing health information to improve health, strengthen health systems, and inform health policy decisions (Graham, Logan et al., 2006; Straus, Tetroe et al. 2009). For the purposes of this chapter, we adopt the definition of knowledge translation developed by the Canadian Institutes of Health Research: a "dynamic and iterative process that includes synthesis, dissemination, exchange, and ethically sound application of knowledge to improve the health of" populations, among other goals (CIHR 2009). This definition has been adopted by WHO, who have highlighted the importance of the "know–do" gap (WHO 2006). Bridging this gap is now being treated as a priority by the European Commission, which has recognized that it requires multiple approaches, not only for the dissemination of health information, but also for its meaningful application by various audiences, from practitioners to policy-makers (European Commission 2008).

An important component of knowledge translation is how knowledge is brokered among both those who produce health information and those who use it. Knowledge brokering includes two key processes: the methods for packaging health information so that it is easily accessible and ready for use (information-packaging mechanisms) and the methods for interactively sharing health information (interactive knowledge-sharing mechanisms) (Lavis, Catallo et al. 2013c, 2013d; Lavis and Catallo 2013).

For the BRIDGE Project, we defined information-packaging mechanisms to include "information products in a variety of media that are focused at least in part on health systems information and that are intended to support policymaking" (Lavis, Catallo et al. 2013d). The outputs can take the form of "policy briefs, issue notes, research summaries, policy dialogue reports, research reports, presentations, audio or video podcasts, videos, blogs, impact summaries, newsletters, annual reports, and cartoons and other visual media, among others" (Lavis, Catallo et al. 2013d).

Interactive knowledge-sharing mechanisms refer to the "mediating interactions that are focused at least in part on health systems information and that are intended to support policymaking" (Lavis, Catallo et al. 2013c). The interactions can take the form of "policy dialogues, personalized briefings, training workshops, online briefings or webinars, online discussion forums, formalized networks, informal discussions, and presentations" (Lavis, Catallo et al. 2013c).

The public health context for knowledge brokering

Policy-makers and stakeholders in public health work in a variety of settings within traditional health systems but also in areas such as education, social care, and transportation. Most empirical findings, including those presented in this chapter, relate to public health organizations operating with some connection to health systems. However, similar findings likely apply to those working outside of them (WHO 2011). A number of key concepts and resources for knowledge brokering in the area of public health can be identified.

Evidence-informed public health

One such concept is evidence-informed public health. This term refers to the process of using valid, reliable, and generalizable sources of evidence (or information, for the purpose of this chapter) in public health decision-making. Moving beyond "evidence-based public health", which many feel emphasizes research evidence only, "evidence-informed public health" acknowledges more explicitly the multitude of factors that influence public health decisions, including local institutional constraints, the interests of stakeholders, and the preferences of the public (Ciliska, Thomas et al., 2008). The approach of evidence-informed public health can benefit decision-makers by critically discerning and questioning sources of health information, avoiding the misuse of information, and placing information in the context of the many other factors that influence decision-making (Oxman, Lavis et al. 2009). This approach also involves being transparent about what type of health information was used and setting out the reasons for its selection. Evidence-informed public health also has been described as a call to identify and address widespread public health problems, assess the effectiveness of interventions, understand local contexts, and demonstrate political and fiscal accountability (Armstrong, Waters et al. 2006).

Sources of public health information

Various types and sources of health information can prove useful for decision-making in public health. Different types of health information are needed to understand public health problems, options to address them, and implementation strategies (Lavis, Oxman et al. 2009; Oxman, Lavis et al. 2009). Much of our understanding about public health problems derives from routine public health data, such as those based on disease surveillance. However, when considering policy and programme options or implementation strategies, high-quality systematic reviews are a crucial source of information. Systematic reviews are becoming more common, including consideration of governance, financial and service delivery arrangements within health systems (Lavis, Oxman et al. 2009; Lavis, Wilson et al. 2009). Systematic reviews attempt to answer research questions through an explicitly defined process of searching the literature and appraising and synthesizing research evidence determined to be of high quality (Cochrane Collaboration 2010). If systematic reviews are not available, primary research (e.g. randomized controlled trials or cohort studies) can be an important source of health information.

Knowledge brokering and the factors that influence the use of health information

While knowledge brokers are often thought of as individuals or organizations (Ward, House et al. 2009), knowledge brokering itself is a complex process that incorporates specific mechanisms to optimize the use of health information in decision-making. In the BRIDGE Project, we considered the use of information-packaging or interactive knowledge-sharing mechanisms to bridge the worlds of policy-makers and researchers. There are a number of reasons for a possible disconnect between these two worlds. For example, many researchers and other stakeholders may want to communicate the urgency of public health problems. They use health information to shed light on the problems and highlight the lack of action, with the aim of initiating a political response. Policy-makers may be on the receiving end of dozens or hundreds of such efforts, most of which will focus on problems and not what is known about options for addressing these problems and about implementation considerations. Policy-makers may then perceive such efforts as "noise instead of music" (Lavis, Permanand et al. 2013b). Policy-makers may also identify a discordance between what is being produced by researchers and other stakeholders and what policy-makers themselves believe, value and hold as political goals and strategies (Aaserud, Lewin et al. 2005; Hennink and Stephenson 2005; Hughes 2007; Madden, King et al. 2009; Waddell, Lavis et al. 2005).

There are other reasons for the disconnect between the worlds of research and policy. One often cited challenge is that health information is rarely made available in a timely fashion and in a format that meets the needs of policy-makers (Petticrew, Whitehead et al. 2004; Waddell, Lavis et al. 2005; Armstrong, Waters et al. 2007; Oxman, Lavis et al. 2007; Jewell and Bero 2008; Schur, Berk et al. 2009). Often, policy-makers work to very short deadlines and need quick access to information. They also require support to find and adapt health information that addresses policy questions rather than research-driven ones. A second challenge is the lack of opportunities for policy-makers and researchers or other stakeholders to come together and engage in dialogue about a pressing public health problem, options for addressing it, and key implementation considerations (Lavis, Ross et al. 2002; Hennink and Stephenson 2005; Waddell,

Lavis et al. 2005; Armstrong, Waters et al. 2007; Oxman, Lavis et al. 2007; Jewell and Bero 2008; Campbell, Redman et al. 2009; Lavis, Catallo et al. 2013c).

Studies that examine decision-makers' preferences for health information provide additional insights regarding the factors that are particularly important in the area of public health. Regional public health decision-makers in Canada reported a need to have access to systematic reviews (Dobbins, Jack et al. 2007) and accorded priority to ease of access (Dobbins, Rosenbaum et al. 2007). They also pointed out that information needed to be relevant to their needs and they preferred information that clearly set out the implications for public health policy and practice from a trustworthy and competent source (Dobbins, Rosenbaum et al. 2007). Moreover, the public health decision-makers indicated that having one-to-one interactions with researchers would help with knowledge brokering, in particular in identifying ways to translate research findings into policy and practice, and would significantly influence the use of evidence by decision-makers (Dobbins, Jack et al. 2007).

These findings are consistent with a systematic review carried out as part of the BRIDGE Project (Catallo, Lavis et al. 2013). We found the following factors promoting or inhibiting the use of health information among policy-makers (both in public health and other domains):

- Interactions between researchers and policy-makers were found to increase (and a lack of interactions to decrease) the prospects for the use of health information in policy-making, especially when these interactions were based on informal relationships (Lavis, Ross et al. 2002; Hennink and Stephenson 2005; Lavis, Davies et al. 2005; Armstrong, Waters et al. 2007; Oxman, Lavis et al. 2007; Jewell and Bero 2008; Campbell, Redman et al. 2009).
- Timely access to health information increased (and a lack of timeliness decreased) the prospects for its use in policy-making (Petticrew, Whitehead et al. 2004; Lavis, Davies et al. 2005; Armstrong, Waters et al. 2007; Oxman, Lavis et al. 2007; Jewell and Bero 2008; Schur, Berk et al. 2009).
- Accordance between health information and the political beliefs, values, interests, and goals of policy-makers and stakeholders increased (and discordance decreased) the prospects for the use of information in policy-making (Aaserud, Lewin et al. 2005; Hennink and Stephenson 2005; Lavis, Davies et al. 2005; Hughes 2007; Madden, King et al. 2009).

Activities to support knowledge brokering

A continued challenge to knowledge brokering is the gap between those who produce and prepare information and those who use it. Studies have found that the passive dissemination of health information among decision-makers is only marginally effective in supporting the adoption of research findings in decision-making (Grimshaw, Shirran et al. 2001; Kerner 2006).

Knowledge-brokering organizations (see the next section for more details) can consider four types of activities to promote the use of research. These include (Lavis, Lomas et al. 2006):

- efforts to "push" health information towards public health policy-makers and stakeholders;
- efforts to "facilitate user pull" of summarized health information;
- efforts by users to undertake "user pull";
- efforts to support the "exchange" of health information between public health decision-makers and information producers.

These activities can be used by knowledge-brokering organizations in combination with innovative information-packaging and interactive knowledge-sharing mechanisms. For example, optimally packaged information can be the focus of all four types of activities.

"Push efforts" aim to bring information to policy-makers and stakeholders and can use "intermediaries", such as knowledge brokers, who communicate health information for use in public health decision-making (Lavis, Lomas et al. 2006). In public health, one example of a "push effort" might be to identify actionable messages arising from a good-quality systematic review and to fine-tune these messages, so that different types of public health decision-makers can use them. Often, organizations rely on the skills of intermediaries who can help shape key messages and determine strategies for sharing health information in ways that suit various public health audiences (Lavis, Robertson et al. 2003).

Turning to "efforts to facilitate user pull", knowledge-brokering organizations can make health information available when policy-makers need it and in a form they can use (Lavis, Lomas et al. 2006), such as through a "one-stop shop" for health information in a defined domain or a policy dialogue that is convened in response to an urgent request. Examples of the former include Health Evidence (a one-stop shop for systematic reviews of the effects of public-health interventions) and Health Systems Evidence (a one-stop shop for systematic reviews, economic evaluations and many other types of health information about governance, financial and delivery arrangements, and implementation strategies within health systems) (Lavis, Permanand et al. 2013a, 2013b). Health Systems Evidence is available in five languages that are widely spoken in Europe (English, French, Portuguese, Russian, and Spanish). An example of the latter is the policy dialogues organized by the European Observatory on Health Systems and Policies that are requested over time-frames of weeks and months (Lavis, Catallo et al. 2013c).

"User pull" efforts can take several forms (Lavis, Lomas et al. 2006). Knowledge brokers and decision-makers located within public health organizations could employ self-assessment tools to assess their capacity to acquire, assess, adapt, and apply health information (Canadian Health Services Research Foundation 2005). Alternatively, they could develop (or help to develop) the capacity of policy-makers and stakeholders to find and use health information (Lavis, Robertson et al. 2003). They could also create mechanisms to prompt policy-makers to use health information, as in a requirement that cabinet submissions (i.e. documents used by governments to obtain approval for a new or existing policy, programme or funding allocation) explicitly outline the health information that supports the anticipated public health action or implementation strategy (Lavis, Lomas et al. 2006).

Finally, "exchange efforts" involve knowledge-brokering organizations creating opportunities for policy-makers and stakeholders to discuss public health challenges with researchers. Knowledge-brokering organizations may be located in a variety of organizational contexts, including the research world (e.g. a university research centre), the policy-making world (e.g. a government strategy unit) or the interface between the two worlds (e.g. an independent think tank) (Lavis, Jessani et al. 2013e). A skilled knowledge-brokering organization will recognize that it needs to use a variety of strategies to engage policy-makers, such as through personal and ongoing interactions, where both parties contribute their expertise to address policy questions (Lavis, Lomas et al. 2006; Lomas 2000, 2007). The knowledge broker could also facilitate a two-way dialogue between public health researchers and policy-makers that focuses on the relevant health information and the full range of other factors to clarify a particular problem, frame options to address the problem, and identify implementation considerations.

Knowledge-brokering organizations in the area of public health: findings of the BRIDGE Project

As part of the BRIDGE Project, the study team identified country correspondents in 31 European countries (the then 27 EU member states, plus Iceland, Liechtenstein, Norway, and Switzerland) who identified potential knowledge-brokering organizations, used explicit criteria to assess whether organizations were eligible for inclusion in the project, and extracted data from the websites of eligible organizations using a common data collection tool. The aim was to identify organizations with at least a partial focus on public health, describe the knowledge-brokering mechanisms they used, and identify innovative knowledge-brokering mechanisms. More details about the methods used in the BRIDGE study are given elsewhere (Lavis and Catallo 2013).

Of the 404 knowledge-brokering organizations in Europe that were considered for inclusion in the study during the September 2009 to March 2010 period, 163 organizations met the eligibility criteria. Four were global organizations, 17 focused on a grouping of European countries (such as the EU or the European Region of the World Health Organization), while the rest focused on the national or sub-national level. We did not include knowledge-brokering organizations that focused primarily on taking political positions (e.g. political advocacy organizations) or solely on clinical or public health issues that had no broader health system connection (e.g. health technology assessment agencies that prepare reports about whether to introduce new vaccinations), or organizations that primarily collect and collate data or that primarily target audiences other than policy-makers within Europe. We also did not include organizations that do not put most of their products in the public domain.

Overall, 87 organizations were identified from the BRIDGE website review as having at least a partial public health mandate. Most organizations viewed national and sub-national politicians ($n = 83$) and civil servants ($n = 82$) as their primary target audience for knowledge-brokering activities. While public health organizations generally made information products available on their websites, they largely relied on more traditional mechanisms, such as reports and newsletters. The organizations were less likely to use interactive knowledge-sharing mechanisms.

Beginning with information-packaging mechanisms, organizations used a variety of traditional and innovative mechanisms. Traditional examples included:

- reports (excluding systematic reviews), such as research reports, working papers, policy studies, country profiles, and health sector reviews, which were the information products most frequently made available on the organizations' websites ($n = 131$);
- newsletters, which were less frequently made available, but were still fairly common ($n = 44$);
- annual reports, which were the third most common type of information product ($n = 17$).

Innovative information products presented public health information in an easy-to-read manner, but few based their findings on systematic reviews or offered online commentaries or briefings.

In terms of information-packaging mechanisms, public health organizations:

- regularly targeted policy-makers as a key audience for information products ($n = 68$);
- developed information products from research projects (i.e. primary research) ($n = 55$) or from a collation of research-related products ($n = 43$), although few were based on systematic reviews ($n = 18$);
- focused on a policy problem ($n = 61$), although fewer examined options to address the problem ($n = 52$) or implementation considerations ($n = 44$);
- created information products that used accessible language ($n = 56$), but slightly less often followed a graded-entry format ($n = 46$) or explicitly highlighted decision-relevant information ($n = 44$).

Few information-packaging mechanisms were accompanied by online commentaries or briefings about the information product by members of the target audience ($n = 3$), although more offered an option to sign up for an e-mail alert/listserv when new products were posted online ($n = 29$).

Innovative examples of information-packaging included summaries of reports (excluding systematic reviews) ($n = 20$) and issue notes ($n = 12$). Other innovative forms of information-packaging mechanisms included summaries of journal articles or systematic reviews, thematically focused compendiums of summaries (although only one was identified), policy briefs, and reports of policy dialogues (Box 18.1).

Box 18.1   Examples of innovative information-packaging mechanisms

Study summary

A study summary can be a summary of findings from a single study. A good example is the research summaries developed by the Personal Social Services Research Unit (http://www.pssru.ac.uk) in the United

Kingdom. These summaries provide a summary of scientific reports, including research aims, key findings, and future directions.

Systematic review summary

A document that summarizes the findings from a systematic review is known as a systematic review summary. The SUPporting POlicy Relevant reviews and Trials (SUPPORT) collaboration (http://www.support-collaboration.org/index.htm) provides systematic review summaries, some of them related to public health topics, such as whether iron supplementation during pregnancy improves maternal and perinatal health outcomes. A SUPPORT summary provides key background information needed to understand the findings of a systematic review, a summary of what the review searched for and found, a detailed summary of the main findings (including an assessment of the evidence underpinning those findings), and an assessment of the relevance of the review (including considerations of local applicability, equity, cost-effectiveness, and the need for monitoring and evaluation). Another example is the structured summaries prepared by the Health Evidence Network (HEN), hosted by the WHO Regional Office for Europe, although not all HEN summaries are summaries of systematic reviews.

Thematically focused compendium of summaries

A compendium of summaries is a thematically focused grouping of summaries of articles or reports that describes findings from single studies, systematic reviews or both. By bringing together a range of perspectives on one issue, a compendium offers a collection of insights in a single document. This approach can save a great deal of effort for people interested in a particular issue, provide them with an opportunity to look across time or jurisdictions, and help them identify a nascent network of others interested in the same issue. An example is the compendium of summaries prepared by the Organization for Health Research and Development in the Netherlands (http://www.zonmw.nl/en/). The compendium, which the organization calls a "knowledge synthesis", draws together a set of summaries about projects it has funded, with the aim of identifying ways to save money while retaining quality.

Policy brief

A policy brief is a report that begins with a policy issue and synthesizes the relevant research evidence about the underlying problem, options to address it, and implementation considerations. Identifying such information products can be challenging, because many are called policy briefs but do not meet this definition, while others meet the definition but are called by a different name (Health Systems Evidence, for example, calls them "evidence briefs for policy"). A series of policy briefs that fits our definition is the one prepared by the HEN, hosted by the WHO Regional Office for Europe. An example is a policy brief on how health systems can respond to population ageing. Another example of a policy brief looks at integrated care for those with chronic illness; it is the first in a planned series by the Norwegian Knowledge Centre for the Health Services (http://www.kunnskapssenteret.no/Home).

Policy dialogue report

A policy dialogue report describes the insights derived from a policy dialogue where policy-makers, stakeholders, and researchers deliberate about a policy issue, ideally informed by a policy brief circulated beforehand and organized in a way that allows for the sharing of tacit knowledge and real-world views and experiences. These reports go well beyond standard meeting reports, and at their best have the potential to generate profound insights about how an issue might be approached by a range of stakeholders. An example is the series of policy dialogue reports prepared by the Estonian think-tank Praxis Centre for Policy Studies (http://www.praxis.ee).

Source: Adapted from Lavis, Catallo et al. (2013d)

In terms of knowledge-sharing mechanisms, most public health organizations in Europe relied on traditional rather than interactive mechanisms, such as presentations to an audience that included policy-makers and stakeholders (for example, at conferences), meetings with expert presentations, seminars, and workshops ($n = 73$). Also reported, although less frequently so, were networks to oversee a research project (in contrast to working groups convened by government) ($n = 4$).

There were also innovative examples of interactive knowledge-sharing mechanisms, some of which were used more often than traditional mechanisms on occasion:

- training workshops that help policy-makers to build the skills they need for finding and applying health information to policy issues ($n = 14$);
- personalized briefings that involve a formalized interaction between the knowledge-brokering organization and the policy-maker ($n = 12$);
- online discussion forums with open access, such as blogs, Facebook, and Twitter ($n = 9$).

However, few of these interactive knowledge-sharing mechanisms were timed to relate explicitly to policy-making processes or requests from policy-makers, and few appeared to involve a true dialogue between policy-makers and the knowledge-brokering organization. In terms of how interactive knowledge-sharing mechanisms were organized and supported, public health organizations:

- regularly targeted other stakeholders ($n = 59$) and policy-makers ($n = 48$) as a key audience for information products;
- developed mechanisms, such as activities for setting the research agenda ($n = 4$) or collating research-related products ($n = 34$), in response to an issue

raised by policy-makers ($n = 33$), but few were based on systematic reviews ($n = 8$) or primary research ($n = 27$);

- less frequently used mechanisms to address a policy problem or objective ($n = 36$), or to identify policy options ($n = 42$) or implementation considerations ($n = 33$);
- irregularly timed mechanisms to relate to a policy-making process ($n = 19$);
- involved a closed list of invitees ($n = 19$), with limited previous circulation of products ($n = 4$) and rules about how comments would be attributed ($n = 2$);
- provided presentations by an expert ($n = 41$), but more rarely used an interactive format, such as a question-and-answer session with an expert ($n = 28$), policy-maker commentaries with expert input ($n = 16$), or a dialogue where each participant has the opportunity to contribute equally ($n = 19$);
- mostly offered in-person interactions ($n = 45$), while few developed products based on these interactions ($n = 19$), or offered the option to sign up for an e-mail alert/listserv when new products were posted online ($n = 13$).

More innovative forms of interactive knowledge-sharing mechanisms included online discussion forums, online briefings or webinars, training workshops, personalized briefings, and policy dialogues (Box 18.2).

Box 18.2 Examples of innovative interactive knowledge-sharing mechanisms

---

Online discussion forums

An online discussion forum offers policy-makers and stakeholders an opportunity to interact with researchers and knowledge brokers. A blog is one type of online discussion forum, with a good example being the PRAXIS blog series from the above-mentioned Praxis Centre for Policy Studies. This series, written in Estonian, discusses current research results as they relate to health systems issues. A public health-related example is the blog that discusses comprehensive social protection for an ageing population. Another organization, providing a blog series on many topics related to health promotion, is the Joseph Rowntree Foundation in the United Kingdom (http://www.jrf.org.uk/). Blogs include, for example, a discussion of health in neighbourhoods and the impact of poverty on health.

Online briefings or webinars

An online briefing or webinar is a web-based presentation by a researcher or knowledge broker that allows policy-makers and stakeholders to interact in real time about the issues raised in the presentation. A good example is the online briefing series set up by the King's Fund in the United Kingdom (http://www.kingsfund.org.uk/). These events involve webcasts of breakfast meetings or seminars featuring policy-makers, other stakeholders and researchers, with audio and video recordings of the briefings later made available through the King's Fund website. While the events are webcast, it is not always possible for remote participants to ask questions of the speakers in real time; however, responses to Twitter postings can be fed back to speakers in the form of questions.

Training workshops

A training workshop is a session that aims to help policy-makers and stakeholders to enhance their skills in finding and using health information. A good example is a training workshop, the first in a planned series, offered by the Norwegian Knowledge Centre for the Health Services. The workshop draws heavily on the SUPporting POlicy Relevant reviews and Trials (SUPPORT) tools for evidence-informed policy-making (Lavis, Oxman et al. 2009) and covers how to find and use health information to clarify a problem, frame options to address it, and identify implementation considerations (Lavis 2009; Lavis, Wilson et al. 2009). A different kind of training is offered by the European Centre for Disease Prevention and Control (ECDC), such as through the European Programme for Intervention Epidemiology Training, a two-year fellowship programme for public health workers and decision-makers to build capacity in epidemiology.

Personalized briefings

A personalized briefing is a formal in-person presentation and discussion of health information on an issue prioritized and framed by policy-makers and stakeholders. The National Institute for Health and Welfare in Finland is an example of an organization that provides personalized briefings to the national parliament or a parliamentary committee.

Policy dialogues

A policy dialogue convenes policy-makers, stakeholders, and researchers to deliberate about a policy issue. As mentioned above, the European Observatory on Health Systems and Policies organizes a series of policy dialogues.

Source: Adapted from Lavis, Catallo et al. (2013c)

Working with country correspondents and extracting data from websites proved to be an efficient way to identify and preliminarily characterize knowledge-brokering organizations in public health in Europe. Our approach also benefited from the use of explicit eligibility criteria, a data-collection tool, a validation step for eligibility assessments, and the involvement of two individuals in each step of the process. An obvious downside of our approach was that websites sometimes do not tell the "whole story". Some organizations with only a partial mandate for public health, for example, may carry out more public health activities than indicated on their website. We may in particular have missed interactive knowledge-sharing activities that were not well documented on the websites of organizations. Another weakness of our approach was that some data collection elements, in particular those carried out by 1–2 individuals per country, had a subjective dimension to them.

Conclusion: next steps for knowledge brokering in public health

This chapter has highlighted many areas where knowledge-brokering organizations in public health in Europe are doing well and areas where further opportunity awaits. We hope it will stimulate a discussion about ways to create, refine, and support the wider use of information-packaging and interactive knowledge-sharing mechanisms for public policy-makers and stakeholders.

The identification of knowledge-brokering organizations active in public health in Europe could be a first step towards establishing a network of like-minded organizations that learn from each other, including with regard to innovative knowledge-brokering mechanisms. Such learning would benefit from an empirical investigation of the impact of innovative mechanisms on public health decision-making.

Areas on which organizations might focus include the more innovative information-packaging mechanisms that are derived from higher-quality sources of health information, such as systematic reviews, primary research or a collation of research-related products. However, they will also need to make sure to address important public health issues of interest to policy-makers. With regard to interactive knowledge-sharing mechanisms, more innovative mechanisms might focus on similar sources of health information to inform a two-way exchange on issues relevant to public health. For both mechanisms (information-packaging and knowledge-sharing), organizations might consider a greater focus on helping to identify a public health problem or policy objective, and providing options to address it and potential implementation considerations. While a number of the knowledge-brokering organizations we examined used websites, they might consider ways for making better use of their web-based platform, such as through providing online briefings about their information-packaging mechanisms that target policy-makers and stakeholders, posting products that arise from interactive knowledge-sharing mechanisms, and offering the option to sign up for e-mail updates when new information products are released.

Note

1   The BRIDGE Study Team included Josep Figueras, Mark Leys, David McDaid, Gabriele Pastorino, Govin Permanand, and John-Arne Røttingen. The research leading to the results presented in this chapter received funding from the European Community's Seventh Framework Programme (FP7/2007-2013) under grant agreement No. 223473. Sole responsibility lies with the authors, and the European Commission is not responsible for any use that may be made of the information contained here.

References

Aaserud, M., S. Lewin, S. Innvaer, E. J. Paulsen, A. T. Dahlgren, M. Trommald, L. Duley, M. Zwarenstein and A. D. Oxman (2005). "Translating research into policy and practice in developing countries: a case study of magnesium sulphate for pre-eclampsia." *BMC Health Services Research* **5**: 68.

Armstrong, R., E. Waters, B. Crockett and H. Keleher (2007). "The nature of evidence resources and knowledge translation for health promotion practitioners." *Health Promotion International* **22**(3): 254–260.

Armstrong, R., E. Waters, H. Roberts, S. Oliver and J. Popay (2006). "The role and theoretical evolution of knowledge translation and exchange in public health." *Journal of Public Health* **28**(4): 384–389.

Campbell, D. M., S. Redman, L. Jorm, M. Cooke, A. B. Zwi and L. Rychetnik (2009). "Increasing the use of evidence in health policy: practice and views of policy makers and researchers." *Australia and New Zealand Health Policy* **6**: 21.

Canadian Health Services Research Foundation (2005). *Is Research Working for You? A self-assessment tool and discussion guide for health services and policy organizations.* Ottawa, Canadian Health Services Research Foundation.

Canadian Institutes of Health Research (CIHR) (2009). *About Knowledge Translation* [http://www.cihr-irsc.gc.ca/e/29418.html, accessed 25 January 2011]. Ottawa, CIHR.

Catallo, C., J. N. Lavis and M. Ellen (2013). "What past research tells us about knowledge brokering: a systematic review and a scoping review." In J. N. Lavis and C. Catallo, Eds. *Bridging the Worlds of Research and Policy in European Health Systems.* Copenhagen, WHO Regional Office for Europe on behalf of the European Observatory on Health Systems and Policies.

Ciliska, D., H. Thomas and C. Buffet (2008). *An Introduction to Evidence-informed Public Health and a Compendium of Critical Appraisal Tools for Public Health Practice.* Hamilton, ON, National Collaborating Centre for Methods and Tools.

Cochrane Collaboration (2010). *What is the Difference between a Protocol and a Review?* [http://www.cochrane.org/faq/what-difference-between-protocol-and-review, accessed 30 May 2011].

Culyer, A. J. and J. Lomas (2006). "Deliberative process and evidence-informed decision-making in health care: do they work and how might we know?" *Evidence and Policy* **12**(31): 357–371.

Dobbins, M., S. Jack, H. Thomas and A. Kothari (2007). "Public health decision-makers' informational needs and preferences for receiving research evidence." *Worldviews on Evidence-Based Nursing* **4**(3): 153–163.

Dobbins, M., P. Rosenbaum, N. Plews, M. Law and A. Fysh (2007). "Information transfer: what do decision makers want and need from researchers?" *Implementation Science* **2**: 20.

European Commission (2008). *Scientific Evidence for Policymaking.* Brussels, European Commission, Directorate-General for Research (EUR 22982 EN).

Graham, I. D., J. Logan, M. B. Harrison, S. E. Straus, J. Tetroe and W. Caswell (2006). "Lost in knowledge translation: time for a map?" *Journal of Continuing Education in the Health Professions* **26**(1): 13–24.

Grimshaw, J., L. Shirran, R. Thomas, G. Mowatt, C. Fraser, L. Bero, R. Grilli, E. Harvey, A. Oxman and M. A. O'Brien (2001). "Changing provider behaviour: an overview of systematic reviews of interventions." *Medical Care* **39** (Suppl. 2): II2–II45.

Hennink, M. and R. Stephenson (2005). "Using research to inform health policy: barriers and strategies in developing countries." *Journal of Health Communication* **10**: 163–180.

Hoffman, S. J., J. N. Lavis and S. Bennett (2009). "The use of research evidence in two international organizations' recommendations about health systems." *Healthcare Policy* **5**(1): 66–86.

Hughes, C. E. (2007). "Evidence-based policy or policy-based evidence? The role of evidence in the development and implementation of the illicit Drug Diversion initiative." *Drug and Alcohol Review* **26**: 363–368.

Jewell, C. J. and L. Bero (2008). "'Developing good taste in evidence': facilitators and hindrances to evidence-informed policymaking in state government." *Milbank Quarterly* **86**(2): 177–208.

Kerner, J. F. (2006). "Knowledge translation versus knowledge integration: a 'funders' perspective." *Journal of Continuing Education in the Health Professions* **26**(1): 72–80.

Lavis, J. N. (2009). "How can we support the use of systematic reviews in policymaking?" *PLoS Medicine* **6**(11): e1000141.

Lavis, J. N. and C. Catallo, Eds. (2013). *Bridging the Worlds of Research and Policy in European Health Systems*. Copenhagen, WHO Regional Office for Europe on behalf of the European Observatory on Health Systems and Policies.

Lavis, J. N., C. Catallo, N. Jessani, G. Permanand, A. Zierler and the BRIDGE Study Team (2013c). *Learning from One Another: Enriching interactive knowledge-sharing mechanisms to support knowledge brokering in European health systems*. Policy Summary 8 (BRIDGE series). Copenhagen, WHO Regional Office for Europe on behalf of the European Observatory on Health Systems and Policies.

Lavis, J. N., C. Catallo, G. Permanand, A. Zierler, and the BRIDGE Study Team (2013c). *Matching Form to Function: Designing Organizational Models to Support Knowledge Brokering in European Health Systems*, Policy summary 9 (BRIDGE series). Brussels: European Observatory on Health Systems and Policies.

Lavis, J. N., C. Catallo, G. Permanand, A. Zierler, and the BRIDGE Study Team (2013d). *Communicating Clearly: Enhancing Information-Packaging Mechanisms to Support Knowledge Brokering in European Health Systems*. Policy summary 7 (BRIDGE series). Brussels: European Observatory on Health Systems and Policies.

Lavis, J. N., H.T.O. Davies, A. D. Oxman, J.-L. Denis and K. Goiden-Biddle (2005). "Towards systematic reviews that inform health care management and policy-making." *Journal of Health Services Research and Policy* **10**(S1): 35–48.

Lavis, J. N., N. Jessani, C. Catallo, G. Permanand, A. Zierler and the BRIDGE Study Team (2013e). *Matching Form to Function: Designing Organizational Models to Support Knowledge Brokering in European Health Systems*. Policy summary 9 (BRIDGE series). Brussels: European Observatory on Health Systems and Policies.

Lavis, J. N., J. Lomas, M. Hamid and N. K. Sewankambo (2006). "Assessing country-level efforts to link research to action." *Bulletin of the World Health Organization* **84**(8): 620–628.

Lavis, J. N., A. D. Oxman, S. Lewin and A. Fretheim (2009). "SUPPORT Tools for evidence-informed health Policymaking (STP)." *Health Research Policy and Systems* **7**(Suppl. 1): I1 [http://www.health-policy-systems.com/content/pdf/1478-4505-7-S1-I1.pdf].

Lavis, J. N., G. Permanand, C. Catallo and the BRIDGE Study Team (2013a). *How can Knowledge Brokering be Advanced in a Country's Health System?* Policy Brief 17 (BRIDGE Series). Copenhagen, WHO Regional Office for Europe on behalf of the European Observatory on Health Systems and Policies.

Lavis, J. N., G. Permanand, C. Catallo and the BRIDGE Study Team (2013b). *How can Knowledge Brokering be Better Supported Across European Health Systems*. Policy Brief 16 (BRIDGE Series). Copenhagen, WHO Regional Office for Europe on behalf of the European Observatory on Health Systems and Policies.

Lavis, J. N., D. Robertson, J. M. Woodside, C. B. McLeod and J. Abelson (2003). "How can research organizations more effectively transfer research knowledge to decision makers?" *Milbank Quarterly* **81**(2): 221–248.

Lavis, J. N., S. E. Ross, J. E. Hurley, J. E. Hohenadal, G. L. Stoddart, C. A. Woodward and J. Abelson (2002). "Examining the role of health services research in public policymaking." *Milbank Quarterly* **80**(1): 125–154.

Lavis, J. N., M. G. Wilson, A. D. Oxman, J. Grimshaw, S. Lewin and A. Fretheim (2009). "SUPPORT Tools for evidence-informed health Policymaking (STP). 5. Using research evidence to frame options to address a problem." *Health Research Policy and Systems* **7**(Suppl. 1): S5 [http://www.health-policy-systems.com/content/7/S1/S5].

Lomas, J. (2000). "Using 'linkage and exchange' to move research into policy at a Canadian foundation: encouraging partnerships between researchers and policy makers is the goal of a promising new Canadian initiative." *Health Affairs* **19**(3): 236–240.

Lomas, J. (2007). "The in-between world of knowledge brokering." *British Medical Journal* **334**(7585): 129–132.

Madden, L., L. King and A. Shiell (2009). "How do government health departments in Australia access health economics advice to inform decisions for health? A survey." *Australia and New Zealand Health Policy* **6**: 6.

Oxman, A. D., J. N. Lavis and A. Fretheim (2007). "Use of evidence in WHO recommendations." *The Lancet* **369**(9576): 1883–1889.

Oxman, A. D., J. N. Lavis, S. Lewin and A. Fretheim (2009). "SUPPORT Tools for evidence-informed Policymaking (STP). 1. What is evidence-informed policymaking?" *Health Research Policy and Systems* **7**(Suppl. 1): S1 [http://www.health-policy-systems.com/content/7/S1/S1].

Petticrew, M., M. Whitehead, S. J. Macintyre, H. Graham and M. Egan (2004). "Evidence for public health policy on inequalities: 1: The reality according to policymakers." *Journal of Epidemiology and Community Health* **58**: 811–816.

Schur, C. L., M. L. Berk, L. E. Silver, J. M. Yegian and M. J. O'Grady (2009). "Connecting the ivory tower to main street: setting research priorities for real-world impact." *Health Affairs* **28**(5): w886–w899.

Straus, S., J. Tetroe and I. D. Graham (2009). "Knowledge to action: what it is and what it isn't." In *Knowledge Translation in Health Care: Moving evidence to practice*. S. Straus, J. Tetroe and I. D. Graham, Eds. Chichester, Wiley-Blackwell Publishing.

Waddell, C., J. N. Lavis, J. Abelson, J. Lomas, C. A. Shepherd, T. Bird-Gayson, M. Giacomini and D. R. Offord (2005). "Research using children's mental health policy in Canada: maintaining vigilance amid ambiguity." *Social Science and Medicine* **61**: 1649–1657.

Ward, V., A. House and S. Hamer (2009). "Knowledge brokering: the missing link in the evidence to action chain?" *Evidence and Policy* **5**(3): 267–279.

World Health Organization (WHO) (2004). *The Mexico Statement on Health Research* [www.who.int/rpc/summit/agenda/Mexico_Statement-English.pdf, accessed 25 January 2011]. Geneva, WHO.

World Health Organization (WHO) (2006). *Bridging the "Know–Do" Gap*. Meeting on knowledge translation in global health [http://www.who.int/kms/WHO_EIP_KMS_2006_2.pdf, accessed 1 June 2011]. Geneva, WHO.

World Health Organization (WHO) (2011). *Health Impact Assessment: The determinants of health* [http://www.who.int/hia/evidence/doh/en/, accessed 24 April 2011]. Geneva, WHO.

chapter nineteen

Drawing the lessons

Bernd Rechel, Martin McKee

Introduction

As the introduction to this book has noted, public health in Europe has achieved tremendous successes, but much more needs to be done and, in some countries, previous gains are being eroded by governments with more individualistic ideologies or the adoption of austerity policies. This concluding chapter brings together some of the key lessons that emerge from the contributions to this volume. It does not aim to be exhaustive, but rather seeks to inform the debate on where public health in Europe needs to go next.

Improving our knowledge base

One major conclusion that permeates many chapters of this book is that there are large gaps in our knowledge on almost all aspects of public health systems and structures in Europe. Even some basic data from health information systems are often lacking. As set out in Chapter 3, the problems are greatest in the poorer countries of the region, giving rise to widespread variation in the availability and quality of information on health and its determinants. Even in high-income countries in western Europe there is considerable scope for improving the coverage and, especially, comparabiity of vital statistics (Mathers, Fat et al. 2005). Furthermore, as Chapter 11 pointed out, even the richer countries often fail to collect routine information that can track social inequalities and when they do, data are under-utilized and there is often little capacity to analyse them. What is especially concerning is that some countries are using austerity to justify political decisions to reduce the data they now collect.

Worryingly, the funding of public health in Europe is an area that is still shrouded in much mystery (Rechel, Brand et al. 2013). As Chapter 14 has argued, even basic information on the levels of public health financing is missing or unreliable. While a global standard of health accounts was published in 2011 (OECD/Eurostat et al. 2011), facilitating shared data collection on health expenditure by the OECD, the European Commission, and the WHO Regional Office for Europe, much expenditure on public health falls outside the activities captured by these accounts (de Bekker-Grob, Polder et al. 2007), and those data that are reported often lack credibility. Chapter 15 shows that there is also very little known about the size, scope, and effectiveness of the public health workforce in Europe. Without this information, it will be very challenging to step up efforts to improve public health in the region.

Knowledge on public health structures, services, and activities is also insufficient. Although the WHO Regional Office for Europe has supported evaluations of some public health services, so far these cover only a fraction of European countries. Furthermore, many of these assessments have remained in draft form only, and the quality and objectivity of assessments differs greatly. A study of public health capacity in the EU funded by the European Commission promised to be another source of information, but it did not cover all facets of public health in depth. The country reports of the European Observatory on Health Systems and Policies complement the picture, but despite exhaustive efforts the information they provide on public health structures varies considerably. Furthermore, much of the information in these and other reports is based on self-reported and non-validated data (Rechel and McKee 2012).

The limited research on the scope and effectiveness of public health operations in Europe has been noted, both with regard to occupational health and safety programmes (WHO 2002) and public health more generally (Rechel and McKee 2012). Far more systematic research has been undertaken in the United States, where the Centers for Disease Control (CDC) has led a National Public Health Performance Standards Programme, but even there it has been noted that research to guide public health practice has been insufficient (Scutchfield, Bhandari et al. 2009).

Ultimately, public health structures will have to be assessed according to the improvements in population outcomes they achieve (Brand, Schroder et al. 2006). However, it is exactly this information that seems to be almost entirely missing. Not only are there very few assessments of the effectiveness of disease prevention programmes in the medium term, as was noted in Estonia (Koppel, Leventhal et al. 2009), but broader evaluations of organizational reforms are generally lacking (Maier and Martin-Moreno 2011). Crucially, empirical evidence on the effectiveness or efficiency of different public health structures is so far missing, with uncertainties surrounding the impact, effectiveness, and efficiency of different governing structures and financing arrangements (Mays, Smith et al. 2009). This is particularly so for governance structures for intersectoral working, with very limited knowledge about the effectiveness of different mechanisms, as noted in Chapter 12.

Finally, there is a need to strengthen public health research. As described in Chapter 17, capacities as well as priorities differ widely across European countries, as do levels of government support. Unfortunately, the first round of the EU's new Horizon 2020 programme contains very little on public health, instead focusing on support for Europe's technology industry. Yet, even where knowledge exists (e.g. on how to reduce smoking), it is often not applied, so that much public health research is not translated into practice. Knowledge brokering and a better understanding of the influences on policy-makers and the process by which they reach decisions (see Chapter 18) can help to bridge this gap between knowledge and practice.

Addressing diversity

Another key conclusion that emerges from the contributions to this book is the wide diversity that exists in public health systems and operations across Europe, affecting organization, governance, provision, and financing. This applies to environmental health services (see Chapter 6), nutrition policies (see Chapter 7), screening programmes (see Chapter 9), intersectoral governance structures (see Chapter 12), the use of health impact assessments (HIAs; see Chapter 13), the public health workforce (see Chapter 15), and public health leadership (see Chapter 16).

As described in Chapter 5, occupational health and safety is one area of public health where differences across countries are particularly striking. While in countries such as Finland and France every enterprise is legally required to provide occupational health services, in other countries this only applies to large- and medium-size enterprises, while some countries have no legal requirements for occupational health services at all (WHO 2007).

Chapter 14 has set out the great diversity that exists in the organization and financing of public health in Europe, both within and outside the health sector. One of the main ways in which countries differ is how far responsibility has been devolved to sub-national levels, which in large part reflects the size of the country and its population, and the underlying constitutional, political, and administrative framework. There is also diversity with regard to how countries address the vertical and horizontal integration of public health activities across different programmes, sectors, and levels of care. Just as with health financing generally, countries in Europe also differ greatly in the financing of public health, including the share of total health expenditure devoted to public health and the mechanisms in place for raising revenues. According to the WHO Global Health Expenditure database, expenditure on prevention and public health varied in 2011 from 0.53% of total health expenditure in Cyprus to 6.33% in Serbia (WHO 2012a), although both extremes are somewhat implausible.

The contributions to this book also highlight differences in public health operations within countries, in particular in federal or decentralized systems. This was noted with regard to screening practices in countries such as Spain (García-Armesto, Abadía-Taira et al. 2010), Belgium (Gerkens and Merkur 2010), Denmark (Strandberg-Larsen, Nielsen et al. 2007), and Italy (Lo Scalzo, Donatini et al. 2009). Substantial variations also exist in some countries with regard to the funding for public health, as was noted for example in Italy (Lo Scalzo, Donatini et al. 2009).

Any attempt to improve public health in Europe will have to be cognisant of these substantial differences across and within countries and the underlying factors behind them, such as widely varying levels of socio-economic development, different historical and cultural contexts, diverse public health capacities, and different political priorities attached to public health. These differences have particular consequences for measures that involve intersectoral action. Improvements will have to be tailored to the situation in the country or sub-national unit in question, but the differences also suggest that there is substantial scope for cross-country learning, in particular among countries with similar trajectories and levels of development.

Some of the chapters in this book indicate how strategies can be modified to fit different contexts. The chapter on screening discusses a cascade concept (Zavoral, Suchanek et al. 2009) that allows the frequency, diagnostic methods, and target populations of screening programmes to be adapted to fit the financial and professional resources available in a particular country. In resource-poor settings, it is possible, initially, to create less ambitious programmes that can then be extended gradually, as the health benefits to the population become clear. A similar model is presented in the chapter on occupational health and safety, with four stages of development, depending on the needs, capacities, and trajectories of individual countries or enterprises. The most basic level aims to lower the threshold for initiation and establish basic occupational health services. This can then provide the basis for developing services further.

Tackling health inequities

A closely related point is the importance of addressing health inequities. Not only do public health operations differ widely across countries, but so does the health of the population (WHO 2011b). Within all European countries, people in lower social classes are more likely to be exposed to social and environmental factors with a detrimental effect on their health, including poorer living conditions, greater exposure to traffic and noise, and feelings of stress and lack of control (Eurofound 2012). In many countries, they also are more likely to have unhealthy diets (see Chapter 7), and to smoke, consume alcohol, and have low levels of physical activity (see Chapter 11). As described in Chapter 11, this "social gradient", which can be defined as "a stepwise or linear decrease in health that comes with decreasing social position" (Marmot 2004), has been found in all European countries (CSDH 2008).

A 2008 report by the Commission on the Social Determinants of Health argued that tackling the social determinants of health would narrow the health gap between and within countries worldwide (CSDH 2008). The new European health policy, Health 2020 (WHO 2012b), adopted by the WHO Regional Office for Europe in 2012, also emphasizes the need to address the social determinants of health, as does a European review of social determinants of health (Marmot, Allen et al. 2012). Tackling health inequities between and within European countries by means of actions on the social determinants of health should therefore be one of the most important missions of European public health, although it faces many political challenges. As Chapter 11 has argued, there is a need for both universal policies acting along the social gradient, albeit with greater intensity at the poorer end (proportionate universalism), as well as targeted programmes addressing the needs of particularly vulnerable groups. Effective policies include income redistribution, improvement of childhood conditions, safer work environments, and promotion of social inclusion (Mackenbach and Bakker 2003).

Stepping up intersectoral action

Inersectoral action is key to tackling health inequalities (WHO 2011b). Many of the determinants of health lie outside the responsibilities of ministries of health. Several contributions to this book have provided examples of the role that other sectors can play. Chapter 14 cited tobacco control efforts that go far beyond the traditional health sector to involve agriculture, trade, education, fiscal policy, and law enforcement, at the local, national, and global level (Allin, Mossialos et al. 2004). Chapter 6 described how environmental determinants of health are shaped by those responsible for housing, transport, agriculture, and employment, going far beyond health systems. Chapter 12 argued that most entry points for alcohol control policies fall within the remit of finance ministries and those responsible for trade, transport, education, economic development, criminal justice, and social welfare.

The need to involve other sectors in tackling the social determinants of health has long been recognized. Article 1 of the 1978 Alma Ata Declaration noted that attaining the "highest possible level of health [. . .] requires the action of many other social and economic sectors in addition to the health sector" (WHO 1978). The 1986 Ottawa Charter for Health Promotion (WHO, Health and Welfare Canada et al. 1986) emphasized the need for healthy public policies, including those on transport, education, and the economy. The same approach is reflected in the Health in All Policies (HiAP), first advocated by the Finnish presidency of the European Council in 2006 (Stahl, Wismar et al. 2006), and in the Rio Political Declaration on Social Determinants of Health, adopted during the World Conference on Social Determinants of Health in 2011 (WHO 2011c, 2013b; Leppo, Olilla et al. 2013).

How can these ambitious aims be achieved? A first strategy emerging from the contributions to this book is coalition-building across sectors. Chapter 6 has described how partnerships between public health and practitioners in other sectors have facilitated the design and implementation of interventions that reduce the environmentally induced disease burden. Another example is given in Chapter 5, where close collaboration between ministries of labour and health (and in some cases environment and emergency response) in some former Soviet countries helped to improve occupational health and safety, partly through better collaboration between multiple inspectorates (such as for labour, the environment, technical issues or mining). Chapter 16 recalls processes of coalition-building in Ireland that achieved a ban on smoking in public and at workplaces through the collaboration of politicians, the public, and the media, acting against powerful opposition from the tobacco industry and its front organizations in the hospitality sector.

A second strategy for boosting intersectoral action is to identify shared objectives with other ministries and sectors. As Chapter 6 shows, collating evidence by sector can mobilize support outside ministries of health. A review summarizing all disease outcomes that would benefit from interventions within the housing sector, for example, can capture the attention of decision-makers in the housing sector (Braubach, Jacobs et al. 2011). It also helps to set an agenda for policy within that sector (Keall, Ormandy et al. 2011). Crucially, it is important to demonstrate the benefits that will accrue to other sectors. Where a policy can be shown to boost health and education, tax revenues or economic growth, it will be much easier to gain support outside the health sector.

The use of health impact assessments (HiAs) is another strategy that can support intersectoral action. Endorsed by the 2009 World Health Assembly in a Resolution on Social Determinants of Health (WHO 2009), HiAs aim to identify the potential health consequences of policies, projects, programmes, and plans (Blau, Ernst et al. 2006). As described in Chapter 13, they can integrate health considerations into non-health policies, increase the awareness of health in areas outside the health sector, and help to establish healthy public policy as a goal shared by all sectors. Although strongly advocated within the EU, few EU member states have used HiA extensively, indicating substantial scope for greater progress.

A final strategy emerging from the contributions to this book is to put in place intersectoral governance structures. Chapter 12 describes the various forms these structures can take. Delegated finance, for example, pools resources outside of government. Examples include the health promotion foundations in Switzerland and Austria, which have helped to increase health promotion expenditure of other sectors (Schang, Czabanowska et al. 2012; Schang and Lin 2012).

Crucially, the multiplicity of actors and the large number of sectors involved requires strong public health leadership (see Chapter 16). Often, this will involve ministries of health, but single persons, institutions, local or national governments, and international agencies can also take on a leadership role (WHO 2011a, 2012b; Kickbusch and Behrendt 2013).

Implementing international commitments

International and European legal instruments and political commitments provide important reference points for strengthening public health at the national level. Much could be achieved by implementing these commitments. An example is the above-mentioned 2009 World Health Assembly Resolution on Social Determinants of Health, but there are many more, such as the WHO Framework Convention on Tobacco Control, which is legally binding on those countries that have ratified it (although there are no sanctions for infringements of governments). Chapter 7 also discusses the European Charter on Counteracting Obesity, and the Second WHO European Action Plan on Food and Nutrition Policy. These documents have given rise to a number of national action plans, although more needs to be done to translate these plans into practice. One of the major challenges is that resolutions such as those of the World Health Assembly are only "morally binding" and deliberately written in a style permitting diverse "translations" or interpretations. This helps greatly in ensuring that governments agree to a resolution but can undermine meaningful implementation.

As described in Chapter 4, the International Health Regulations (IHR) define core public health capacity obligations for all states parties for disease surveillance, detection, assessment, and response at all levels. States parties have committed themselves to improving their national and sub-national capacity and a range of monitoring tools is available to assess whether IHR core capacities are met.

Chapter 5 describes some of the key international instruments for occupational health and safety, including the 1996 Global Strategy on Occupational Health for All, the Global Plan of Action on Workers' Health 2008–2017, ILO conventions, the European Social Charter by the Council of Europe, and EU directives on safety and health at work. The ultimate goal set out in many of these documents is universal coverage of all workers in all occupations with occupational health services. Recognizing that many workers in small and medium-sized enterprises and informal sectors are rarely covered by occupational health services, the ILO and WHO have come to embrace the concept of basic occupational health services as a more feasible starting point that can be scaled up later on (Rantanen 2005).

Chapter 9 noted how the EU and the WHO Regional Office for Europe recommend organized, population-based screening programmes for cervical, breast, and colorectal cancers (Council of the European Union 2003; WHO Regional Office for Europe 2011). Yet, by 2007, only 22 of the then 27 EU countries had implemented population-based screening programmes for breast cancer, 15 for cervical cancer and 12 for colorectal cancer (Arbyn, Anttila et al. 2008). Progress has been particularly slow in countries of the former Soviet Union (Maier and Martin-Moreno 2011).

EU directives require countries to enact legislation (as, if they fail to do so, the directives have direct legal force after two years). Chapter 5 has set out how the process of EU accession led to strengthening occupational health and safety in the new EU member states. This has helped to strengthen the legal basis for action, although population coverage still leaves much to be desired. There has also been progress in other areas of public health covered by EU legislation, such as tobacco control, food safety, and environment and health.

Enhancing collaboration

Collaboration between international, national, and sub-national actors is crucial for strengthening public health capacities and action. This begins with health information systems. Although some harmonization has been achieved in Europe, through the efforts of the WHO Regional Office for Europe with its European Health for All database, as well as work by Eurostat and the Organisation for Economic Co-operation and Development (OECD), more can be achieved to align data collection systems, avoid overlaps and duplications, and improve data quality. Crucially, this also applies to the collaboration between international organizations. Until very recently, Eurostat, WHO, and OECD published diverging data on health expenditure in European countries. They have now embraced a common System of Health Accounts (OECD, Eurostat et al. 2011), which allows harmonized data reporting. EU-level surveys using the same set of indicators, such as the European Union Statistics on Income and Living Conditions (EU-SILC) or the European Community Household Panel (ECHP), are also an important source of public health information that is largely comparable across countries. Other examples are the WHO Childhood Obesity Surveillance Initiative, a surveillance system with 17 European countries participating by 2010 (see Chapter 7), and the survey on Health Behaviour in School-Aged Children (HBSC), now covering 43 countries in Europe and North America. Finally, cooperation is also important in the area of public health research, with many projects supported by the European Commission's Framework Programme.

International organizations and European networks can play a particularly useful role in facilitating information exchange. Examples include the networks on public health emergencies, such as the EU's Early Warning and Response System (EWRS) and the WHO system of information exchange under the International Health Regulations (IHRs). Furthermore, as Chapter 4 describes for public health emergency responses, international organizations such as the EU and WHO are also involved in a variety of activities to strengthen public health capacity across Europe.

The sub-national, local level also matters. Initiatives such as Healthy Cities demonstrate how action on the social determinants of health, including the local environment, can be crucial for public health. As described in Chapters 6 and 13, involving communities and civil society in decision-making processes and linking health to development is a particularly promising way for successful multisectoral action and HIAs.

Integrating public health into health care

Several chapters of this book discuss ways of integrating public health into health care. Chapter 5 argued that the integration of occupational health services into primary health care is an important means of expanding occupational health services for all workers. Chapter 7 argues that primary health care needs to play a part in obesity prevention efforts. Chapter 14 revealed how many preventive services are provided in healthcare settings. This includes immunizations, screening or health checks, and the notification of communicable diseases (Saltman, Allin et al. 2012). Countries that seem to have achieved a better integration of public health services into primary care include Denmark, Estonia, Finland, Portugal, Slovenia, Spain, and Sweden (Glenngård, Hjalte et al. 2005; Barros and de Almeida Simoes 2007; Strandberg-Larsen, Nielsen et al. 2007; Vuorenkoski, Mladovsky et al. 2008; Koppel, Leventhal et al. 2009; García-Armesto, Abadía-Taira et al. 2010; Anell, Glenngård et al. 2012). Those in secondary care also increasingly recognize their role in public health, such as in the Health-Promoting Hospital initiative (Whitehead 2004).

Enhancing public health capacity

Ensuring a well-trained workforce for public health is one of ten essential public health operations (EPHOs). However, as Chapter 15 has argued, the boundaries and quantity of the public health workforce in Europe are rather elusive. There is a clear case for a more formal recognition of its role, as well as adequate educational facilities and a clear set of competencies. The newly established Agency for Accreditation of Public Health Education in Europe may help to improve educational standards (Otok et al., 2011).

Chapter 6 illustrated how public health training still differs substantially across countries. Examining the area of environmental health, it finds that there is no common curriculum. Finnish physicians working in this area tend to have been trained in occupational health. In the Netherlands, a specialization in environmental health for physicians was established in the late 1980s and other professionals trained in environmental health or biomedical sciences were added in the 1990s. In Belgium, a mix of professionals, ranging from psychologists to biologists, are working in environmental health (Public Health Services Gelderland Midden 2011). Training content also differs greatly across countries. In one European country, professionals may receive training in toxicology, but not in risk communication, while the reverse may be true in the neighbouring country (Public Health Services Gelderland Midden 2011). This indicates that there is substantial scope for increased collaboration and harmonization in Europe in environmental health, but also more widely. It will be even more important (not least in times of austerity) to create employment opportunities for public health professionals, an area of major concern throughout Europe, but particularly in many countries in central and eastern Europe and the former Soviet Union.

Coping with the financial crisis

The financial and economic crisis that started in 2007 is a recurrent concern in the contributions to this book. It is already having a major impact on the social determinants of health, through rising levels of unemployment and social inequality, as well as, in some countries, decreasing government expenditure on social protection, health systems, and public health. Unemployment, and in particular youth unemployment, has reached very high levels in some southern European countries. As described in Chapter 6, one of the areas of public health that has already been negatively affected is occupational health and safety, as some countries have deregulated labour laws, making occupational health and safety provisions less stringent. The experience in other parts of the world (Min, Min et al. 2010) suggests that cutting back on occupational safety and health during an economic crisis is likely to have a sustained negative effect. Some countries in Europe have also cut back on public health programmes more generally (Aluttis, Chiotan et al. 2013).

Countries in Europe differ in terms of the social protection they afford their populations to deal with the consequences of the economic crisis (European Commission 2010). While some countries, such as Italy and Kyrgyzstan, have adopted measures to protect low-income groups from the effects of the economic crisis (WHO 2009), other countries are scaling down social protection systems, which is likely to result in widening social and health inequalities.

Making the economic case for public health action

Health is a human right, aside from the strong moral obligations to promote health. However, in the current economic context, it will be more vital than ever to demonstrate the economic case for public health action. A growing number of public health interventions are being recognized as cost-effective in the medium and long term. Chapter 5 has argued that investing in workplace prevention yields substantial economic benefits for employers, despite the fact that most economic costs of occupational injury and disease fall on other actors (Kankaanpää, van Tulder et al. 2008). An international study covering 15 countries found that companies expected on average a benefit of 2.2 currency units for every unit invested in workplace prevention (International Social Security Association 2011). Chapter 6 has argued that many environmental health interventions are as cost-effective as other types of health-sector interventions (Prüss-Üstün and Corvalán 2006). The effectiveness of controlling environmental determinants of disease has, for example, been shown with regard to air quality, in terms of both the reduced burden of disease and the economic costs and benefits. Furthermore, interventions reducing housing-related health burdens are often among the most cost-effective (DiGuiseppi, Jacobs et al. 2010; OECD 2010; WHO 2013a).

Embracing a broad vision of public health

Public health in many European countries is evolving from a focus on sanitary supervision and the prevention of infectious diseases to encompass the main threats to population health, acting through health promotion, disease prevention, and intersectoral action (see Chapters 10–14). However, substantial differences still exist across European countries in the terminology and conceptualizations of public health (Kaiser and Mackenbach 2008). A major conclusion from the contributions to this book is that, to successfully address the determinants of poor health in Europe, a broad vision of public health is required that embraces the values of ecological sustainability, social justice, and political engagement.

Chapter 6 has made a strong case for an ecologically sustainable model of social and economic development. It has argued that the current economic model, based on the use of non-renewable resources and the primacy of economic growth, undermines the biosphere, biodiversity, and environmental health (Bothamley, Ditiu et al. 2008; Max-Neef 2010). What is instead needed is an economy that only consumes as much as the natural environment can produce (McMichael, Smith et al. 2000; Daly 2005). This will be of benefit to both the environment and human health (Haines 2012).

Most actions that reduce greenhouse gas emissions, including in the areas of transport, household energy, food and agriculture, and electricity generation, have public health benefits (Haines, McMichael et al. 2009). Furthermore, many unhealthy activities are carbon-intensive (NHS Sustainable Development Unit 2010). Some of the causes of the growing burden of obesity, for example, are directly related to the excessive use of energy, such as in the consumption of meat and other energy-dense foods produced by industrial food production systems (Neff, Parker et al. 2011). Reducing greenhouse gas emissions through reductions in private car use and increased active travel (walking and cycling), on the other hand, benefits both the climate and population health. Low carbon technologies, strategies, and lifestyles have ancillary or collateral benefits for health, the so-called "health co-benefits". In some cases, the health benefits partly or fully offset the costs for implementing these policies (Haines 2012). The task for public health will be to demonstrate these benefits and help usher in more sustainable models of economic and social development.

Public health also needs to be concerned with social justice and greater equality (Hastings 2012). This was well recognized in the nineteenth century when the discipline of public health emerged. As Chapter 16 recalls, Rudolph Virchow (1821–1892), the founder of the discipline of social medicine, noted that "medicine is a social science, and politics is nothing else but medicine on a large scale" (Brown and Fee 2006). Many of these concerns were taken up again more than 100 years later by the Commission on the Social Determinants of Health, which argued that addressing the social determinants of health requires social justice, social protection across the life course, and a more equitable distribution of power, wealth, and resources (CSDH 2008). The pursuit of democracy and the rule of law are also critical for public health (Bothamley, Ditiu et al. 2008), not least because populations tend to be healthier in countries with greater political freedom, independent of economic factors (Franco, Alvarez-Dardet et al. 2004). Yet, there are still countries in the WHO European Region where the population does not enjoy effective political participation and engagement (Rechel and McKee 2007).

All too often, public health focuses on individual risk factors, which can divert attention from underlying political and economic determinants of health and the role of power and politics (Stuckler, Basu et al. 2010). One of the challenges in a growing number of European countries is how a powerful neoliberal agenda is promoting cutbacks in welfare states and placing blind faith in the role of markets (McKee and Stuckler 2011). Coupled with the restraints on state budgets that have been exacerbated by the current economic crisis, there is a major danger that health inequalities in Europe will increase further and that the corrective role of the state will be further diminished. This not only damages the prospects of those in less advantaged social positions, but harms societies as a whole. More equal societies do better on a range of social and health indicators (Haines, McMichael et al. 2009). As Chapter 5 has argued, the impact of these political and economic pressures is already visible in the area of occupational health and safety, such as in Georgia, where the government terminated all occupational safety and health-related inspection services and minimum safety requirements, leading to a series of workplace accidents. In many other countries in central and eastern Europe and the former Soviet Union, the privatization or collapse of public companies, as well as the growth in the number of self-employed people and of the informal sector, have led to more hazardous working conditions. The role of public health is to press for more equitable societies that afford every member the possibility to reach their full potential.

Public health needs imagination and the vision of a fairer, more sustainable world that is conducive to the health of the population. Importantly, it needs to insist that "things could be different and better" (Adorno 1951). This not only requires being critical of the powers that be, but also taking on vested interests, and increasingly, the major corporations that act as vectors for disease (Hastings 2012; Mindell, Reynolds et al. 2012). Working towards an ecologically sustainable future and a more equitable distribution of power, wealth, and resources is deeply political and will have to overcome substantial resistance.

Powerful multinational corporations are one of the main sources of resistance. As set out in Chapter 16, this is apparent in the history of tobacco control efforts. Even after the health risks of smoking became well established, it took decades for governments to pass effective measures. Although much has been achieved, there is still a substantial way to go in many European countries to make smoking a thing of the past.

While there is also much to do in relation to alcohol (in itself an energy-rich food, similar to sugar in its impact on the human body), it is diet, the third major risk factor for non-communicable disease, where the greatest progress is needed in the coming years, in order to address growing levels of obesity. While the ban on smoking in public places has become widely accepted in most European countries, public health is much further behind when addressing the causes of obesity. There is now growing evidence that excessive sugar consumption, especially in sugar-rich beverages, is at the root of the problem (Lustig, Schmidt et al. 2012; Basu, McKee et al. 2013; Basu, Stuckler et al. 2013), and, at population level, the availability of sugar can explain diabetes prevalence rates (Basu, Yoffe et al. 2013). However, while the consumption of tobacco and alcohol are regulated by governments to protect public health, sugar consumption is not (Lustig, Schmidt et al. 2012).

Progress will depend on forging successful alliances against the short-term interests of big food companies. This will not be easy. In 2006, Coca-Cola spent more on marketing its soft drinks than the biannual budget for WHO (Bothamley, Ditiu et al. 2008). Leading food corporations, such as Coca-Cola and McDonald's, have also been successful in associating themselves with sports events and physical activity, such as the 2012 Olympic Games in London, blaming inadequate physical activity, rather than sugar consumption, for rising levels of obesity (Dorfman and Yancey 2009; Basu, Stuckler et al. 2013). This is grossly misleading. For a large fast food meal (containing a double cheeseburger, chips, a soft drink, and a dessert) to be burnt off, consumers would need to run a full marathon (Ebbeling, Pawlak et al. 2002). A range of policy options are available, including taxation of sugar-sweetened beverages and foods that contain any form of added sugars, and controls on advertising and marketing (Lustig, Schmidt et al. 2012; Mytton, Clarke et al. 2012). Going beyond sugar, serious attempts to address the obesity epidemic will also need to tackle the excessive consumption of meat, as well as the global system of food production, trade, and agriculture (see Chapter 7). Not only are people in richer countries eating too much, but in 2009 one billion people in the world were undernourished (Carolan 2011). This underlines the importance of addressing public health problems in Europe in their global context.

Making it happen

How can the required change be brought about? The contributions to this volume suggest that research evidence on its own is clearly not enough. There is a "know–do" gap (WHO 2005) between knowledge and doing and, once policies have been adopted, there is a gap between policies and implementation (Nichols, Maynard et al. 2009). Policy-making can be a very complex process involving a variety of actors at different levels with different agendas and levels of influence. Historical trajectories and institutional structures matter, but so do actors, ideas, and ideologies. To be successful, public health in Europe will have to engage in strategic leadership, as well as processes of coalition-building and lobbying at the local, national, and international level.

Although the review of the status of public health activities in Europe presented in this book is by necessity incomplete (in particular with regard to countries in the east of the region), it is possible to determine where the need for action is greatest. Both in terms of population health and public health capacities, many of the countries in central and eastern Europe, but in particular the former Soviet countries, fare worst. They will have to invest heavily in all public health functions if they are to close the wide health gap with the rest of Europe (see Chapter 2). The case for doing so can be made on many grounds, from the recognition of health as a human right to the economic argument for a healthy population.

Yet, there is no room for complacency in other European countries. There is an overwhelming need to address the growing challenge posed by chronic disease, both in terms of its absolute level and its inequitable distribution within the population. Four risk factors stand out: poor diet, tobacco and alcohol consumption, and inadequate physical activity. Much more needs to be done to address tobacco and hazardous alcohol consumption and increase levels of physical activity, but it seems that changing people's diets will be one of the most difficult challenges in the coming years. There is a clear role for stronger government regulation of the amount of fat and sugar in food and drinks. Public health professionals can contribute to this goal by gathering the necessary evidence, advocating for change, forging political alliances, and overseeing implementation. In this way, they have the opportunity to demonstrate the many benefits public health can bring to society.

While civil society, communities, and individuals also have important contributions to make, it is ultimately governments that must accept their responsibility to secure and enhance the health of their populations by means of appropriate national health policies. Within Europe, governments have signed up to a new European policy framework, Health 2020, and the European Action Plan for Strengthening Public Health Capacities and Services. Now it is up to them to make these fine words a reality.

References

Adorno, T. W. (1951). *Minima Moralia: Reflections on a damaged life*. London, Verso.

Allin, S., E. Mossialos, M. McKee and W. Holland (2004). *Making Decisions on Public Health: A review of eight countries.* Copenhagen, WHO on behalf of the European Observatory on Health Systems and Policies.

Aluttis, C., C. Chiotan, K. Michelsen, C. Costongs and H. Brand (2013). *Review of Public Health Capacity in the EU.* Luxembourg, European Commission Directorate General for Health and Consumers.

Anell, A., A. Glenngård and S. Merkur (2012). "Sweden: health system review." *Health Systems in Transition* **14**(5): 1–159.

Arbyn, M., A. Anttila, J. Jordan, G. Ronco, U. Schenck, N. Segnan, H. G. Wiener, A. Herbert, J. Daniel and L. von Karsa, Eds. (2008). *European Guidelines for Quality Assurance in Cervical Cancer Screening*, 2nd edition. Luxembourg, Office for Official Publications of the European Communities.

Barros, P. P. and J. de Almeida Simoes (2007). "Portugal: health system review." *Health Systems in Transition* **9**(5): 1–142.

Basu, S., M. McKee, G. Galea and D. Stuckler (2013). "The relationship of soft drink consumption to global overweight, obesity and diabetes: a cross-national analysis of 75 countries." *American Journal of Public Health* **103**(11): 2071–2077.

Basu, S., D. Stuckler, M. McKee and G. Galea (2013). "Nutritional determinants of worldwide diabetes: an econometric study of food markets and diabetes prevalence in 173 countries." *Public Health Nutrition* **16**(1): 179–186.

Basu, S., P. Yoffe, N. Hills and R. H. Lustig (2013). "The relationship of sugar to population-level diabetes prevalence: an econometric analysis of repeated cross-sectional data." *PLoS ONE* **8**(2): e57873.

Blau, J., K. Ernst, M. Wismar, F. Baro, M. Blenkus, K. von Bremen, R. Fehr, G. Gulis, T. Kauppinen, O. Mekel and K. Nelimarkka (2006). "The use of health impact assessment across Europe." In *Health in All Policies.* T. Stahl, M. Wismar, E. Ollila, E. Lahtinen and K. Leppo, Eds. Helsinki, Ministry of Social Affairs and Health: 209–230.

Bothamley, G. H., L. Ditiu, G. B. Migliori, C. Lange and TBNET Contributors (2008). "Active case finding of tuberculosis in Europe: a Tuberculosis Network European Trials Group (TBNET) survey." *European Respiratory Journal* **32**: 1023–1030.

Brand, H., P. Schroder, J. Davies, I. Escamilla, C. Hall, K. Hickey, E. Jelastopulu, R. Mechtler, W. Yared, J. Volf and B. Weihrauch (2006). "Reference frameworks for the health management of measles, breast cancer and diabetes (type II)." *Central European Journal of Public Health* **14**(1): 39–45.

Braubach, M., D. E. Jacobs and D. Ormandy (2011). *Environmental Burden of Disease Associated with Inadequate Housing: Methods for quantifying health impacts of selected housing risks in the WHO European Region.* Bonn, WHO European Centre for Environment and Health, WHO Regional Office for Europe.

Brown, T. M. and E. Fee (2006). "Rudolf Carl Virchow." *American Journal of Public Health* **96**(12): 2104–2105.

Carolan, M. (2011). *The Real Cost of Cheap Food.* London, Earthscan.

Commission on Social Determinants of Health (CSDH) (2008). *Closing the Gap in a Generation: Health equity through action on the social determinants of health.* Final Report of the Commission on Social Determinants of Health. Geneva, WHO.

Council of the European Union (2003). Council recommendation of 2 December 2003 on cancer screening. *Official Journal of the European Union* **2003/878/EC**(L327): 34–38.

Daly, H. E. (2005). "Economics in a full world." *Scientific American* **293**(3): 100–107.

de Bekker-Grob, E., J. Polder, J. P. Mackenbach and W. Meerding (2007). "Towards a comprehensive estimate of national spending on prevention." *BMC Public Health* **7**: 252.

DiGuiseppi, C., D. E. Jacobs, K. J. Phelan, A. D. Mickalide and D. Ormandy (2010). "Housing interventions and control of injury-related structural deficiencies: a review of the evidence." *Journal of Public Health Management and Practice* **16**(5 Suppl.): S34–S43.

Dorfman, L. and A. Yancey (2009). "Promoting physical activity and healthy eating: convergence in framing the role of industry." *Preventive Medicine* **49**(4): 303–305.

Ebbeling, C., D. Pawlak and D. Ludwig (2002). "Childhood obesity: public-health crisis, common sense cure." *The Lancet* **360**(9331): 473–482.

Eurofound (2012). *Fifth European Working Conditions Survey.* Luxembourg, Publications Office of the European Union.

European Commission (2010). *Joint Report on Social Protection and Social Inclusion 2010.* Brussels, European Commission.

Franco, A., C. Alvarez-Dardet and M. Ruiz (2004). "Effect of democracy on health: ecological study." *British Medical Journal* **329**: 1421–1423.

García-Armesto, S., M. Abadía-Taira, A. Durán, C. Hernández-Quevedo and E. Bernal-Delgado (2010). "Spain: health system review." *Health Systems in Transition* **12**(4): 1–295.

Gerkens, S. and S. Merkur (2010). "Belgium: health system review." *Health Systems in Transition* **12**(5): 1–266.

Glenngård, A., F. Hjalte, M. Svensson, A. Anell and V. Bankauskaite (2005). *Health Systems in Transition: Sweden.* Copenhagen, WHO Regional Office for Europe on behalf of the European Observatory on Health Systems and Policies.

Haines, A. (2012). "Sustainable policies to improve health and prevent climate change." *Social Science and Medicine* **74**(5): 680–683.

Haines, A., A. McMichael, K. Smith, I. Roberts, J. Woodcock, A. Markandya, B. Armstrong, D. Campbell-Lendrum, A. Dangour, M. Davies, N. Bruce, C. Tonne, M. Barrett and P. Wilkinson (2009). "Public health benefits of strategies to reduce greenhouse-gas emissions: overview and implications for policy makers." *The Lancet* **374**(9707): 2104–2114.

Hastings, G. (2012). "Why corporate power is a public health priority." *British Medical Journal* **345**: e5124.

International Social Security Association (ISSA) (2011). *The Return on Prevention: Calculating the costs and benefits of investments in occupational safety and health in companies.* Geneva, ISSA.

Kaiser, S. and J. Mackenbach (2008). "Public health in eight European countries: an international comparison of terminology." *Public Health* **122**(2): 211–216.

Kankaanpää, E., M. van Tulder, M. Aaltonen and M. De Greef (2008). "Economics for occupational safety and health." *Scandinavian Journal of Work, Environment and Health Supplement* **5**: 9–13.

Keall, M. D., D. Ormandy and M. G. Baker (2011). "Injuries associated with housing conditions in Europe: a burden of disease study based on 2004 injury data." *Environmental Health* **10**: 98.

Kickbusch, I. and T. Behrendt (2013). *Implementing a Health 2020 Vision: Governance for health in the 21st century. Making it happen.* Copenhagen, WHO Regional Office for Europe.

Koppel, A., A. Leventhal and M. Sedgley, Eds. (2009). *Public Health in Estonia 2008: An analysis of public health operations, services and activities.* Copenhagen, WHO Regional Office for Europe.

Leppo, K., E. Olilla, S. Pena, M. Wismar and S. Cook, Eds. (2013). *Health in All Policies: Seizing opportunities, implementing policies.* Helsinki, Ministry of Social Affairs and Health.

Lo Scalzo, A., A. Donatini, L. Orzella, S. Profili, A. Cicchetti, l. S. Profi and A. Maresso (2009). "Italy: health system review." *Health Systems in Transition* **11**(6): 1–216.

Lustig, R. H., L. A. Schmidt and C. D. Brindis (2012). "The toxic truth about sugar." *Nature* **482**: 27–29.

Mackenbach, J. P. and M. J. Bakker (2003). "Tackling socioeconomic inequalities in health: analysis of European experience." *The Lancet* **362**(9393): 1409–1414.

Maier, C. B. and J. M. Martin-Moreno (2011). "Quo vadis SANEPID? A cross-country analysis of public health reforms in 10 post-Soviet states." *Health Policy* **102**(1): 18–25.

Marmot, M. (2004). *Status Syndrome*. London, Bloomsbury.

Marmot, M., J. Allen, R. Bell, E. Bloomer, P. Goldblatt and Consortium for the European Review of Social Determinants of Health and the Health Divide (2012). "WHO European review of social determinants of health and the health divide." *The Lancet* **380**(9846): 1011–1029.

Mathers, C., D. Fat, M. Inoue, C. Rao and A. Lopez (2005). "Counting the dead and what they died from: an assessment of the global status of cause of death data." *Bulletin of the World Health Organization* **83**(3): 171–177.

Max-Neef, M. (2010). "The world on a collision course and the need for a new economy." *Ambio* **39**(3): 200–210.

Mays, G. P., S. A. Smith, R. C. Ingram, L. J. Racster, C. D. Lamberth and E. S. Lovely (2009). "Public health delivery systems." *American Journal of Preventive Medicine* **36**(3): 256–265.

McKee, M. and D. Stuckler (2011). "The assault on universalism: how to destroy the welfare state." *British Medical Journal* **343**: d7973.

McMichael, A. J., K. R. Smith and C. F. Corvalan (2000). "The sustainability transition: a new challenge." *Bulletin of the World Health Organization* **78**(9): 1067.

Min, K., J. Min, J. Park, S. Park and K. Lee (2010). "Changes in occupational safety and health indices after the Korean economic crisis: analysis of a national sample, 1991–2007." *American Journal of Public Health* **100**(11): 2165–2167.

Mindell, J., L. Reynolds, D. Cohen and M. McKee (2012). "All in this together: the corporate capture of public health." *British Medical Journal* **345**: e8082).

Mytton, O., D. Clarke and M. Rayner (2012). "Taxing unhealthy food and drinks to improve health." *British Medical Journal* **344**: e2931.

Neff, R. A., C. L. Parker, F. L. Kirschenmann, J. Tinch and R. S. Lawrence (2011). "Peak oil, food systems, and public health." *American Journal of Public Health* **101**(9): 1587–1597.

NHS Sustainable Development Unit (2010). *Saving Lives, Saving Money, Securing the Future*. Sustainability, Health and the NHS Factsheet. London, NHS Sustainable Development Unit.

Nichols, A., V. Maynard, B. Goodman and J. Richardson (2009). "Health, climate change and sustainability: a systematic review and thematic analysis of the literature." *Environmental Health Insights* **3**: 63–88.

OECD (2010). *Obesity and the Economics of Prevention: Fit not fat*. Paris, OECD.

OECD/Eurostat/WHO (2011). *A System of Health Accounts*, 2011 edition [http://www.who.int/nha/sha_revision/sha_2011_final1.pdf, accessed 28 January 2013]. Paris, OECD.

Prüss-Üstün, A. and C. Corvalán (2006). *Preventing Disease through Healthy Environments: Towards an estimate of the environmental burden of disease*. Geneva, WHO.

Public Health Services Gelderland Midden (2011). *Training of Professionals in Environment and Health*. Luxembourg, European Commission Directorate General for Health and Consumers.

Rantanen, J. (2005). "Basic occupational health services – their structure, content and objectives." *Scandinavian Journal of Work, Environment and Health* **1**: 5–15.

Rechel, B., H. Brand and M. McKee (2013). "Financing public health in Europe." *Gesundheitswesen* **75**: e28–e33.

Rechel, B. and M. McKee (2007). "The effects of dictatorship on health: the case of Turkmenistan." *BMC Medicine* **5**: 21.

Rechel, B. and M. McKee (2012). Preliminary Review of Institutional *Models for Delivering Essential Public Health Operations in Europe.* Copenhagen, WHO Regional Office for Europe.

Saltman, R., S. Allin, E. Mossialos, M. Wismar and E. van Ginneken (2012). "Assessing health reform trends in Europe." In *Health Systems, Health, Wealth and Societal Well-being.* J. Figueras and M. McKee, Eds. Maidenhead, Open University Press: 209–246.

Schang, L., K. Czabanowska and V. Lin (2012). "Securing funds for health promotion: lessons from health promotion foundations based on experiences from Austria, Australia, Germany, Hungary and Switzerland." *Health Promotion International* **27**(2): 295–305.

Schang, L. and V. Lin (2012). "Delegated financing." In *Intersectoral Governance for Health in All Policies.* D. McQueen, V. Lin, M. Wismaret, Eds. Copenhagen, WHO Regional Office for Europe on behalf of the European Observatory for Health Systems and Policies.

Scutchfield, F., M. Bhandari, N. Lawhorn, C. Lamberth and R. Ingram (2009). "Public health performance." *American Journal of Preventive Medicine* **36**(3): 266–272.

Stahl, T., M. Wismar, E. Ollila, E. Lahtinen and K. Leppo, Eds. (2006). *Health in All Policies: Prospects and potentials.* Copenhagen, WHO Regional Office for Europe on behalf of the European Observatory on Health Systems and Policies.

Strandberg-Larsen, M., M. Nielsen, S. Vallgårda, A. Krasnik, K. Vrangbæk and E. Mossialos (2007). "Denmark: health system review." *Health Systems in Transition* **9**(6): 1–164.

Stuckler, D., S. Basu and M. McKee (2010). "Public health in Europe: power, politics, and where next?" *Public Health Reviews* **32**(1): 213–242.

Vuorenkoski, L., P. Mladovsky and E. Mossialos (2008). "Finland: health system review." *Health Systems in Transition* **10**(4): 1–168.

Whitehead, D. (2004). "The European Health Promoting Hospitals (HPH) project: how far on?" *Health Promotion International* **19**(2): 259–267.

World Health Organization (WHO) (1978). *Declaration of Alma-Ata,* International Conference on Primary Health Care, Alma-Ata, USSR, 6–12 September 1978. Geneva, WHO.

World Health Organization (WHO) (2002). *Good Practice in Occupational Health Services: A contribution to workplace health.* Copenhagen, WHO Regional Office for Europe.

World Health Organization (WHO) (2007). *Workers' Health: Global plan of action.* Geneva, WHO.

World Health Organization (WHO) (2009). *Reducing Health Inequities through Action on the Social Determinants of Health,* Sixty-second World Health Assembly, 22 May 2009. Geneva, WHO.

World Health Organization (WHO) (2011a). *Governance for Health in the 21st Century: A study conducted for the WHO Regional Office for Europe.* Copenhagen, WHO Regional Office for Europe.

World Health Organization (WHO) (2011b). *Interim Second Report on Social Determinants of Health and the Health Divide in the WHO European Region.* Copenhagen, WHO Regional Office for Europe.

World Health Organization (WHO) (2011c). *Rio Political Declaration on Social Determinants of Health,* Rio de Janeiro, Brazil, 21 October 2011. Geneva, WHO.

World Health Organization (WHO) (2012a). *Global Health Expenditure Database* [http:// apps.who.int/nha/database/DataExplorer.aspx?ws=0&d=1, accessed 20 May 2012]. Geneva, WHO.

World Health Organization (WHO) (2012b). *Health 2020: Policy framework and strategy.* Copenhagen, WHO Regional Office for Europe.

World Health Organization (WHO) (2013a). *The Case for Investing in Public Health.* A public health summary report for EPHO 8. Copenhagen, WHO Regional Office for Europe.

World Health Organization (WHO) (2013b). *Helsinki Statement on Health in All Policies,* adopted at the 8th Global Conference on Health Promotion, Helsinki, Finland, 10–14 June 2013. Geneva, WHO.

WHO, Health and Welfare Canada and Canadian Public Health Association (1986). *Ottawa Charter for Health Promotion: An International Conference on Health Promotion. The move towards a new public health,* 17–21 November 1986, Ottawa, Ontario, Canada [http://www.phac-aspc.gc.ca/ph-sp/docs/charter-chartre/pdf/ charter.pdf, accessed 11 March 2013].

World Health Organization (WHO) Regional Office for Europe (2011). Regional Committee for Europe: Resolution EUR/RC61/12 – Action plan for implementation of the European Strategy for the Prevention and Control of Noncommunicable Diseases 2012–2016, Baku, Azerbaijan, 15 September 2011. Copenhagen, WHO Regional Office for Europe.

Zavoral, M., S. Suchanek, F. Zavada, L. Dusek, J. Muzik, B. Seifert and P. Fric (2009). "Colorectal cancer screening in Europe." *World Journal of Gastroenterology* **15**(47): 5907–5915.

Index

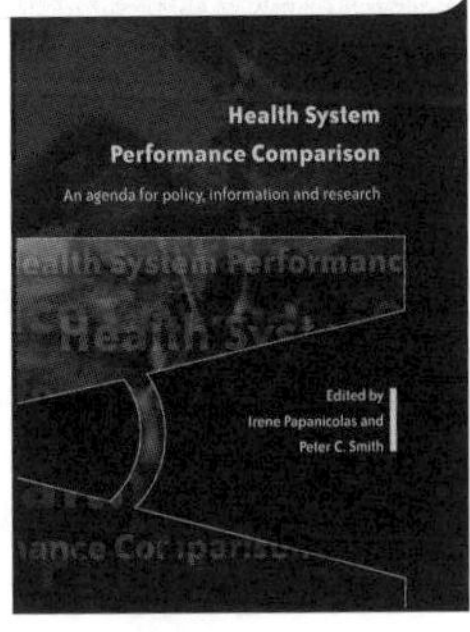

HEALTH SYSTEM PERFORMANCE COMPARISON
An Agenda for Policy, Information and Research

Irene Papanicolas and Peter C. Smith

9780335247264 (Paperback)
April 2013

eBook also available

This timely and authoritative book offers an important summary of the current developments in health system performance comparison. It summarises the current state of efforts to compare systems, and identifies and explores the practical and conceptual challenges that occur. It discusses data and methodological challenges, as well as broader issues such as the interface between evidence and practice.

Key features:

- Assesses the strengths and limitations of existing conceptual frameworks for thinking about health systems and assessing performance
- Examines the existing indicators in use, the gaps and limitations
- Identifies methodological weaknesses in existing performance measurement initiatives, and assesses the scope for future improvements

www.openup.co.uk

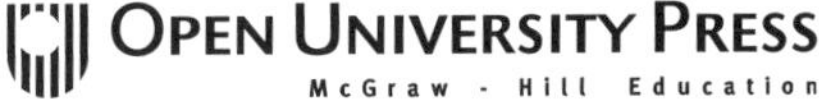

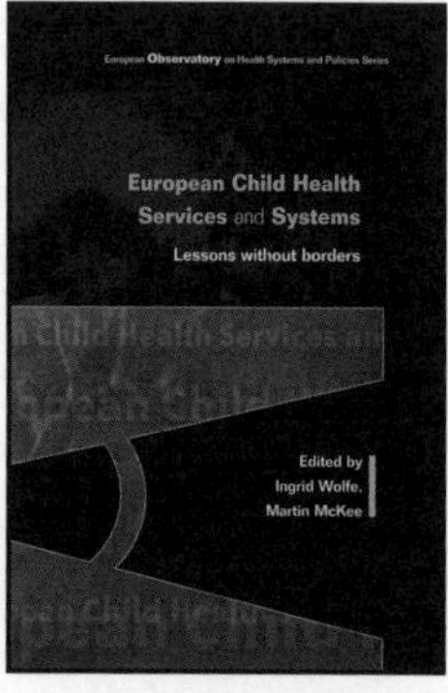

EUROPEAN CHILD HEALTH SERVICES AND SYSTEMS
Lessons without Borders

Ingrid Wolfe and Martin McKee

9780335264667 (Paperback)
December 2013

eBook also available

Taking a child-centric view on understanding how health services and systems work the book aims to contribute towards improving children's health through deepening the understanding of children's health services.

Focusing primarily on the western European countries the book draws on research conducted with child health leaders in ten countries: Austria, Britain, Finland, France, Israel, Italy, Netherlands, Norway, Poland, and Sweden.

Key features:

- Service integration and coordination
- Public health measures
- Enhancing the quality of care for children

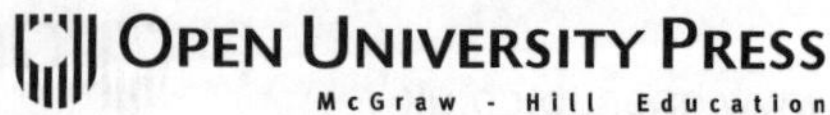

www.openup.co.uk